Cystic Fibrosis Care: a Practical Guide

For Elsevier

Commissioning Editor: Heidi Harrison
Development Editor: Siobhan Campbell
Production Manager: Morven Dean
Design: George Ajayi

Cystic Fibrosis Care: a Practical Guide

Edited by

Allison Peebles MCSP

Senior Cystic Fibrosis Physiotherapist, Southampton General Hospital, Southampton, Hants

Judi Maddison RGN RSCN MSc

Cystic Fibrosis Nurse Specialist, Southampton General Hospital, Southampton, Hants

Joan Gavin BSc(Hons) SRD MPhil

Cystic Fibrosis Dietitian, Southampton General Hospital, Southampton, Hants

Gary Connett DCH MRCP MD FRCPCH

Consultant Respiratory Paediatrician, Southampton General Hospital, Southampton, Hants

Foreword by

Andrew Bush MD FRCP FRCPCH

Professor of Paediatric Respirology, Royal Brompton Hospital, London, UK

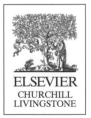

ELSEVIER
CHURCHILL
LIVINGSTONE

EDINBURGH LONDON NEW YORK OXFORD PHILADELPHIA ST LOUIS SYDNEY TORONTO 2005

ELSEVIER
CHURCHILL
LIVINGSTONE

ISBN 0 443 10003 9

British Library Cataloguing in Publication Data
A catalogue record for this book is available from the British Library.

Library of Congress Cataloging in Publication Data
A catalog record for this book is available from the Library of Congress.

Note
Medical knowledge is constantly changing. As new information becomes
available, changes in treatment, procedures, equipment and the use of
drugs become necessary. The author/contributors and the publishers have
taken great care to ensure that the information given in this text is accurate
and up to date. However, readers are strongly advised to confirm that the
information, especially with regard to drug usage, complies with the latest
legislation and standards of practice.

The Publisher

 your source for books,
journals and multimedia
in the health sciences
www.elsevierhealth.com

The
Publisher's
policy is to use
**paper manufactured
from sustainable forests**

Printed in China

Contents

Contributors

Dr June Abay BM FRCPCH
Consultant Paediatrician, Southampton General Hospital, Southampton, Hants

Dr R. Mark Beattie MB BS BSc(Hons) MRCP FRCPCH
Consultant Paediatric Gastroenterologist, Southampton General Hospital, Southampton, Hants

Dr Peter R Betts MD FRCP FRCPCH
Consultant Paediatric Endocrinologist, Southampton General Hospital, Southampton, Hants

Ms Amanda Bevan BSc(Hons) MRPharmS DipClinPharm
Directorate Pharmacist – Child Health, Southampton General Hospital, Southampton, Hants

Dr Mary Carroll MD FRCP
Consultant Adult Respiratory Medicine, Southampton General Hospital, Southampton, Hants

Mr Matthew Coleman MD MRCOG MRCP(UK)
Consultant in Obstetrics & Gynaecology, Southampton General Hospital, Southampton, Hants

Dr Gary Connett DCH MRCP MD FRCPCH
Consultant Respiratory Paediatrician, Southampton General Hospital, Southampton, Hants

Dr Joanna Fairhurst MA MRCP FRCR
Consultant Paediatric Radiologist, Southampton General Hospital, Southampton, Hants

Mrs Clare Forsyth BSc(Hons – Nursing) RGN
Cystic Fibrosis Nurse Specialist, Southampton General Hospital, Southampton, Hants

Mrs Joan Gavin BSc(Hons) SRD MPhil
Cystic Fibrosis Dietitian, Southampton General Hospital, Southampton, Hants

Mr D. Mervyn Griffiths MCh FRCS
Consultant Paediatric Surgeon/Senior Lecturer in Paediatric Surgery, Southampton General Hospital, Southampton, Hants

Dr Sucheta Iyengar MD MBBS
Specialist Registrar in Obstetrics and Gynaecology, Southampton General Hospital, Southampton, Hants

Dr Graeme Jones MRCP MRCPath
Consultant in Medical Microbiology, Southampton General Hospital, Southampton, Hants

Dr Julian Legg MA FRCPCH MD
Consultant Respiratory Paediatrician, Southampton General Hospital, Southampton, Hants

Dr Anneke Lucassen DPhil SRCP
Consultant in Clinical Genetics, Southampton General Hospital, Southampton, Hants

Mrs Judi Maddison RGN RSCN MSC
Cystic Fibrosis Nurse Specialist, Southampton General Hospital, Southampton, Hants

Mrs Allison Peebles MCSP
Senior Cystic Fibrosis Physiotherapist, Southampton General Hospital, Southampton, Hants

Dr Simon Pennell BM BA
General Practitioner, Southbourne Surgery,
17 Beaufort Road, Bournemouth

Mr Christopher J. Randall FRCS
Consultant Otolaryngologist, Southampton General
Hospital, Southampton, Hants

Dr Fiona Regan MB ChB MRCP
Specialist Registrar in Paediatrics, Southampton
General Hospital, Southampton, Hants

Dr Karen Temple MD FRCP
Consultant in Clinical Genetics, Southampton
General Hospital, Southampton, Hants

Dr Claire Turner MRCP
Specialist Registrar in Clinical Genetics, Southampton
General Hospital, Southampton, Hants

Dr Valerie Walker BSc(Hons) MD Chb FRCPath FRCPCH
Consultant in Chemical Pathology, Southampton
General Hospital, Southampton, Hants

Dr Lee Wisby BM BSc MRCPCH
Specialist Registrar in Paediatrics, Southampton
General Hospital, Southampton, Hants

Dr Catherine Wood MB ChB FRCA
Consultant Paediatric Anaesthetist, Southampton
General Hospital, Southampton, Hants

Foreword

It is a great honour to be asked to write the foreword to this book, and it was a great pleasure to read it. The well established and respected cystic fibrosis team at Southampton have produced a volume that is at once both deceptively simple, and yet packed with useful information and tables. The reader will find a thorough, up to date overview of all the relevant aspects of the multi-disciplinary care of this complex, multi-system disease. The text is easy to read, clearly illustrated, with boxes to highlight the key points, but it is also a source of useful reference tables, to which many of us will return again and again to check the failing memory. The book reflects the realities of modern day practice, namely a true multi-disciplinary approach, with all team members having things to teach, as well as to learn from others.

The concept of the 'expert patient' is nowhere better developed than in the world of cystic fibrosis. However, although patients rapidly become experts, they too have to learn; and I suspect that many newly (and not so newly) diagnosed families will gain a lot from this book. Not least valuable is the final chapter of how to access useful organisations for families and professionals.

Sooner rather than later, the patient usually becomes the main teacher of the team. The wealth of information on the internet, and the attendant ease of communication, means that the patient entering the clinic has never been better informed. This can be very daunting for the new team member, who may feel out of their depth. Trying to learn about CF quickly can lead to information overload from the internet, and a lack of balance from overexposure to a few small, well-meaning but sometimes vociferous and over-enthusiastic groups whose view of evidence based medicine was well summarised many years ago by W.S. Gilbert: 'I m'Lords, embody the law'. The wood can be well and truly obliterated by the trees.

There is thus a clear need for a 'woods' book – a clear, concise and balanced overview, which will be both a practical guide for immediate problem solving, and the necessary stable foundation for delving into the cutting edge research in this field. It should surprise no-one that the editors and their team of authors have produced exactly this. The book will complement local and parochial guidelines (who specifically to ask about a particular problem, and more importantly, who not to ask), and the more detailed large volumes and reviews. It is essentially a *practical* book, with practical help offered by a team with years of priceless hands on experience. Although of course no two doctors will ever agree about everything, this volume charts an approach which will be in broad agreement with all but the most extremist.

Very few people, no matter how experienced, will read this book from cover to cover and close it without having learned something; and most of those who have not got anything out of it will be from the ranks of the unteachable. I recommend it without reservation to all members of the cystic fibrosis team, but in particular to those who are new in the field. Our main teachers are our patients, and there can be no substitute for years of hands on experience; but tapping into the expertise represented here can only be of help to all who want to improve the standards of care in the cystic fibrosis clinic.

Andrew Bush MD FRCP FRCPCH
Professor of Paediatric Respirology
Consultant Paediatric Chest Physician
Royal Brompton Hospital

Chapter **1**

Organisation of CF services: From national levels of care to home care

Judi Maddison

INTRODUCTION

Once diagnosed, the child and their family become part of the vast CF world. Participation varies enormously. Some choose only to have contact with their CF Team whilst others become actively involved with national charities and seek out new therapies. Forces outside of the local centre can impact significantly on treatment and lifestyle choices (Figure 1.1).

THE NATIONAL PERSPECTIVE

Good local care is essential and everyone should have access to a regional specialist centre. The UK Clinical Standards Advisory Group (CSAG) has defined the levels of care that can be provided by hospitals according to clinic size and the services available. These are:

Level 1 – A national resource centre

These have large clinics and fulfil a tertiary role for complex problems including those who might benefit from heart-lung transplantation. They provide national education and training and are an important resource.

Level 2 – A major specialist centre

These provide a regional service for over 100 patients. CF is a major specialist interest and the centre provides training, undertakes research and acts as a resource for smaller units.

Figure 1.1 The Cystic Fibrosis pyramid.

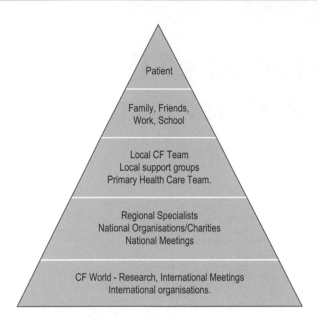

Patient

Family, Friends, Work, School

Local CF Team
Local support groups
Primary Health Care Team.

Regional Specialists
National Organisations/Charities
National Meetings

CF World - Research, International Meetings
International organisations.

Level 3 – local specialist centres

These care for around 35–40 patients (possibly including some adults) and provide specialist CF clinics. There is some specialist interest amongst the staff but numbers are often insufficient for a dedicated specialist team.

Level 4 – local hospital

These generally care for fewer than 20 patients who are usually seen in general clinics or the occasional special CF clinic, and provide general day-to-day local care.

It is recommended that the minimum number of patients to develop and maintain a specialist team is 50. Staffing levels are recommended in CSAG as per 50 patients in full care. Ratios are halved for shared care patients.

All individuals should have regular access to a level 1 or 2 centre. This can be provided through shared care. How this is arranged varies according to local facilities and geography. All new diagnoses should be referred to a level 1 or 2 unit and local service arrangements organised by the specialist centre. Whilst many prefer the convenience of a local hospital, regular input and support from a specialist centre is essential for modern care.

ESSENTIAL SERVICE CRITERIA (as defined by CSAG)

The following must be provided by level 1 and 2 centres:

- Appropriate numbers of medical and paramedical staff with relevant experience
- Dedicated outpatient clinics and facilities with sufficient time for discussion with the families
- Appropriate in-patient facilities, including side rooms, with sufficient staff to allow carers respite from daily care

- Clinical and laboratory investigations
- Other relevant specialist services for referrals as appropriate
- Referral to centres for assessment for organ transplantation
- Agreement over the provision of medication and equipment in the primary care setting.

THE REGIONAL PERSPECTIVE

Shared care

This has developed as a means of providing specialist care for a large number of individuals. Its aim is to reduce the need to travel long distances, and to provide local expertise and community support. Shared care normally involves referral from a level 3 or 4 centre to a level 1 or 2 centre (although in remote districts it may be from a level 4 to a level 3 centre). Shared care can be provided in different formats.

Annual assessment

Individuals receive most of their care from a level 3 hospital under a single consultant and attend a level 1 or 2 centre for annual assessment. Following this process a report is sent to the local consultant and GP. This defines the current clinical status and details treatment recommendations and expectations for the coming year. Ideally the assessment is carried out by level 1 or 2 staff visiting the local hospital thus providing an opportunity to teach and update the local carers. It is important to ensure all necessary investigations can be undertaken locally to an acceptable standard.

Alternating visits

Individuals attend their local level 3 or 4 and level 1 or 2 centres alternately. Good communication (possibly including patient held health records) is important to avoid conflicting advice. This system can be problematic if clinics are staffed by many different doctors. Joint notes should be considered.

Local joint clinics

Individuals attend their local clinic and a level 1 or 2 specialist team attends regularly. This can reduce the families' need to travel although they might still need to attend the regional centre for specific investigations.

THE SPECIALIST CF TEAM

Daily management is usually directed by a specialist team, based at the nearest CF centre, plus input from an extended number of health professionals. A multidisciplinary approach is essential. Team members must meet regularly because:

- CF is a complex multi-system disorder requiring diverse knowledge and understanding.
- Families have a high level of knowledge and increasing expectations that need to be met.
- Advances are rapid and treatment protocols change regularly.

The members of the CF Team are detailed in Table 1.1.

Table 1.1   Members of the CF Team.

Medical Personnel	• Primary Care Physicians • Paediatricians & Physicians (Respiratory Endocrinology and Gastroenterology) • Surgeons (ENT, GI and Transplant) • Gynaecologists and Obstetricians
Nursing	• Hospital Staff • Community Nurses • Clinical Nurse Specialists and Nurse Consultants
Physiotherapy	• Specialist Respiratory Physiotherapist • Community Physiotherapists
Dietetics	• Specialist Dietitian
Psychological Support	• Child Guidance/Adult Support Teams • Psychiatrists
Social/Supportive	• Social Workers • Chaplains/Religious Support • Family and Friends • Administrative Staff

Close co-ordination is vital. Many teams are devolved but others work better with clear leadership. Individual roles often overlap and good communication avoids duplication. A dedicated secretary or administrator is invaluable for large centres. Such personnel can usefully co-ordinate team activities, maintain the patient database and provide an initial point of contact for all referrals.

A team approach ensures:

- Multidisciplinary expertise is brought to all aspects of care
- Better knowledge of individual families
- Continuity; especially when team members change
- Families have a specific point of contact and know who to talk to
- Knowledge of treatment advances and the ability to apply these in daily management.

Team meetings   Regular team meetings are important to:

- Plan ongoing care for individuals.
- Assess the impact and effectiveness of current treatment.
- Update on psycho-social issues affecting the family.
- Provide opportunities for teaching.
- Discuss research and new treatment protocols.

Whilst team meetings would normally only include the specialist team, consideration must be given to involving wider team members such as those in related specialities, the community and other units. It often needs considerable effort to keep lines of communication open. Written reports can be helpful for those unable to attend meetings.

ORGANISATION OF LOCAL SERVICE

- Funding services
- Isolation policies
- Outpatient follow up clinics
- Annual assessments
- Inpatient care
- Home care.

Funding services

The way CF services are funded varies between regions. 'Postcode' prescribing and disparities in access to services are ongoing concerns. Ensuring unified care for all is extremely difficult. Banding patients according to treatment needs and providing funding on this basis for the next financial year works well in some centres. Unfortunately, regional differences in prescribing patterns have caused problems with introducing this nationally.

Isolation policies

For many years those growing *B. cepacia* or MRSA have been managed in strict isolation from other CF patients (CF Trust 1994). Recently there have been concerns about the possibility of cross infection with highly transmissible strains of *P. aeruginosa*. Some centres have many infected with identical strains of pseudomonas and these organisms can be multi-resistant. Most clinics address these issues using some form of cohorting or isolation policy.

Cohorting out-patients into groups according to their most recent microbiology result carries the risk of cross infection before current microbiology is known. This can be practically difficult with frequently changing microbiological status and changing sensitivities of chronic pseudomonas isolates. Decisions about when a patient can be declared clear of an organism and transfer between clinics are debatable. There are no clear guidelines.

Many clinics opt for a total isolation policy. When individuals attend the outpatient department, they are allocated a side room, instead of sitting in the waiting area. They remain in this room throughout the clinic visit and CF Team members come to them. Rooms are cleaned between patients. Staff observe strict hygiene precautions and instruments such as stethoscopes and pulmonary function machines are cleaned between use. Toys are removed from rooms and parents are asked to bring toys from home to occupy their child.

In-patients are allocated side rooms. They are asked to remain in them and not use communal ward areas during their stay. Computer gaming systems and small items of gym equipment can provide entertainment, encourage physical fitness and minimise boredom. Internet access can enable communication with others. Staff should have control over which websites are accessed. Normal visiting rules should apply for non-CF visitors.

Whilst a total isolation policy might seem harsh, and discourages contact between CF families, it should minimise the spread of multi-resistant organisms. Treating everyone similarly prevents individuals who harbour particular organisms from feeling like outcasts from the rest of the local CF community.

Irrespective of what policies are used it is important that all clinics perform regular microbiological surveillance of new isolates of *P. aeruginosa* to detect the spread of transmissible organisms within their patient population. Identification of *B. Cepacia* and unusually resistant pseudomonads should be confirmed by a reference laboratory.

Out-patient follow up clinics (CF Trust 1994)

Clinic services provide the basis for good care (Wood & Piazza 1988). Clinic visits should:

- Enable early identification and treatment of any health deterioration
- Assess adherence to recommended treatment regimes
- Assess the impact of any changes in care
- Facilitate ongoing communication
- Provide ongoing education and support.

Follow up should be:

- In a dedicated clinic where all team members can attend
- Two monthly when well and more often at other times
- Well co-ordinated and efficient to prevent unnecessary waiting
- Easily accessible with systems for urgent review and self-referral
- Individually tailored. Dedicated adolescent clinics can overcome difficulties with transfer from paediatric to adult services (see Chapter 22).

Clinic visits should include:

- Height (for children) and weight measurements plotted on growth charts (see Chapter 8)
- Preferably sputum or else cough swabs for microbiology (see Chapter 8)
- Review by a paediatrician/physician, dietitian and physiotherapist
- Lung function
- Access to other CF Team members (e.g. social worker, psychologist) as appropriate.

> **Remember**
>
> Consistent height and weight measurements and good microbiological specimens are vital. A dedicated clinic nurse can ensure the efficient running of clinics.

Team meetings at the end of clinics enable useful discussion about those seen and ensure all team members are aware of changes in management. A letter outlining current status, medication and changes in treatment should be sent to the GP and any other centre with whom there is shared care. It is considered good practise to send copies of correspondence to the family.

The annual assessment

This should:

- Review and document the past year's events
- Examine all aspects of needs
- Screen for complications
- Formulate a treatment plan for the coming year
- Provide ongoing education.

Every centre performs annual assessments differently and practise continues to evolve. Most are in two parts – initial investigations and fact finding followed by feedback and recommendations for the following year. Many specialist nurses have developed nurse-led clinics to undertake the investigative part. This gives families time with non-medical team members to discuss issues they might not think are relevant to medical staff. It also allows for individualisation of the assessment process.

The use of a standard proforma facilitates comparisons within and between patients. Assessments include:

History

Accurate documentation of respiratory status, gastrointestinal and nasal symptoms and treatment. An opportunity to discuss any concerns. Some centres will include a brief past history, including method of diagnosis and dates of significant events.

Examination

Including documentation of respiratory and ENT signs, abdominal findings, nutritional status and, when appropriate, pubertal staging.

Microbiological review

- Cough swab or whenever possible sputum sent for culture and sensitivity testing to include screening for atypical mycobacteria, fungae and *B. cepacia* (see Chapter 8)
- Review microbiological cultures over the past year with attention to treatment given for positive isolates
- Dates of first isolates of particular organisms.

Imaging

- Chest X-ray (lateral +/− PA films) formally scored (see Chapter 9). Some centres will now perform annual chest CT scans.
- Liver ultrasound (see Chapter 12).

Lung function

- Lung function including bronchodilator response using spirometry as a minimum – this is generally achievable from around the age of 4 years (see chapter 8)
- Oxygen saturation
- Exercise tolerance testing – to assess aerobic capacity and level of fitness (see Chapter 5)
- A review of inhaler techniques if used (see Chapter 5)
- Capillary blood gases if there are severe respiratory complications and FVC < 40% predicted
- Equipment review.

Blood tests   The following will screen for known complications and should be considered according to age and well being:

- Full Blood Count – screening for anaemia and eosinophilia
- Biochemical profile including liver and renal function
- Prothrombin time
- Screening for glucose intolerance. HbA1c and fasting glucose have limited value. Formal glucose tolerance test is recommended for all children over 10 years (see Chapter 11)
- Vitamin A, Vitamin E, red cell Vitamin E (see Chapter 7). Some clinics also monitor Vitamin D levels.
- Indices of aspergillus sensitisation; i.e. IgG fungal precipitins, aspergillus specific RASTs and total IgE (see Chapter 4)
- Iron status
- Pseudomonas serology
- Serum immunoglobulins and C-reactive protein
- Hepatitis virology and alpha 1 antitrypsin phenotype should be established for detectable liver disease.

Dietetic review   See Chapter 7.

Physiotherapy review   See Chapter 5.

Genetics
- Ensure that genotype has been determined, and send blood for the detection of rare mutations where appropriate (see Chapter 3).
- Ensure the family are aware of the services available for antenatal diagnosis and cascade screening of the extended family.

Psycho-social (Taylor 1996)   The impact of the disease treatment can have far reaching effects on the whole family and should be considered before introducing new therapies. A home visit prior to assessment provides an opportunity to discuss issues families might find difficult to bring up in the clinic setting. Visiting the home enables a better understanding of individual beliefs and needs.

Topics that might be discussed include:

- Understanding of the disease and its treatments
- Areas causing concern
- Family circumstances that might adversely affect treatment
- Financial situation; ensuring receipt of appropriate allowances
- Sexuality and fertility (see Chapter 16)
- Attitudes towards death and dying including open discussion about beliefs and expectations.

Planning a strategy   When assessment results are available there should be a multi-disciplinary team meeting to discuss findings and plan a strategy for the coming year. The full report should be made available to community staff, GP and shared care teams.

It is our practise to send uncensored copies of the report together with a glossary of commonly used medical terms to the family. The annual assessment is useful for the family:

- It provides written documentation about progress.
- It acknowledges their efforts in trying to maintain good health.
- It enables correction of misunderstandings or factual errors.
- It can be a useful document to take when travelling abroad.

PATIENTS IN HOSPITAL

There is increasing emphasis on providing home treatment but there are occasions when admission to hospital is necessary. Some regard an admission as a failure and it is useful to emphasise the positive aspects of inpatient stays.

> **Remember**
>
> All admissions provide an opportunity to examine and review treatment as well as updating education.

Reasons for admission

- New diagnosis: this can usefully ensure the initiation of high standards of adequately supervised care
- Acute respiratory or gastrointestinal complications
- Planned admission for routine therapy or related surgery
- Non-CF related admission
- Terminal/respite care.

> **Remember**
>
> Mechanisms should be in place to ensure that the CF Team are notified of all admissions irrespective of whether these are for CF related problems.

Planning admission

Discuss:

- The reason for admission
- Targets to be achieved
- Treatment and investigations
- Approximate length of stay
- The impact of treatment changes.

Families need to be involved in all decisions about treatment (CF Trust 1994). Medical staff should explain treatment clearly and discuss all available options.

The following infection control measures should be mandatory for all personnel:

- Meticulous hand-washing after every contact
- Single room nursing
- No sharing of equipment
- Appropriate cleaning of nebulisers (see Chapter 5).

For spirometry we recommend:

- Individual filtered mouthpieces or 'bag in the box' technique.
- Limit the measurement of flow volume loops to the expiratory manoeuvre.

Ward accommodation

Ward accommodation should consist of:

- Individual room
- Available oxygen and air supply, for nebulising medication and providing supplemental oxygen where appropriate
- Adequate ventilation, for example air flow/conditioning, or at least near a window that opens when using nebulised antibiotics (exhausting exhaled antibiotics via an open window prevents local environmental contamination)
- A bed that tips for postural drainage during physiotherapy
- Facilities for a parent to be resident
- Play equipment.

Admissions with respiratory exacerbations

An admission should be seen as an opportunity to optimise regular treatment and assess overall health. We recommend:

- Overnight monitoring of oxygen saturation for at least the first night of admission to detect the occurrence of nocturnal hypoxaemia. Give oxygen to maintain saturations of at least 92%.
- Pre- and 2 hour post-prandial measurements of capillary blood glucose for at least 24 hours to detect the development of glucose intolerance.
- Assessment of response to MDI and/or nebulised bronchodilators to determine the optimal use of inhaled therapy during admission.
- Intensification of airway clearance techniques as needed.
- Regular weighing and monitoring of oral intake to determine the need for oral supplements and/or enteral feeding.

Daily routine

Families often have fixed treatment regimes and find it stressful when ward routines differ. Nursing staff should discuss this on admission and agree an appropriate routine. Children should be encouraged to maintain their schooling.

Remember

Repeated hospital admissions can be socially isolating, and make it difficult to 'fit in' after discharge. Maintaining contact with family, friends and the school should be encouraged.

Discharge planning

Forward planning should include:

- Liaison between hospital and community staff
- Provision of treatment and equipment required at home
- Arranging follow-up
- A home visit prior to discharge can identify potential problems.

If a major change in treatment has been introduced, such as gastrostomy, discharge arrangements should commence prior to admission. Community staff should be involved during the inpatient stay and agree a suggested discharge date, before the family is notified.

INTRAVENOUS HOME CARE SERVICES

The aims of home care are to:

- Prevent repeated hospital admission
- Minimise disruption to normal life.

Advantages of home care

- Family preference
- Better placed for support from family and friends
- Conscientious timing of treatment
- Reduced risk of hospital acquired infection
- Home cooking
- Cost savings.

Disadvantages of home care

- Decreased medical and physiotherapy input
- Increased family stress
- Delay receiving emergency help
- Fewer educational opportunities
- Fewer opportunities for 'fine tuning' of medical treatments.

> **Remember**
>
> Home care should never be primarily a money saving strategy. Careful consideration is essential before allowing treatment to be undertaken at home (Maddison, Walsh & Peebles 1996).

Key points to successful home care

- Prior assessment
- Thorough training
- Liaison with community staff
- Easy access to back-up services
- Adequate resources to provide necessary equipment.

ASSESSING SUITABILITY FOR HOME CARE (Wynn 1992)

Initial assessments should be carried out in the home (see Figure 1.2). Families should be aware of the extent of treatment required and be willing and able to carry it out (see Figure 1.3).

Basic requirements

- Good compliance
- Suitable, safe environment including storage facilities
- Basic amenities, for example running water, lighting, refrigerator
- Telephone
- Transport facilities.

Figure 1.2 Home assessment: environment.

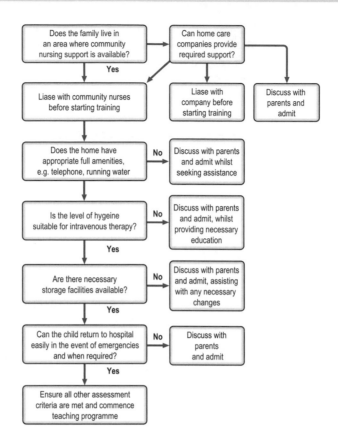

Figure 1.3 Home assessment: parents.

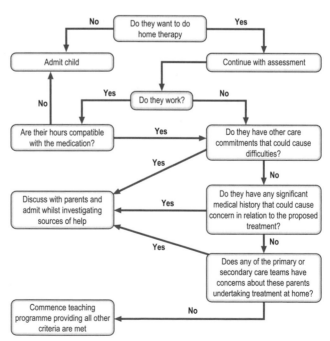

Figure 1.4   Home care: an algorithm for assessment.

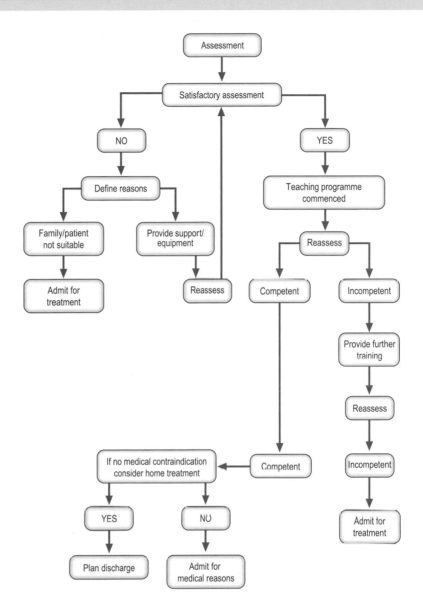

Contraindications to home care

- Poor compliance
- Family reluctance
- Carers need respite
- Need for further assessment or training.

TEACHING SKILLS FOR CARERS

Families must complete a comprehensive teaching programme (CF Trust 1995). This should occur in hospital and should never be rushed to facilitate early discharge. Teaching home care skills must address the items shown in Table 1.2.

It is advisable to issue anaphylaxis kits to those undertaking intravenous antibiotics at home. The most commonly used injectable adrenaline is the

Table 1.2 Teaching programme checklist.

Explanation about treatment	• what it is, for example name and dose of antibiotic • why it is being given • frequency of dosing • expected outcome
Hygiene needs associated with the treatment	• hand washing or use of gloves • storage of feeds (if applicable) • preparation on clean surfaces
Storage and disposal of equipment	• where and how to store it • use of sharps boxes (if applicable) • domestic rubbish vs. clinical waste
Trouble-shooting and problem solving	• what to do in the event of a problem • common problems and how to solve them • who to contact • important do's and don'ts
Side effects or complications of treatment	• anaphylaxis kits and their use (for example, with use of parenteral antibiotics) • what to look for • appropriate actions • when to seek help
Demonstration and learning	• observe staff performing treatment • practise with supervision and support • demonstrate ability to undertake treatment at a satisfactory level of competence

'Epi-Pen' and this is available on prescription. Written instructions about its use and the actions to take in an emergency must be given.

Every part of the teaching programme should be documented and on completion the carer and staff should sign that it has been successfully completed.

There should be regular visits to:

- Assess adherence.
- Monitor the patient's condition and assess the need for further intervention.
- Ensure the carer's continued ability to cope and provide support.

Families should be aware that a course of treatment at home is not just the administration of intravenous antibiotics. It must include intensification of physiotherapy and nutrition.

Remember

A family's ability to undertake home treatment should be continually reviewed, particularly if home circumstances change.

USE OF HOME CARE COMPANIES

There are numerous home care companies providing assistance for home treatment including enteral feeding.

The services offered vary according to the contracts between individual health authorities and the companies. Companies are generally more expensive than the use of hospital supplied medication but they can offer families the opportunity to be at home when community nursing is insufficient to provide the necessary support. Families using home care companies for treatment must still fulfil all the inclusion criteria listed above.

References

CF Trust 1994 A statement on B cepacia. Bromley

CF Trust 1994 The care of patients with CF – A patients charter. Bromley

CF Trust 1995 Home intravenous therapy and CF – advice for patients, parents and carers. Bromley

CF Trust BPA and British Thoracic Society 1996 Recommendations of a working group: clinical guidelines for CF care. Royal College of Physicians, London.

Maddison J, Walsh A, Peebles A 1996 A model of care for patients undergoing home intravenous antibiotics.

Poster presentation. International CF Conference, Jerusalem

Taylor B 1996 Parents as partners in care. Paediatric Nursing 8(4)

Wood R E, Piazza F 1988 Survival in CF: correlation with treatment in 3 CF centres. 10th International CF Congress, Sydney

Wynn S 1992 The CF nurse specialist and home intravenous antibiotics, training, supervision. The Medicine Group, London

Chapter 2

Diagnosis

Valerie Walker, Gary Connett

INTRODUCTION

One of the most important principles of care is early detection and treatment of complications to prevent irreversible damage. Whilst screening should achieve this for the majority, a small number of individuals will escape detection. Clinicians should remain vigilant and consider the possibility of CF when confronted with the diverse manifestations suggesting the diagnosis.

PRESENTATION – INDICATIONS FOR A SWEAT TEST

Pulmonary

- Chronic or recurrent wet coughing, pneumonia or bronchiolitis
- Purulent expectoration of sputum
- Difficult 'asthma'
- Unexplained haemoptysis
- Nasal polyps
- Chronic sinusitis.

Gastrointestinal

- Meconium ileus, meconium plug syndrome, abnormal bowel or peritoneal calcification on fetal ultrasound scanning
- Failure to thrive
- Frequent or large, greasy/shiny, offensive stools – steatorrhoea
- Pistachio green stools – protein malabsorption
- Rectal prolapse
- Atypical gastro-oesophageal reflux

Figure 2.1 Rapid skin wrinkling.

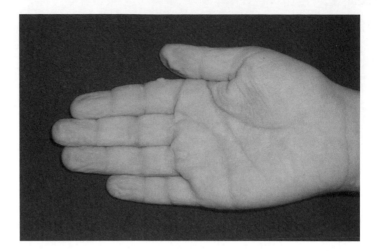

- Biliary cirrhosis, portal hypertension
- Hypoproteinaemia, anaemia and oedema with ascites
- Prolonged jaundice, neonatal hepatitis syndrome.

Other
- Pseudo-Bartter's Syndrome
- Heat exhaustion
- Male infertility
- Salty taste when kissed
- Sibling with CF
- Delayed puberty/short stature
- Male infertility, congenital bilateral absence of the vas deferens
- Parental suspicions
- Appendicitis – as suggested by histology.

CF individuals typically have rapid skin wrinkling, readily demonstrated by immersing their hands in water for a short period (Figure 2.1). A bulging fontanelle or facial palsy can occur as a result of Vitamin A deficiency. Vitamin K deficiency can result in INR prolongation and abnormal bleeding.

In unscreened populations, CF typically presents with gastro-intestinal and/or respiratory symptoms (see Table 2.1). Asthma is a common diagnostic label to explain respiratory symptoms in early childhood that might be due to CF. Gastrointestinal symptoms are also commonly attributed to other causes such as toddler diarrhoea. CF children presenting with failure to thrive will invariably have steatorrhoea on faecal fat testing. Conversely some children with malabsorption thrive initially as a result of increasing their food intake. Parent-held records provide useful diagnostic information about parental anxieties and poor postnatal growth.

Remember

A history of abnormal stools might not be reported by inexperienced parents. Careful questioning is necessary to elicit an accurate bowel history.

Table 2.1 Percentage distribution of presenting features in an unscreened CF population.

Presenting feature	%
Meconium ileus	15
Respiratory	25
Gastrointestinal	30
Respiratory and gastrointestinal	15
Family history	10
Other	5

Delayed diagnosis typically occurs in the following scenarios:

- Presentation with gastro-intestinal symptoms with little or no respiratory symptoms
- Atypical presentation
- Ethnic minorities: CF has been diagnosed in most racial groups
- Less severe phenotype: 'the patient looks too healthy'
- Poor sweat test technique
- Misinterpretation of sweat test result (see below).

In the majority of cases the diagnosis of CF is straightforward and based on the presence of either typical features or positive screening tests plus a positive sweat test and/or the identification of two CF gene mutations. Some cases are less straightforward (Wallis 1997). For example, individuals homozygous for the $3849 + 10\,kbC \rightarrow T$ mutations results in severe lung disease and normal sweat electrolytes (Highsmith 1994). There are also individuals with a typical CF phenotype but no identifiable CF mutations after CFTR gene sequencing. This suggests that there are genes at other loci affecting the clinical presentation. Despite such reservations the sweat test remains the gold standard for confirming the diagnosis and such occurrences are very rare (NCCLS 2000).

SWEAT TESTING

In normal term babies, sweat electrolytes are high in the first 48 hours of life, and fall to low values within 7 days. Pre-term babies might not sweat in the first 2 weeks of life. Sweat sodium and chloride are normally low in early childhood. Both rise progressively up to around 12 years of age and then stabilise. In CF, sodium and chloride remain high postnatally. Sodium increases further with age, but by a relatively small amount. Chloride levels do not change significantly. Chloride concentrations of CF and normal populations are more widely separated than sodium, especially in older subjects. Chloride is therefore a more discriminating analyte (Kirk 1992, LeGrys 1996).

Demonstration of raised sweat chloride is the primary diagnostic test for CF. Raised values for sweat sodium, conductivity and osmolality provide supportive evidence, but should not be used without chloride for diagnosis.

Pilocarpine iontophoresis is the only acceptable sweat test procedure. In the Gibson and Cooke method, sweat is collected onto filter paper and then eluted for analysis (Gibson & Cooke 1959). With the Wescor Macroduct® system, sweat is collected into a coiled capillary tube from which it is sampled directly for analysis (see Chapter 8).

Sweat requirement

Sweat electrolyte concentrations are related to the rate of sweating. They are *low* at *low* sweat rates.

A rate exceeding $1 \, g/m^2$ of stimulated skin per minute is required.

The minimum amount of sweat depends on the size of the electrode, the stimulation area and the duration of collection.

> **Example**
>
> Gibson and Cooke method: Collection onto a 5 cm × 5 cm filter paper for 30 min needs at least 75 mg of sweat.
>
> Wescor Macroduct® system: a 30 min collection needs at least 15 ul.

It is *not* permissible to pool paired samples if the individual sweat weight or volumes are insufficient.

The main action of the stimulated glands is in the first 15 minutes. Collection should be for 20–30 minutes. Longer collection times require more sweat and there is an increasing risk of error from evaporation.

With the Gibson and Cooke procedure, sweat is often collected from both arms. This is not essential, but discrepant values indicate contamination, evaporation or laboratory errors.

Interpretation

Chloride levels for a well-conducted test with adequate sweat:

<40 mmol/L	normal
40–60 mmol/L	borderline/equivocal
>60 mmol/L	consistent with CF
>150 mmol/L	non-physiological-contamination or error

When both arms are tested

If chloride <60 mmol/L: results should agree to within 10%
If chloride >60 mmol/L: results should agree to within 15%

Conductivity

<60 mmol/L	CF unlikely
60–90 mmol/L	equivocal further investigation needed
>90 mmol/L	consistent with CF
>170 mmol/L	probably non-physiological

Until more data are available, chloride must be measured as well.

Comments on interpretation

Chloride is >60 mmol/L in around 98% of individuals with CF.
Chloride is <60 mmol/L in 1–2% of individuals with CF (confirmed on repeat testing) (see Figure 2.2).

Figure 2.2   The effect of age on sweat chloride in normal controls 0, and patients with CF. ▲ > 70 mmol/L, □ < 70 mmol/L (Kirk 1992).

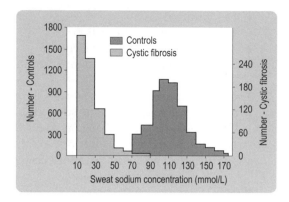

Figure 2.3   Effect of age on Sweat Sodium Concentrations (Gibson & Cooke 1959).

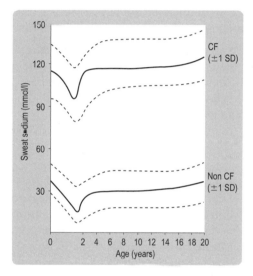

Heterozygotes have significantly higher sweat chlorides than homozygous normal subjects (Farrell & Koscik 1996). Concentrations in early life are below the CF cut-off level. However, it is not uncommon for adult heterozygotes to have values >60 mmol/L.

Some healthy adolescents and adults also have sweat chloride >60 mmol/L (Kirk 1992).

Spurious results

These are usually a result of poorly conducted tests. Other causes include:

False negatives

- Insufficient sweat
- Unusual CF mutations (1–2% of individuals with CF)
- Oedema
- Hypochloraemic alkalosis.

False positives

- Sample evaporation
- Contamination, including Munchausen by proxy
- Analytical errors
- Eczema and other skin rashes

- Dehydration
- Protein/calorie malnutrition
- Adrenal or thyroid insufficiency
- Some rare inherited metabolic disorders.

The interpretation of equivocal tests in older children can be clarified by carrying out a fludrocortisone suppression test.

Oral fludrocortisone ($3\,mg/m^2/day$) for 2 days causes a decrease in sweat sodium in normals but not in CF. However, there are no reports about the effect on chloride and the test is not widely used.

GENOTYPING

Regional services will screen for gene mutations common to the local population when requested. Genotyping is highly specific but sensitivity is low because of the large number of CF gene mutations. Genotyping can be useful in the following situations:

- For confirmatory diagnosis in neonates presenting with meconium ileus (There are often difficulties obtaining adequate sweat samples for analysis in the first 2–3 weeks of life)
- When repeat sweat tests are not diagnostic but there is a strong clinical suspicion
- In all individuals with a confirmed diagnosis (i.e. confirmatory sweat test or nasal PD).

Sampling for genetic testing

- For adults and older children: 10 mls blood in EDTA bottle.
- For neonates and infants: minimum volumes of 0.5 mls blood in EDTA bottle. Guthrie card dried blood spots are used in neonatal screening programmes.
- Mouth brush samples can also be analysed; obtained by brushing the buccal mucosa with a sterile brush and sending in a dry container.

National references laboratories can screen for rare mutations not picked up on routine local testing. Information about ethnicity and phenotype might usefully increase the chances of identifying specific mutations. An up-to-date registry of all identified mutations is available at http://www.genet.sickkids.on.ca/cftr.

One of the common diagnostic problems is the child with clinical features suggesting CF, an indeterminate sweat test and only one identifiable gene mutation. In such cases the sweat test should be repeated in a regional centre and blood sent to screen for rare mutations. If results are still indeterminate, detailed clinical evaluation and ancillary testing for evidence of CFTR dysfunction such as nasal potential difference measurements might be appropriate (see below).

NASAL POTENTIAL DIFFERENCE (Alton 1990)

Individuals with CF have a more negative potential difference (PD) across their respiratory epithelium compared with normal controls. This can be measured in cooperative subjects using a probe placed in the nasal cavity. The PD response to the instillation of drugs and ionic solutions can be measured using a second probe in the opposite nostril. The test requires technical expertise and is best performed in an experienced laboratory with a validated test protocol and their own reference values. Children under the age of 7 years are unlikely to cooperate and might require sedation if tests are to be carried out in this age group. Results can be affected by the following:

- Recent viral infection
- Previous nasal surgery
- Allergic rhinitis and polyps
- Precise anatomic location of measurement.

Nasal PD testing can usefully exclude pulmonary CFTR dysfunction in individuals who might previously have been misdiagnosed as having CF on the basis of a false positive sweat test.

IMMUNE REACTIVE TRYPSIN (IRT)

IRT measured from dried blood spots (collected on Guthrie cards in the UK) is 2–5 times higher in neonates with CF than normal controls. Levels decrease after 1–2 months. There is a high false positive rate and IRT measurements are only of value when used as a part of a newborn screening programme.

TESTS FOR MALABSORPTION

See Chapter 8.

ATYPICAL CF

With an ever increasing number of CF genes, it has been recognised that some conditions caused by two CFTR mutations, for example bilateral absence of the vas deferens, do not meet diagnostic criteria for CF. This has lead to the concept of CFTR-related disease (see Chapter 3). Some experts have suggested the concept of 'pre-CF' for individuals with a CF genotype but no discernable disease as might, for example, be identified through newborn screening programmes (Bush & Wallis 2000). Careful consideration needs to be given about how best to tailor appropriate levels of care and surveillance for these different phenotypes. Detailed evaluation of late presenting atypical cases is necessary to assess the extent of end organ damage and to exclude important differential diagnoses.

Clinical evaluation of atypical cases

Respiratory

- Sputum/cough swab for culture of CF related pathogens
- Chest X-ray and chest CT scan to look for bronchiectasis
- Consider fibre-optic bronchoscopy
- Paranasal sinus CT to look for polyps/sinus related disease.

Pancreatic function

- Faecal elastase
- Abdominal ultrasound
- Faecal fat assessment.

Male genitalia

- Clinical examination
- Ultrasound scan
- Semen analysis if appropriate.

Investigations for the differential diagnosis of respiratory illness

- Immunological work up
- Allergy work up
- Reflux studies
- Ciliary studies.

WHO classification of CF and related disorders

The World Health Organization classifies CF and related disorders into 12 different groups (WHO 2000). The morbidity and prognosis varies considerably. This classification usefully clarifies the diagnosis of CFTR-related disease according to different phenotypes for insurance purposes, to address medico-legal issues and to ensure the appropriate provision of care packages (Rosenstein 2002).

- Classical CF pancreatic insufficient (PI)
- Classical CF pancreatic sufficient (PS)
- Atypical CF
- CF other specified
- CF not otherwise specified
- Isolated obstructive azoospermia*
- Chronic pancreatitis*
- Allergic bronchopulmonary aspergillosis (ABPA)*
- Disseminated bronchiectasis*
- Diffuse panbronchiolitis*
- Sclerosing cholangitis*
- Neonatal hypertrypsinogenemia.
  *at least one CFTR mutation identified

All health care professionals need to be alert to the possibility of CF in their patients. Continued vigilance is necessary for the early identification of those cases that will be missed through neonatal screening. A good working knowledge of the wide range of presenting phenotypes is essential. CF carers need to repeatedly review the possibility of false positive diagnoses in their well patients.

References

Alton E W, Currie D, Logan S R et al 1990 Nasal potential difference: a clinical diagnostic test for CF. European Respiratory Journal 3:922–926

Bush A, Wallis C 2000 Time to think again – CF, like cancer is not an 'all or none' disease. Pediatric Pulmonology 30:139–144

Farrell P M, Koscik R E 1996 Sweat chloride concentrations in infants homozygous or heterozygous for F508 CF. Pediatrics 97:524–528

Gibson L E, Cooke R E 1959 A test for concentration of electrolytes in sweat in CF of the pancreas utilizing pilocarpine by iontophoresis. Pediatrics 23:545–549

Highsmith W E, Burch L H, Zhou Z et al 1994 A novel mutation in the CF gene in patients with pulmonary disease but normal sweat chloride concentrations. New England Journal of Medicine 331:974–80

Kirk J M, Keston M, McIntosh I et al 1992 Variation of sweat sodium and chloride with age in CF and normal populations: further investigations in equivocal cases. Annals of Clinical Biochemistry 29:145–152

LeGrys V A 1996 Sweat testing for the diagnosis of CF: practical considerations. Journal of Pediatrics 129:892–897

NCCLS 2000 Sweat testing: sample collection and quantitative analysis: approved guidelines-second edition. NCCLS document C34-A2 (ISBN 1-56238-407-4), Wayne PA, Pennsylvania

Rosenstein B J 2002 CF: new dilemmas for an older disorder. Pediatric Pulmonology 33:83–84

Report of a joint WHO/ICF(M)A/ECFTN meeting 2000 Classification of CF and related disorders. Stockholm, Sweden (www.cfww.org/WHO-index.asp)

Wallis C 1997 Diagnosing CF: blood sweat and tears. Archives of Diseases Childhood 76:85–91

Chapter 3

Genetics

Claire Turner, Karen Temple, Anneke Lucassen

INTRODUCTION

The identification of the CF gene in 1989 and research into its function and malfunction, has expanded knowledge of the disease process and opened up new therapeutic possibilities. Over subsequent years the sensitivity of genetic testing has improved as increasing numbers of CF gene mutations have been identified. This has enabled more accurate genetic diagnosis of individuals and screening of families and populations. The disease spectrum has broadened as it has become clear that some mutations are associated with a milder phenotype than the classical disease.

INHERITANCE

CF shows a Mendelian autosomal recessive inheritance (Figure 3.1). Affected individuals have two copies of a mutated CF gene, one inherited from either parent. 'Carriers' have one copy of a mutated CF gene. Carrier status does not appear to affect the health of the individual.

Population risks

Mutations of the CF gene are most common in those of white European origin. However CF has been described in almost all racial groups. In the UK the incidence is 1 in 2500 births. The carrier risk is therefore approximately 1:25 ($1/25 \times 1/25 \times 1/4 = 1/2500$).

Figure 3.1 Autosomal recessive inheritance. Carrier parents have a 1:4 risk of an affected offspring per pregnancy; Unaffected offspring have a 2:3 risk of being a carrier.

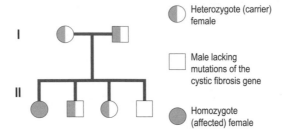

Heterozygote (carrier) female

Male lacking mutations of the cystic fibrosis gene

Homozygote (affected) female

Table 3.1 The percentage of all mutations of the CF gene found to be the delta F508 mutation in different European populations.

Country	% delta F508
Netherlands	88
UK	79
Denmark	78
Ireland	75
France	75
Germany	65
Poland	55
Italy	50
Turkey	30

THE GENE AND ITS MUTATIONS

- Located on the long arm of chromosome 7 at 7q31–q32 the CF gene is 250 kilobases in length.
- The gene has 27 exons and encodes the 'Cystic Fibrosis Transmembrane Conductance Regulator' (CFTR), a protein of 1,480 amino acids.
- CFTR codes for a chloride channel present on the apical membrane of exocrine epithelial cells. This is involved in salt and water balance across epithelial surfaces.
- The first mutation identified was a deletion of three adjacent base pairs at the 508th codon of the gene: ΔF508.
- In north European communities, the ΔF508 mutation accounts for about three quarters of all mutations (and thus in the UK about half are homozygous for ΔF508), but its frequency varies significantly between populations (Worldwide survey 1990). Among Ashkenazi Jews ΔF508 accounts for only a third of mutations, whereas W1282X accounts for about a half. (Table 3.1).
- Over 1,200 different mutations of the CFTR gene have been identified to date. Most are individually rare, confined to a few families, and account for 1–3% of the CF mutations among the local population (Worldwide survey 1994). Most diagnostic laboratories in the UK routinely look for about 30 of the commonest mutations, but this varies and testing for rarer mutations can be requested.

Mutations can be divided into 5 broad classes (Table 3.2).

Up-to-date information about CF mutations can be found at the website http://www.genet.sickkids.on.ca/cftr

Table 3.2 Classes of CFTR mutations.

Class	Effect on CFTR	Types of Mutation	CF patients (Europe)(%)	Potential Therapy
I	Defective synthesis of message causing absence of CFTR	Premature stop codon (either nonsense or frame shift (i.e. W1282X or G542X)	7	Aminoglycosides Gene transfer
II	Abnormal CFTR produced which fails to leave endoplasmic reticulum	Amino acid deletion (i.e. ΔF508) or missense mutation	85	Butyrates, Gene transfer
III	Abnormal CFTR causing disruption of activation and regulation at cell membrane	Missense mutation (i.e. G551D)	<3	Genistein, Gene transfer
IV	Abnormal CFTR, reducing chloride conductance	Missense; mutation (i.e. R117H or R347P)	<3	Milrinone, Gene transfer
V	Reduced or absent synthesis of CFTR due to decreased splicing of normal CFTR	Missense mutation or Splice site mutation (i.e. A445E or 5T)	<3	Gene transfer

Note:
1. There is overlap between different classes of mutation. For example, the ΔF508 mutation can cause reduced chloride channel opening time as well as abnormal CFTR processing.
2. Sometimes the CFTR mutation can be modified by another mutation or polymorphism on the same allele. See genotype phenoytpe correlations below.

FACTORS DETERMINING DISEASE EXPRESSION

Three factors contribute to the variability of the CF phenotype:

- The individual's specific pair of CFTR mutations (i.e. CF genotype).
- The rest of the genome. These might directly compensate for CFTR absence or dysfunction or else modify the pathogenic consequences.
- The environment, including therapeutic interventions.

Genotype/phenotype correlations

(i.e. the correlation between specific gene mutations and the clinical picture.)

- Genotype correlates most strongly with pancreatic exocrine insufficiency and sweat chloride concentrations. There is generally poor correlation with pulmonary function (The cystic fibrosis genotype/phenotype consortium 1993, Zielenski 2000).
- The classic CF phenotype (pancreatic involvement in infancy, chronic pulmonary disease, abnormal sweat electrolytes, and absent vas deferens in males), is usually caused by disruption of CFTR synthesis through frame shift or nonsense mutations and includes classes I, II and III (see Table 3.2). These are 'severe' mutations and the genotype is usually associated with complete loss of CFTR chloride channel function.
- Compound heterozygotes for 'severe' and 'mild' (classes IV and V) mutations, tend to have preservation of pancreatic function.
- Recently more subtle CFTR modifying factors have been identified. For example, the pathogenicity of the R117H mutation is modified by the number of polythymidine (polyT) residues within intron 8 (see Box).

Thymidine residues in intron 8 and the R117H mutation

The length of the polythymidine tract in intron 8 is polymorphic i.e. 5, 7 or 9 thymidine residues (5T, 7T and 9T). The number of thymidine residues affects the efficiency of the splice-acceptor site in intron 8 of the CFTR gene. The 5T allele is associated with the least efficient usage of the splice-acceptor site reducing the amount of mature, functional CFTR protein. This alteration is variably described in the literature as a polymorphism or a mutation. When the mutation R117H is in-cis (i.e. in series) with 5T rather than 7T or 9T, it is more pathogenic. The occurrence of 5T alleles in series with other CFTR gene sequence variants might also result in atypical (mild) CF phenotypes.

Modifier genes

- Complex interactions between CFTR and several modifier genes explain some of the variation in respiratory phenotype (Acton & Wilmott 2001).
- Several candidate loci have been studied, for example the mannose-binding lectin, glutathione-S-transferase, transforming growth factor-beta1, tumour necrosis factor-alpha, beta-2-adrenergic receptor, and HLA class II antigens (Merlo & Boyle 2003).

CFTR-RELATED DISEASES

As knowledge about CFTR mutations increases, a spectrum of diseases caused by CFTR mutations distinct from CF have been characterised. These, usually milder phenotypes, are referred to as 'CFTR-related disease'.

Congenital bilateral absence of the vas deferens

50–82% of otherwise healthy male subjects investigated for azoospermia who have congenital absence of the vas deferens have CFTR mutations. Ten per cent have biallelic CFTR mutations. One of these is usually an R117H mutation or a 5T(5 Thymidine) splicing mutation (Chillon 1995, Anguiano 1992). Although those affected are usually asymptomatic, they might be at increased risk of bronchiectasis in later life.

In male infertility, other abnormalities reported to be possibly associated with CFTR mutations include unilateral absence of the vas deferens, idiopathic epididymal obstruction and asthenospermia (reduced sperm motility).

Chronic pancreatitis

13–37% of subjects with idiopathic chronic pancreatitis (i.e. excess alcohol ingestion excluded) have at least one CFTR mutation. The 5T mutation is particularly prevalent in this sub group (Sharer 1998, Cohn 1998).

Idiopathic disseminated bronchiectasis

Those affected should be screened. An overrepresentation of CFTR mutations, particularly 5T, has been found in this group (Noone 2000, Girodon 1997). In one study the percentage of children with diffuse bronchiectasis and at least one CFTR mutations was 41% (Ninis 2003).

Chronic rhinosinusitis (CRS)

CFTR mutations occur more frequently with ΔF508 being the most common (Wang 2000).

Allergic bronchopulmonary aspergillosis (ABPA) in asthmatics

This is also associated with an increased frequency of one or more CFTR mutations.

DETECTING CFTR MUTATIONS

There are two main indications for CFTR mutation testing:

- Diagnosis (prenatal and postnatal)
- Screening (including carrier screening and presymptomatic testing of neonates).

The use of DNA analysis as a diagnostic tool

Testing for approximately 30 mutations yields in the region of 90% of mutations. Of affected individuals in the UK:

- Over 99% have 1 or more detectable mutations
- 81% (90/100 × 90/100) have 2 detectable mutations.

When a regional laboratory is unable to detect two CF mutations and the clinical diagnosis warrants confirmation, nominated laboratories will perform a more extensive mutation search. In the future this will be performed by the UK National Genetics Testing Network (www.doh.gov.uk/genetics/gtn.htm).

Situations in which CF mutations are not detected but when CF may still be suspected include:

- Parents are first cousins
- Non caucasian families
- Mild disease.

When only one or no identifiable mutations are identified, further diagnostic confirmation with sweat testing and/or nasal potential difference, if not already done, should be arranged.

In neonates at risk of CF, DNA analysis can be a useful diagnostic tool if sweat testing is not feasible. Consider the diagnosis in:

- meconium ileus
- inspissated bile syndrome
- parents known to be carriers but no prenatal diagnosis performed.

> **Remember**
>
> In neonates, cord blood sampling avoids venepuncture but needs forward planning.

The use of DNA analysis for carrier screening

DNA analysis is the only reliable way of identifying carriers.

For white Europeans, when a laboratory has screened for approximately 30 common mutations:

- Testing yields approximately 90% of mutations so 10% of carriers tested have mutations that are not identified.
- If no mutations are identified the risk of being a carrier is approximately 1/240. This is calculated using Bayes' theorem and is described in most modern genetic textbooks (Bayes 1958).

Risk calculations should be modified according to ethnic group and the number of mutations screened for.

Cascade screening

This is the selected screening of extended family members of an index case.

- If the genotype of the index case is known, accurate carrier testing of blood relatives is possible.
- If individuals are screened before conceiving children, carrier status can usefully inform reproductive decisions. Careful counselling is required. Over time, screened carriers have poor recall of information (Axworthy 1996).
- When the index case has no identified mutations, linkage analysis can be used to predict risks for family members. This requires DNA from several family members and can fail if there are no informative genetic markers or if the family structure is inappropriate.

PREDICTING RISK: EXAMPLES

Carrier status risk for unaffected siblings of index cystic fibrosis case

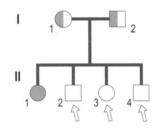

Figure 3.2 Assuming the siblings (II2, II3 and II4) are clinically unaffected there is an individual 2/3 risk of carrying a CF gene.

Carrier status for unaffected sibling of known carrier

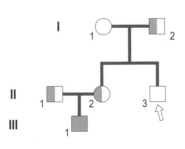

Figure 3.3 Sister II2 has an affected child III1. She and her partner II1 are obligate carriers. II2 has inherited a mutated CF gene from her father I2. Her brother, II3, will have a 1/2 risk of inheriting the same gene.

Risk to offspring of parent with affected sibling where carrier status is unknown

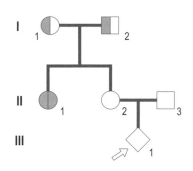

Figure 3.4   Carrier risk for II2 is 2/3 (see Figure 3.2). Carrier risk for her partner II3 if unscreened is 1/25 (population risk). Therefore risk to III1 of having CF = 2/3 × 1/25 × 1/4 = 1/150.

Refining the risk with DNA analysis

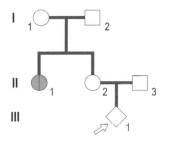

Figure 3.5   If routine screening fails to detect a mutation in the partner II3 his carrier risk is reduced to 1/240. The risk now to III1 of having CF is 2/3 × 1/240 × 1/4 = 1/1440.

Risk to offspring of parent with affected child by previous partner

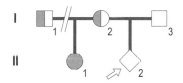

Figure 3.6   I2 is an obligate carrier. I3 is an unscreened, unaffected Caucasian and has a carrier risk of 1/25. Therefore the risk to II2 of being affected is 1 × 1/25 × 1/4 = 1/100.

Risk to offspring of parent with affected child by previous partner where new partner has screened negative for common CF mutations

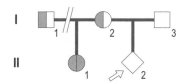
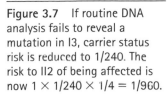

Figure 3.7   If routine DNA analysis fails to reveal a mutation in I3, carrier status risk is reduced to 1/240. The risk to II2 of being affected is now 1 × 1/240 × 1/4 = 1/960.

Carrier screening

'Carrier couples' can be identified at pre-conception or antenatal visits. Pilot studies have shown universal carrier testing to be inefficient and expensive with poor uptake and poor long-term recall of test results (Axworthy 1996, Bekker 1993).

Antenatal screening

Screening pregnant women and their partners provides genetic information at a highly relevant time. Uptake rates are around 70% (Brock 1996).

Detection is limited by false negatives among individuals with rare mutations.

The risk of a CF pregnancy in a couple where both partners test negative for common mutations and have no family history is 1:230,400 ($1/240 \times 1/240 \times 1/4$). When one partner is a heterozygote the risk is 1:960 ($1 \times 1/240 \times 1/4$).

Antenatal screening is sometimes initiated following the identification of features that may be attributable to CF on antenatal fetal anomaly scans e.g. hyperechogenic bowel, especially in the presence of dilated bowel loops or the absence of the gall bladder (Muller 2002). If both parents are found to be carriers, prenatal fetal diagnosis can be considered.

Antenatal screening needs skilled counselling. Not all parents of CF children choose to terminate an affected subsequent pregnancy. The ethical issues surrounding abortion of fetuses affected by a condition with ever increasing life expectancy need consideration.

Two methods of antenatal screening have been trialed (Brock 1996).

Advantages

● Offers the opportunity for cascade screening for carriers.

Disadvantages

● More expensive: 4% of individuals identified as carriers will require counselling
● If paternity has been wrongly attributed.

Figure 3.8   Two step testing.

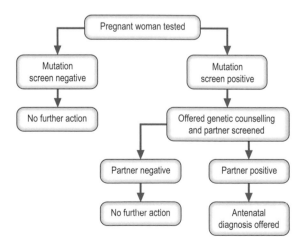

Figure 3.9 Couple testing.

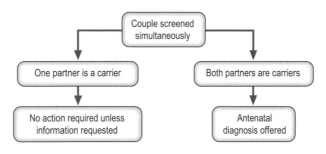

Advantages

- Economical as only 0.1% of couples require counselling.

Disadvantages

- Carrier status not revealed. This may be relevant if there is a change of partner in future pregnancies and for relatives.
- If paternity has been wrongly attributed.

Pre-implantation diagnosis

Pre-implantation testing is available. This might be suitable when known carriers are undergoing in vitro fertilisation (IVF) techniques for an infertility problem or where in utero diagnosis and the prospect of aborting an affected fetus would be unacceptable.

IVF techniques allow removal of one cell at the 6–8 cell, embryo stage for DNA analysis. Only embryos lacking two copies of the mutated gene are replaced. Genotype of both egg and sperm donors must be established.

Because of the technical difficulties (i.e. the need for IVF), the chance of a live born infant using this technique is currently low. Routine screening of sperm or egg donors, or couples undergoing IVF with no family history, is not common practice.

Pre-natal testing

This should be offered to parents when both are carriers. Fetal DNA can be obtained by two techniques:

Chorionic villous sampling (CVS)

- Mutations can be detected from DNA in trophoblast tissue sampled at 10–11 weeks gestation, allowing first trimester termination of an affected fetus.
- Spontaneous miscarriage rates of 1–2% are quoted. Fetal limb and facial abnormalities have occurred following CVS. The risk is minimal if performed after 10 weeks gestation.
- When fetal DNA reveals a female karyotype with one copy of a gene mutation, comparison with maternal DNA will rule out contamination by maternal tissue. Most genetics labs already have stored samples of maternal DNA. If not, a maternal sample should be sent with the CVS sample to minimise delay.

Amniocentesis

- Can be performed from 16 weeks gestation. Depending on the size of the sample, fetal cell culture and DNA analysis can be performed within 2–3 weeks.
- Amniocentesis has spontaneous miscarriage rates of 0.3–1%.

Figure 3.10   Newborn screening.

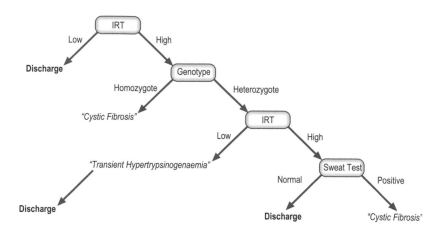

Note: False negatives (missed cases) can occur at any stage.

Neonatal testing (Screening)

The vast majority of CF clinicians are in favour of newborn screening. However, screening can only be beneficial if it is linked to subsequent specialist care.

Advantages of early diagnosis include reduced hospitalisation and decreased levels of care to maintain health (Chatfield 1991). A recent retrospective review also suggested improved growth parameters among those diagnosed neonatally compared to those diagnosed later following symptoms (Siret 2003).

Screening reduces parental stress from delayed diagnosis, allows more positive relationships between families and professionals and engenders a more positive attitude towards the child (Boland & Thompson 1990). Pre-natal diagnosis can be offered for future pregnancies.

Screening programmes using serum immunoreactive trypsin (IRT) measurements alone have a high false positive rate (Hammond 1991). This is improved by combining immunoreactive trypsin assays with DNA analysis of abnormally high results (Ranieri 1991).

A UK-wide neonatal screening programme is planned for 2004 and will follow the 3-stage protocol summarised in Figure 3.10.

PHARMACOGENETICS

New pharmacological treatments are likely to be aimed at specific classes of CFTR mutation. Recent research on the use of aminoglycoside antibiotics suggests that these may be specifically beneficial in Class I CFTR mutations caused by a premature stop codon. Aminoglycosides inhibit ribosomal proofreading allowing insertion of a poorly matched amino acyl-transferase (amino acid attached to the tRNA). When this occurs at the premature stop codon it permits translation to continue to the end of the gene so that a full-length functional CFTR protein can be produced (Wilschanski 2003).

Class II CFTR mutations (including ΔF508) cause impaired trafficking of CFTR. Butyrate compounds impair the molecular chaperones that target the abnormal CFTR for destruction and so may be of benefit.

GENE THERAPY

Gene replacement therapy aims to introduce a normal copy of a gene into cells and restore normal gene function. This is a theoretical possibility for treating related lung disease. The gene product is now well characterised. The idea is to administer the normal gene to the affected lungs using a modified virus or cationic liposome vector. Studies have shown that this can produce detectable mRNA of CFTR but at low levels.

The main problem has been the inefficiency of gene transfer in the lungs. This is mainly due to a series of barriers preventing vector penetration (mucus, lack of apical receptors, immunity). Intracellular mechanisms also hinder effective gene transfer.

Research has focussed on the nasal passages, as a model for lower airway gene transfer. Nasal potential difference measurements are used as a proxy for assessing gene transfer (Alton 1999, Harvey 1999).

References

Acton J D, Wilmott R W 2001 Phenotype of cystic fibrosis and the effects of possible modifier genes. Paediatric Respiratory Reviews 2(4):332–339

Alton E, Stern M et al 1999 Cationic lipid-mediated CFTR gene transfer to the lungs and nose of patients with cystic fibrosis: a double blind placebo controlled trial. Lancet 353:947–954

Anguiano A, Oates R et al 1992 Congenital bilateral absence of the vas deferens. A primarily genital form of cystic fibrosis. Journal of the American Medical Association 267:1794–1797

Axworthy D, Brock D J H et al 1996 Psychological impact of population based carrier testing for cystic fibrosis: 3 year follow-up. Lancet 347:1443–1446

Bayes T 1958 An essay towards solving a problem in the doctrine of chances. Biometrika 45:296–315

Bekker H, Modell M et al 1993 Uptake of cystic fibrosis in primary care: supply push or demand pull? British Medical Journal 306:1584–1586

Boland C, Thompson NL 1990 Effects of newborn screening for cystic fibrosis on reported maternal behaviour. Archives of Diseases in Childhood 65:1240–1244

Brock D J H 1996 Prenatal screening for cystic fibrosis: 5 years experience reviewed. Lancet 347:148–150

Chatfield S, Owen G et al 1991 Neonatal screening for cystic fibrosis in Wales and the West Midlands: clinical assessment after five years of screening. Archives of Diseases in Childhood 66:29–33

Chillon M, Casals T, Mercier B et al 1995 Mutations in the cystic fibrosis gene in patients with congenital absence of the vas deferens. New England Journal of Medicine 332:1475–1480

Cohn J A, Friedman K J, Noone P G et al 1998 Relation between mutations of the cystic fibrosis gene and idiopathic pancreatitis. New England Journal of Medicine 339:653–658

Cystic Fibrosis Genetic Analysis Consortium 1994 Population variation of common cystic fibrosis mutations. Human Mutation 167–177

Girodon E, Cazeneuve C et al 1997 CFTR gene mutations in adults with disseminated bronchiectasis. European Journal of Human Genetics 5:149–155

Hammond K B, Abman S H et al 1991 Efficacy of statewide neonatal screening for cystic fibrosis by assay of trypsinogen concentrations. New England Journal of Medicine 325:769–774

Harvey B, Leopold P et al 1999 Airway epithelial CFTR mRNA expression in cystic fibrosis patients after repetitive administration of a recombinant adenovirus. Journal of Clinical Investigation 104(90):1245–1255

Merlo C A, Boyle M P 2003 Modifier genes in cystic fibrosis lung disease. Journal of Laboratory and Clinical Medicine 141(4):237–241

Muller F, Simon-Buoy B et al 2002 Predicting the risk of cystic fibrosis with abnormal ultrasound signs of foetal bowel: results of a French molecular collaborative study based on 641 prospective case. American Journal of Medical Genetics 110(2):109–115

Ninis V et al 2003 High frequency of T9 and CFTR mutations in children with idiopathic bronchiectasis. Journal of Medical Genetics 40:530–535

Noone P, Pue C et al 2000 Lung disease associated with the IVS8 5T allele of the CFTR gene. American Journal of Respiratory and Critical Care Medicine 162:1919–1924

Ranieri E, Ryall R G et al 1991 Neonatal screening strategy for cystic fibrosis using immunoreactive trypsinogen and direct gene analysis. British Medical Journal 302:1237–1240

Sharer N, Schwarz M, Malone G, et al 1998 Mutations of the cystic fibrosis gene in patients with chronic pancreatitis. New England Journal of Medicine 339:645–652

Siret D, Bretaudeau G et al 2003 Comparing the clinical evolution of cystic fibrosis screened neonatally to that of the cystic fibrosis diagnosed from clinical symptoms: a 10 year retrospective study in a French region (Brittany.) Pediatric Pulmonology 35(5):342–349

The Cystic Fibrosis Genotype/Phenotype consortium 1993 Correlation between genotype and phenotype in patients with cystic fibrosis. New England Journal of Medicine 329:1308–1313

Wang X, Movlan B et al 2000 Mutation in the gene responsible for cystic fibrosis and predisposition to chronic rhinosinusitis in the general population. Journal of the American Medical Association 284:1814–1819

Worldwide survey of the delta F 508 mutation: report from the cystic fibrosis genetic analysis consortium 1994 American Journal of Human Genetics 47:354–359

Wilschanski M, Yahav Y et al 2003 Gentamicin-induced correction of CFTR function in patients with cystic fibrosis and CFTR stop mutations. New England Journal of Medicine 349(15):1433–1441

Zielenski J 2000 Genotype and phenotype in cystic fibrosis. Respiration 67:117–183

Chapter 4

Respiratory care

Gary Connett

INTRODUCTION

Premature death from respiratory failure is the most common outcome for individuals with CF. The prevention, eradication or delay of chronic infection of the lower airways is the most important strategy to postpone this prospect. This can be achieved by the optimal use of antibiotics, appropriate airway clearance techniques, physical fitness and good nutrition.

It is essential that individuals with CF and their physician agree on an aggressive approach to treatment. Effective systems of care should be in place to detect infecting organisms and provide early antibiotic treatment whenever necessary. Frequent follow-up and routine bacteriological surveillance are essential. General measures including avoidance of tobacco smoke and routine influenza vaccination are also important.

RECOGNITION OF RESPIRATORY EXACERBATIONS

There must be a low threshold for obtaining treatment of symptoms as soon as they occur. Any of the following should be considered indicative of a respiratory exacerbation for which treatment is required to prevent worsening lung damage.

Symptoms

- Increased frequency, severity or duration of coughing
- Increased sputum production or change from clear to yellow/green in colour
- Increased breathlessness/decreased exercise capacity
- New or worsening haemoptysis
- Unexplained anorexia or weight loss
- Increased feeling of congestion within the chest.

Signs

- Significant decline in lung function (see Chapter 8)
- New radiological abnormalities
- New lower respiratory tract signs: breathlessness, hypoxia and new signs on auscultation.

Individuals and their carers must be taught and regularly reminded about recognising changes in their respiratory status. Frequent outpatient follow up with accurate recording of lung function is critical for detecting respiratory exacerbations.

OBTAINING AND INTERPRETING MICROBIOLOGICAL SAMPLES

Properly collected and processed specimens of respiratory secretions are essential for determining the appropriate use of antibiotics (see Chapter 8).

What type of specimen should be collected?

If productive of sputum

- Whenever possible obtain a purulent sputum specimen. Sputum is usually reliably indicative of lower respiratory infection.
- On occasions, when individuals have difficulty producing a specimen, physiotherapy might facilitate expectoration.
- If minimally productive, arrange for sputum pots to be available at home so that a specimen can be caught on the rare occasion when expectoration occurs. *Pseudomonas aeruginosa* (*Ps. aeruginosa*) and *Burkolderia sp* can be cultured from samples stored at room temperature for several days after collection. However refrigeration is preferable and ideally samples should be processed within two to three hours to maximise the chances of identifying the full range of CF pathogens.
- Vomit sometimes contains copious amounts of swallowed sputum and is a potential source of respiratory secretions for culture.

The non-productive or uncooperative child

- Specimens from those who cannot expectorate are most easily obtained from deep throat cough swabs.

Figure 4.1 Clubbing is usefully indicative of the progression of bronchiectasis.

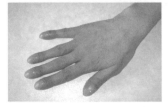

- Children can be trained from the age of 2 years to cough when the swab is placed in the oro-pharynx. These specimens should be collected by an experienced nurse or physician, ideally after a physiotherapy session.
- When deep throat cough swabs yield *Staphylococcus aureus* (*S. aureus*) and/or *Haemophilus influenzae* (*H. influenzae*) there is reasonable sensitivity but these specimens are of poor specificity and false positives are common. Unfortunately the presence of symptoms does not usefully differentiate between true and false positives. Asymptomatic infection can occur and particularly in young children without advanced respiratory complications.
- Deep throat swabs yielding *Ps. aeruginosa* should always be treated. Unfortunately these specimens are less sensitive for this organism and false positives can also occur.
- Sputum induction is possible in non-productive, cooperative individuals (generally aged >5 years) by the inhalation of hypertonic saline (for example 4.8%). A specimen is usually obtained within 1–2 minutes of inhalation. Bronchodilators given prophylactically can reduce the risk of transient bronchospasm as a result of the procedure.
- Laryngeal aspirates can be obtained by suctioning through a soft catheter placed in the supraglottis via the mouth.
- Bronchoalveolar lavage also has a useful role in non-productive children (see Chapter 8).

How often should specimens be collected?

Regular microbial surveillance is essential to:

- Identify infection with *S. aureus* and *H. influenzae*
- Identify the onset of infection with *Ps. aeruginosa*
- Identify aspergillus, which might be significant if there are other indicators of allergic sensitisation
- Identify other rarer pathogens including *Burkholderia cepacia* (*B. cepacia*).

Sensitivity testing usefully indicates appropriate antibiotic choices.

- Specimens should be obtained:
  - monthly throughout infancy or during the first year following diagnosis
  - at least 2–3 monthly thereafter and at every clinic visit
  - as soon as possible after the onset of any increase in lower respiratory symptoms
  - whenever sputum is unexpectedly produced
  - annually to screen for acid-fast bacilli.

Remember

- A negative cough swab does not exclude significant lower respiratory infection. If clinical signs and symptoms are suggestive of infection a 'best guess' antibiotic should be prescribed.
- Consider treatment whenever *S. aureus* and *H. influenzae* are cultured irrespective of whether there is an increase in symptoms.

INVOLVING THE PRIMARY CARE PHYSICIAN IN THE MANAGEMENT OF RESPIRATORY INFECTIONS
(see Chapter 21)

The primary care physician should be included in the care of those with CF as soon as possible after diagnosis. Regular communication with prompt clinic letters including advice about treatment of exacerbations is helpful.

Written guidelines for primary care physicians should emphasize the following:

- The management of respiratory infections in CF is quite different to treatment of respiratory infections in healthy individuals.
- Lower respiratory tract infections may present with worsening symptoms, such as increase in cough or sputum production, and auscultatory findings may be unreliable.
- Sputum or deep throat cough swabs for bacterial culture should always be obtained.
- Antibiotics should always be started promptly and there should be a low threshold for treatment. Treatment should not be delayed for microbiological results. Where there are difficulties getting prompt access to primary health care, a solution is to allow the family to store oral antibiotics at home so that they can initiate treatment independently.

IMMUNOLOGICAL DIAGNOSIS OF PSEUDOMONAS INFECTION

A variety of methods have been developed to detect serum antibodies to pseudomonal antigens. IgG antibodies detected by ELISA can be arranged through the Central Public Health Laboratory (Brett 1992).

- Negative antibodies confirm the absence of *Ps. aeruginosa* infection in support of negative cultures.
- Negative antibodies but positive cultures indicate early infection that might be eradicated after appropriate antibiotics.
- Positive antibodies with negative cultures demand an intensive search for the pathogen using the techniques listed above. (Initial isolates are more likely to occur during viral upper respiratory infections.)
- Rising antibody titres indicate progression of lung damage and the need for more intensive antibiotic treatment.

NOTES ON TREATING SPECIFIC ORGANISMS
Staphylococcus aureus
Prophylactic therapy

Continuous oral beta lactamase resistant penicillins (for example, flucloxacillin) to treat infants diagnosed by newborn screening, decreases cough and the need for in-patient treatment in the first two years of life (Smyth & Walters 2002). The suggestion that this practice causes early infection with *Ps. aeruginosa* has not been substantiated although there is evidence that this might occur after the continuous use of cephalosporins (cephalexin) in similar circumstances (Stutman & Marks 1994).

Prophylactic flucloxacillin to treat those diagnosed following presentation with symptoms is of unproven benefit but potentially achieves similar results to those in screened populations.

Compliance with flucloxacillin prophylaxis can be improved by administering the total daily dose in two or three rather than four divided doses.

The use of continuous antibiotics does not negate the need for regular collection of specimens for bacterial culture and the use of additional antibiotics if there is continued isolation of *S. aureus* in spite of good compliance with prophylactic treatment.

Treatment of infection

S. aureus can be eradicated in many cases although treatment with combinations of antibiotics for up to 4–6 weeks may be necessary. Positive isolates following a course of therapy often represent re-infection with different strains. Those with repeatedly positive cultures probably have chronic infection with the same strain and require continuous treatment.

Isolates of *S. aureus* despite prophylactic flucloxacillin indicates the need for higher doses of flucloxacillin plus an additional anti-staphylococcal antibiotic to eradicate breakthrough infection (see Chapter 24). Additional anti-staphylococcal antibiotics include:

- sodium fusidate
- azithromycin or clarithromycin
- clindamycin
- rifampicin.

Antibiotics should be chosen according to sensitivity testing. Macrolide resistance can occur after repeat antibiotic exposure. This is generally a class effect and also associated with clindamycin resistance.

Unless there is MRSA infection, *S. aureus* isolates generally remain sensitive to flucloxacillin. Higher doses perhaps given intravenously might be of benefit.

Nebulised aminoglycosides can be used as an additional measure to prevent chronic or recurrent infection with *S. aureus* despite maximal doses of oral flucloxacillin.

S. aureus remains an important infecting pathogen in those chronically infected with *Ps. aeruginosa*. Anti-staphylococcal antibiotics must still be prescribed whenever this organism is isolated. Ciprofloxacin alone is insufficient to treat *S. aureus* and additional anti-staphylococcal antibiotics should be given to provide effective therapy.

Individuals not infected with pseudomonas but with an exacerbation of respiratory disease requiring intravenous antibiotics for *S. aureus* infection should receive either a second generation cephalosporin, an aminoglycoside or vancomycin for at least 10–14 days (see Chapter 24).

Haemophilus influenzae

All isolates of non-capsulate strains of *H. influenzae* should be regarded as pathogens and treated. This is a fastidious organism and its growth can be obscured by more rapidly growing pseudomonas species.

A two week course of antibiotics is usually sufficient to treat *H. influenza* but resistance to macrolides and ampicillin commonly occurs necessitating a change to alternative antibiotics.

When persistent bronchiolitic *H. influenzae* infection occurs it is best treated with a prolonged course of intravenous antibiotics, for example cefuroxime, cefotaxime or ceftazidime, until there is sustained improvement in symptoms.

Occasionally, repeated isolates of *H. influenzae*, despite the above measures, should be treated with continuous appropriate oral antibiotics according to sensitivity testing to limit subsequent lung complications.

Pseudomonas aeruginosa

Intermittent infection (non-colonised) (Wood & Smyth 2003)

One of the most important aims of treatment is to delay as long as possible the onset of chronic infection with *Ps. aeruginosa*. Regular microbiological surveillance is important for the early detection of this organism so that antibiotics can be used early to eradicate it.

Pseudomonas rarely causes respiratory symptoms when it first infects the CF lung although it is sometimes first cultured during an intercurrent viral infection. Aggressive treatment of initial isolates is mandatory in all cases. Nebulised colomycin plus oral ciprofloxacin is the most commonly used first line strategy.

All new isolates should be typed by the Central Public Health Laboratory as part of surveillance to detect the occurrence of cross-infection within clinics.

> The Copenhagen CF Centre obtain monthly laryngeal aspirates. They have shown that treating asymptomatic individuals who first isolate pseudomonas with nebulised colomycin plus oral ciprofloxacin for three weeks, delays the onset of permanent infection (Valerius, Koch & Hoiby 1991). Repeat isolates are treated with the same antibiotics for 3 months. This successfully delays the median time to recurrence of this organism from 9 to 18 months (Frederiksen, Koch & Hoiby 1997).

Alternative strategies

- If there are acute respiratory symptoms the individual should be admitted to hospital for intravenous antibiotics – this applies to all children who continue to isolate *Ps. aeruginosa* despite oral ciprofloxacin. Nebulised antibiotics should be given throughout.
- Consider replacing colomycin with preservative-free tobramycin (TOBI) and assess adherence to nebulised antibiotic treatment.
- Consider using nebulised antibiotics indefinitely in those with chest X-ray changes and/or reduced lung function irrespective of whether there are further *Ps. aeruginosa* isolates.
- Monthly follow-up cultures should be performed to identify early any re-infection. If this occurs despite prolonged colomycin and ciprofloxacin consider intravenous antibiotics.
- Pseudomonas antibodies will help determine whether there is chronic infection and the need for more intensive treatment such as regular intravenous antibiotics.

Chronic infection

Those with cultures repeatedly positive for *Ps. aeruginosa* despite the above measures should be considered permanently infected (chronic colonisation). Repeatedly positive pseudomonas antibody titres are also suggestive. There is no consensus about how many positive cultures indicate chronic infection and over what time scale. The subsequent progression of lung damage in those colonised with *Ps. aeruginosa* is highly variable but average life expectancy is reduced compared with those who remain uninfected. There is no consensus about the management of chronic

Table 4.1 Advantages of regular versus as required antibiotics for chronic *Ps. aeruginosa* infection.

Regular IV antibiotics	As required antibiotics
• Routine care for all to maintain stability	• Individualised therapy to maintain stability
• Fewer acute exacerbations	• Decreased emergence of resistant organisms
• Prolonged maintenance of good lung function	• Fewer antibiotic allergy problems*
• Possibly better general health	• Fewer problems with securing IV access
• Possibly increased survival	• Less routine disruption to work/education
	• Decreased costs of treatment

*See Report of the UK CF Trust Antibiotic Group for desensitisation protocols.

infection, but aggressive treatment is always necessary if there is evidence for disease progression such as increased cough, changes in lung function or radiographic abnormalities. Two main options are widely practised:

- Elective courses of intravenous antibiotics irrespective of clinical state at regular intervals, for example three monthly
- Oral or intravenous antibiotic treatment of respiratory exacerbations.

There are advantages and disadvantages with these two approaches (see Table 4.1).

There is no doubt that frequent doses of intravenous antibiotics should be used in individuals with evidence of increasing respiratory problems until stabilized (Breen & Aswani 2003).

The use of continuous nebulised antibiotics

There is no consensus on choice or duration of treatment with nebulised antibiotics for chronic infection (Ryan 2003). Many centres advocate continuous and indefinite treatment with colomycin, preservative-free tobramycin (TOBI) or a combination of both colomycin and an aminoglycoside. Aminoglycosides might usefully provide additional cover in those who continue to have chronic infection with *S. aureus* as well as *Ps. aeruginosa*. Resistance to colomycin is unusual and this drug can be of benefit to individuals given intravenously even after many years of nebulised inhalation.

Choice of anti-pseudomonal antibiotics (see Chapter 24 for drug doses)

Parenteral treatment   A beta lactam in combination with an aminoglycoside is recommended as the first choice. Most recent antimicrobial sensitivity should be used to guide choice. Treatment should be given for at least 10–14 days according to clinical recovery. There is good evidence for the safety and efficacy of intravenous tobramycin given once daily. Occasionally antibiotics might need to be continued for several weeks, but beware of aminoglycoside toxicity.

Oral treatment   Oral ciprofloxacin is commonly used to treat minor exacerbations. Resistance to this antibiotic can occur after repeated exposure in individuals with chronic *Ps. aeruginosa* infection. In vivo benefits might still be achieved and in some centres ciprofloxacin is used in combination with an oral macrolide antibiotic to good effect in these circumstances.

There are no additional benefits from giving ciprofloxacin intravenously except in achieving compliance in those who are unwilling to take the drug orally.

There is accumulating evidence that long-term macrolide antibiotics might be of benefit to individuals with chronic pseudomonas infection (Southern, Barker & Solis 2003). Individual trials should be considered in those with evidence of disease progression despite optimal use of other maintenance therapies. Azithromycin 10 mg/kg/day has been used once daily for three days per week.

Remember

- Repeated usage of ciprofloxacin rapidly leads to the development of resistance particularly when used in insufficient dose.
- Ciprofloxacin monotherapy is not sufficient where there is concomitant *S. aureus* infection.

Resistant organisms

- Repeat sputum cultures should be obtained shortly after initiating treatment to detect the development of resistance and poor response to treatment.
- If bacteria are multi-resistant, useful clinical benefits can still occur due to sub-MIC antibiotic effects on the pathogenicity of *Ps. aeruginosa* organisms. Antibiotics should be chosen on the basis of previous best responses.
- In less severe exacerbations oral chloramphenicol might have useful activity against some strains of organisms.
- Synergy testing is not yet widely available but might identify combinations of antibiotics which are likely to be effective (see Chapter 8).
- Newer carbapenem antibiotics (meropenem) and colomycin can safely be used in higher doses to good effect.

Burkholderia cepacia

B. cepacia is an ubiquitous saprophyte. It causes vegetables to rot but is rarely isolated as a pathogen in non-CF individuals (except in chronic granulomatous disease when *B. cepacia* septicaemia can be fatal).

'Epidemic' strains of *B. cepacia* are more easily transmitted than *Ps. aeruginosa*. The incidence of infection varies widely between CF centres. This is attributed in part to the extent to which transmissible epidemic strains are present and may reflect local infection control policy (see Chapter 1). Most acquire a single strain but secondary infection with epidemic strains can also occur.

Three clinical syndromes have been described:

- No obvious change in respiratory status
- Accelerated respiratory deterioration with fever, weight loss and increased need for in-patient treatment
- Fulminant and rapid decline in respiratory status.

Possible risk factors for the acquisition of *B. cepacia* include:

- Increasing age
- Pre-existing severe lung disease
- The existence of an infected sibling
- Close contact with infected individuals
- Exposure to aminoglycoside antibiotics and inhaled colomycin
- Glucose intolerance or diabetes.

> ### Remember
> - All laboratories should routinely use selective media to identify *B. cepacia* (see Chapter 21).
> - New isolates should be confirmed by a reference laboratory and typed to identify the individual strain and its transmissibility.
> - Strain typing might be predictive of infectivity but is not predictive of virulence and antibiotic resistance.

Treatment (see Chapter 24 for drug doses)

Management of first isolate   There are no established protocols to prevent chronic infection. While transient infection with non-epidemic strains is well documented, this cannot be predicted and aggressive treatment of first isolates is recommended.

- Initial isolates are usually resistant to aminogylcosides, colomycin and ciprofloxacin.
- Organisms are often sensitive to the carbapenem antibiotics and might retain sensitivity to Ceftazidime, although in-vivo effectiveness is variable.
- Sensitivity testing suggests that oral treatment with chloramphenicol, co-trimoxazole or tetracyclines might be of benefit.
- The intravenous carbapenem antibiotics imipenem and meropenem might be of benefit in reducing the virulence of *B. cepacia* when used to treat respiratory exacerbations caused by multi-resistant strains.

Management of chronic infection
- Long term nebulised therapy with ceftazidime or ticarcillin might be of benefit if organisms are sensitive.
- Chronic infection with *B. cepacia* is a relative contraindication to lung transplantation in some centres.

Alternative strategies   High dosage immunotherapy with prednisolone and cyclosporin has been reported to be of benefit in treating fulminant disease in extremes. Discussion with the regional centre is advised.

Infection control measures for epidemic strains   Particularly strict measures should be in place for individuals harboring epidemic strains of this organism (see Chapter 1 for general measures).

- Segregation is of proven benefit in limiting the spread of this organism.
- Those in whom *B. cepacia* is identified should attend a separate outpatient clinic and be kept apart from all other CF individuals, irrespective of their *B. cepacia* status.
- Strict attention must be applied to infection control measures, including the use of separate equipment (stethoscope and vitallograph).
- Hospital admission should be to a separate ward space.
- Social contact with others with CF should be discouraged.

Miscellaneous infections

There are a number of other organisms that should be considered as pathogens when isolated from the CF airway. These include:

- *Stenotrophomonas maltophilia*
- *Alcaligenes faecalis.*

These organisms should be considered as important pathogens and treated aggressively in much the same way as *Ps. aeruginosa* according to sensitivity testing. High dose co-trimoxazole can be effective in eliminating these organisms if sensitive.

There is less certainty about the importance of isolates of the following organisms:

- *Strep. pneumoniae*
- *Enterobacteriaceae*
- coliforms such as *E. coli* and *Klebsiella.*

Viral infection

There is no evidence that viral infections of the respiratory tract are more common in CF. They occur between 1 and 10 times per year (mean of 3.7/year aged <6 and 2.3/year aged >6). They are an important cause of:

- Acute deterioration in respiratory status.
- Accelerated decline in lung function, particularly when frequent.

Management of viral infection

- If coryzal with signs or symptoms of lower respiratory infection a naso-pharyngeal aspirate should be sent for virus isolation.
- Appropriate broad spectrum antibiotics should be prescribed whenever symptoms are severe to prevent secondary bacterial infection.
- CF infants with respiratory syncytial virus (RSV) or adenovirus bronchiolitis are at risk of severe respiratory morbidity. Studies suggest synergism between RSV and *Ps. aeruginosa* infection. Early treatment with nebulised ribavarin according to current treatment protocols is recommended.
- There should be a low threshold for additional antibiotic cover against *Ps. aeruginosa.*

Prevention strategies

- Discuss whether attendance at day care centres is appropriate. Individual social circumstances need to be considered.
- Advise influenza immunisation every autumn.

Methicillin–resistant Staphylococcus aureus

Although recovery of this organism from the airway is not usually associated with worsening lung problems, colonisation presents difficulties in relation to transplantation and cross infection issues.

Infection is usually hospital acquired but family members should be screened. Parents working in hospitals or care institutions can transmit MRSA.

Clearance can occur spontaneously but this usually happens in the first few months.

There are a number of treatment regimes to try and eradicate repeat isolates and antibiotic choices should be dictated by extended sensitivity testing. Rapid emergence of resistance is likely after monotherapy.

Nebulised vancomycin 5 mg/kg up to 150 mg 4 times daily for 1–2 weeks can be effective if used in combination with an oral antibiotic such as doxycycline, chloramphenicol, rifampicin or linezolid (see Chapter 24).

Treated individuals should also use betadine shampoo daily, triclosan 2% soap substitute, bactroban nasal ointment twice daily and corsodyl mouthwash twice daily for a week to eliminate skin and nasal carriage.

Intravenous antibiotics to consider for acute symptoms include teicoplanin, vancomycin and linezolid according to sensitivity testing (see Chapter 24).

Mycobacterial infection

Mycobacterium tuberculosis infection does not occur more commonly in CF. Whenever identified it should be regarded as a pathogen and treated with standard anti-tuberculous chemotherapy.

Increasing numbers of individuals have been identified with atypical (non-tuberculous) mycobacteria in their sputum. Repeated isolates of the same mycobacterial species, particularly with positive direct AFB smears and evidence of a decline in respiratory status, is highly suggestive of infection and indicates the need for specific anti-mycobacterial chemotherapy.

Diagnosis of mycobacterial infection

Clinicians should have a high index of suspicion and consider infection with atypical mycobacteria in those with a decline in respiratory status and poor responses to standard antibiotic therapy.

All sputum producers should have an annual specimen stained for acid-fast bacilli and processed for mycobacterial culture.

Sensitivity testing and identification of atypical isolates should be confirmed by the national reference laboratory.

Whenever possible histopathological evidence for infection should be obtained by bronchoscopic biopsy.

Treatment

Specialist advice should be sought about the most appropriate antibiotic regime to use. Drugs used include clarithromycin, isoniazid, rifabutin, ethambutol and ciprofloxacin.

In most cases treatment should be continued for at least 12–18 months with close monitoring for the potential side effects of therapy.

Contact tracing is not necessary for atypical, non-tuberculous mycobacteria.

Mycoplasma pneumoniae

M. pneumoniae infections occur in epidemics every 3–4 years. There is no seasonal variation in incidence.

Clinical features

Typically children present with fever, cough and malaise of insidious onset. Coryzal symptoms are usually absent. Pharyngitis is a common finding. Respiratory signs may be minimal but in some cases there is troublesome wheeze, particularly if the child has concomitant asthma.

Suggestive non-respiratory manifestations

- Headache
- Abdominal pain
- Maculo-papular rash.

Useful investigations

- Differential white cell count: typically normal; band forms and toxic granulation do not occur.
- Serum cold agglutinins: typically positive when symptoms are moderate or severe.
- Serology titres: less useful being typically low at the onset of disease although a titre of 1:128 or greater suggests recent infection.

Treatment

Macrolide antibiotics should be given for a minimum of two weeks.

ANTI-INFLAMMATORY THERAPY

Neutrophil inflammation occurs shortly after birth in the CF lung. This raises the possibility of an intrinsic CFTR-based defect of inflammatory homeostasis and suggests the need for early intervention with anti-inflammatory therapies.

A number of treatment options are available but there is no consensus on best usage.

Ibuprofen

Ibuprofen in doses of 20–30 mg/kg (adjusted according to plasma levels) has been shown to significantly slow the progression of lung disease in those aged 5–13 years with FEV1 > 60% predicted, over a four-year trial period. The rate of decline in FEV1 was delayed by 59% compared to controls. Treatment was not significantly effective in those above this age range. Lower doses of ibuprofen might have adverse pro-inflammatory effects.

Large variations in ibuprofen metabolism necessitate individual dosing. Close supervision is necessary to detect potentially serious side effects, which have been increasingly reported in follow up studies. The place of ibuprofen in CF treatment is not yet clear (Dezateux & Crighton 2003).

Corticosteroids

These are of benefit in treating allergic bronchopulmonary aspergillosis (see below). A large multi-centre study has suggested that oral prednisolone 1 mg/kg on alternate days benefits those aged 6–14 years with mild to moderate disease and *Ps. aeruginosa* infection (Eigen 1995). Benefits were apparent within 6 months but treatment beyond two years was associated with side effects including growth reduction and increased glucose intolerance. Regular blood pressure monitoring and screening for cataract formation is advisable when oral steroids are used continuously for more than a year.

Some centres are now using corticosteroids during acute infective exacerbations (1 mg/kg/day to a maximum of 30 mg) although the benefits of this approach are not yet clearly established.

Inhaled steroids are undergoing clinical evaluation (Dezateux, Walters & Balfour-Lynn 2003). Their use is mandatory if there is evidence of concomitant asthma but the optimal dose for arresting the lung inflammation of CF has not yet been established.

MANAGEMENT OF RESPIRATORY COMPLICATIONS

Aspergillus and Allergic Broncho-Pulmonary Aspergillosis (ABPA)

There is a complex relationship between the fungus *Aspergillus fumigatus* (Figure 4.2) and the progression of lung disease in CF.

- The organism can be cultured in up to 50% of sputum specimens. In many cases positive cultures are caused by contamination with 'passing' organisms.
- Skin prick tests and serum precipitins are positive in up to 30%. These are indicative of the development of allergy but are not diagnostic of ABPA unless other features are present.
- Allergy to aspergillus tends to develop soon after initial *Ps. aeruginosa* infection.
- Allergy to aspergillus can occur without other signs of atopy
- Positive cultures of aspergillus and allergic sensitisation to the organism are associated with worsening lung disease irrespective of the development of ABPA.

Management issues

Aspergillus avoidance Aspergillus is an ubiquitous organism. It grows particularly well in manure and rotting vegetation. Those who ride should be excused from mucking out the stables. Individuals should avoid areas where there is extensive demolition or building work.

Treatment of aspergillus allergy
- There is no evidence that treating simple allergy to *A. fumigatus* is of benefit.

Figure 4.2 *Aspergillus fumigatus.*

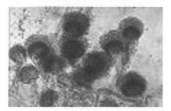

- Those with aspergillus allergy are at risk of ABPA for which corticosteroids are essential.
- Regular monitoring of the allergic status to aspergillus is essential (see Chapter 1). This should occur at annual review and the onset of respiratory exacerbations when ABPA is suspected.

Treatment of ABPA   ABPA is a syndrome with a wide range of lung pathologies including asthma, bronchiectasis, mucoid impaction, and eosinophilic pneumonia. Disease is caused by intense allergic responsiveness to aspergillus antigen without fungal invasion of lung parenchyma.

Typical diagnostic features include:

- Troublesome wheezing
- Fleeting pulmonary shadows
- Blood and sputum eosinophilia
- Raised IgE and/or IgG to *A. fumigatus* (precipitins)
- Positive *A. fumigatus* cultures.

A 4-fold or greater rise in total IgE is highly suggestive and usefully differentiates ABPA from bacterial infection as a cause of acute respiratory illness. IgE values increase on a logarithmic scale (Marchant, Warner & Bush 1994).

Treatment is prednisolone 1 mg/kg/day to a maximum dose of 60 mg daily for at least a month with gradual dose reduction to alternate day treatment according to repeat measurements of total IgE, clinical well being, lung function and resolution of radiographic changes (see Chapter 9).

Many cases will require continued alternate day steroid treatment for up to a year and occasionally longer.

Treatment with inhaled steroids *alone* is of no proven benefit in preventing or treating ABPA.

There is no good evidence that oral itraconazole is of benefit although it is commonly used, especially after relapse. Doses between 100–200 mg twice daily are commonly used. Higher doses have been associated with adrenal suppression and impaired clearance of inhaled corticosteroids. Itraconazole can impair liver function and should not be used if there is significant CF-related liver disease. It can cause decreased clearance of antihistamines. Antacids and H-2 antagonists will decrease absorption.

Sputum clearance is a useful proxy indicator of efficacy. Serum levels can be measured if there is treatment failure although there is uncertainty about what constitutes an adequate therapeutic level. Oral voriconazole has also been used and has better absorption than itraconazole.

Treatment with nebulised amphotericin, 5 mg bd, has anecdotally been shown to reduce the allergen load within the bronchi and might have a useful steroid sparing effect in relapsing cases if tolerated. Relapses are common, particularly if steroid dosages are curtailed too rapidly and necessitate an immediate increase in prednisolone dosage. Delayed diagnosis and treatment will lead to worsening lung disease including proximal bronchiectatic lung damage.

Treatment of pulmonary aspergilloma   Pulmonary aspergillomas (fungus balls) are surprisingly rare despite the common occurrence of cavities with advanced bronchiectasis. Chest X-ray appearances might be suggestive. Surgical treatment has a high morbidity. There is a case report of successful treatment of this condition by percutaneous instillation of amphotericin B via an indwelling catheter (Ryan 1995).

Treatment of invasive aspergillosis Invasive aspergillosis has been considered a rare complication. However, pathological studies have demonstrated parenchymal and/or disseminated infection in up to a fifth of post- mortem cases. It has not been established whether invasive fungal disease is a treatable pre-terminal event in CF (Vivek Bhargava et al 1989).

Bronchial Hyperreactivity and Asthma

Bronchial hyperresponsiveness is common in CF, particularly during intercurrent infection and in those with poor baseline lung function.

Any decrease in lung function on routine spirometry should be retested after bronchodilator inhalation to detect reversible airways obstruction. In moderately severe lung disease bronchodilators should be given by nebuliser.

Some will have atopic asthma as well as CF. These individuals are at risk of more severe lung disease and must be identified so that they can receive aggressive anti-asthma therapy.

The following suggest atopic asthma as an additional cause of respiratory morbidity:

- Exercise induced wheeze
- Persistent nocturnal coughing
- Cough or wheeze following allergen exposure
- Concomitant eczema and/or allergic rhinitis
- Parent or sibling with atopic illness.

Useful investigations include:

- Skin tests to identify provoking allergens
- Measurement of total IgE (plus specific IgE to aspergillus to exclude ABPA presenting with increased wheeze).

Treatment

Avoidance measures

Families should be advised:

- Against acquiring cats and dogs as pets. If sensitized, serious consideration should be given to giving away furry pets already living in the family home.
- To strictly avoid cigarette smoke exposure.
- To keep strong smells out of the home, for example fragrant soaps, shampoos and perfumed lotions.
- To keep windows closed when the outside air is full of exhaust fumes, pollution, dust or pollen from trees and plants.
- To open windows when rooms are hot, stuffy, or when there is smoke from cooking.
- To observe house dust mite avoidance measures for proven sensitivity.

Drug therapy Those with bronchial hyperresponsiveness and atopic asthma will benefit from bronchodilator therapy as symptomatic relief and prior to physiotherapy. Some might benefit from long acting B2-agonists.

- An increase in FEV1 of 10% or more after inhalation of a bronchodilator should be considered a positive response.
- Bronchodilator responsiveness should be regularly assessed to identify paradoxical deterioration in lung function (FEV1 and FEF 25–75) after inhalation.
- Regular peak flow monitoring adds an additional burden and is of little benefit.

Inhaled steroids All those with atopic asthma should receive inhaled steroids in generous doses. Those who continue to have bronchoreversibility despite inhaling regular long-acting β2-agonists might also benefit from inhaled corticosteroids.

- Pre-school children treated by MDI via spacer and mask delivery systems will require at least 200–400 mcg bd of beclometasone or budesonide (half these doses of fluticasone) to achieve benefit.
- Doses of 400 mcg–1 mg daily are advised for older children/adults.
- Repeat spirometry should be use to determine an optimal dose response.
- Doses should be doubled at the onset of any increase in respiratory symptoms.
- Inhaler techniques should be reviewed regularly.
- Drug delivery systems should be tailored to individual requirements.

Persistent infantile wheezing

This is an unusual but potentially serious complication in which respiratory distress occurs despite the appropriate use of antibiotics. Such cases need detailed evaluation including fibre-optic bronchoscopy to exclude tracheo-bronchomalacia and chest CT to more accurately determine the extent of lung damage. A 24-hour pH probe will usefully exclude gastro-oesophageal reflux. If this is demonstrated then consideration should be given to a trial of cow's milk avoidance under dietary supervision to exclude cow's milk protein intolerance as the cause of reflux (see Chapter 6). The benefits of nebulised bronchodilators should be assessed as objectively as possible and if no other cause is found a trial of oral corticosteroids (1–2 mg/kg daily) should be given.

Monthly intravenous immunoglobulin infusions have been used in those with protracted symptoms and has been shown to have useful steroid sparing effects (Balfour-Lynn 2004).

Pneumothorax

Pneumothorax is a rare complication occurring in adolescents and adults with moderate to severe lung disease and is typically caused by rupture of a sub-pleural bleb or bullae adjacent to degenerated pleural tissue. Occurrences are usually unrelated to acute respiratory illness and are recurrent in up to 50% of cases.

- Typical symptoms include sudden onset of dyspnoea, unilateral chest, neck or arm pain and small haemoptysis.
- Clinical signs include hyperresonance and decreased breath sounds.

- Severe dyspnoea, cyanosis and mediastinal shift indicate a tension pneumothorax requiring emergency chest tube drainage prior to X-ray confirmation.
- Investigations should include inspiratory and expiratory films, performed with a physician in attendance whenever the diagnosis is suspected.

Management

Small (<15%) pneumothoraces can be managed conservatively with in-patient observation.

Larger pneumothoraces should be treated with early recourse to closed thoracotomy chest tube drainage and without suction initially.

Up to one third of cases will not settle without pleurodesis and recurrence of non-iatrogenic pneumothoraces is common (>50%). Most experts recommend early referral for apical pleurectomy and limited surgical abrasion. Thoracic surgery might complicate future lung transplantation (see Chapter 19).

Those unfit for anaesthesia might be effectively managed for a prolonged period by attachment of a Heimlich flutter valve to an intercostal chest drain (Edenborough, Hussain & Stableforth 1994).

Advice to those at risk of pneumothoraces

Those with radiographic evidence of apical blebs or bullae (>0.5 cm) should be informed about the symptoms of pneumothorax and advised to seek prompt medical attention should they occur.

Such individuals should avoid high pressure PEP forms of physiotherapy (see Chapter 5).

Advice following pneumothorax

- Positive pressure breathing i.e. through the PEP mask, should be used cautiously if at all.
- Air travel is hazardous and should be avoided.
- Travel to long distances from acute medical services should be avoided.

Pneumomediastinum and sub-cutaneous emphysema

This typically occurs due to alveolar rupture and dissection of air into parenchymal tissues. There is rarely an associated pneumothorax. Treatment consists of adequate oxygen therapy, antibiotics and physiotherapy as indicated.

Massive haemoptysis

Massive life-threatening bleeding occurs due to the rupture of bronchial arteries after bouts of coughing. Those with haemoptysis in excess of 250 mls should be referred for specialist regional care.

- Immediately cross-match and stabilise with blood transfusions if necessary.
- Consider associated clotting disturbances in those with liver disease, particularly if there is thrombocytopaenia associated with hypersplenism.
- Position head down, lying on the side from which bleeding is thought to have originated.

Specialist interventions include bronchoscopy to determine the site of bleeding, angiography and embolisation.

Atelectasis

Frequent careful clinical examination is essential to detect changes in expansion, resonance and breath sounds suggesting atelectasis. Localised wheeze or crackles are suggestive. Chest X-rays should be performed whenever atelectasis is clinically suspected or when there is a poor response to first line treatment of respiratory symptoms. Always consider the possibility of mucous plugging as a complication of ABPA and treat with high dose corticosteroids as appropriate.

Treatment

- Intensive physiotherapy, bronchodilators and antibiotics are essential in all cases.
- Those not responding to these measures should be referred for bronchoscopic lavage and suctioning.
- Surgical resection might be of benefit to those with chronic atelectasis causing considerable morbidity but who maintain good pulmonary function.

Surgical treatment of localised bronchiectasis

A small number develop severe bronchiectasis localised to one lobe. The right upper lobe is most commonly involved. Such individuals might benefit from lobectomy. Detailed pre-operative assessment including high resolution CT scans and radioactive isotope ventilation scans are essential to confirm the localised distribution of lung damage.

Those with persistent, disabling respiratory symptoms, little evidence of bronchiectasis elsewhere and good lung function are those most likely to benefit from surgery. Intensive peri-operative treatment is essential to achieving a good clinical outcome (Lucas 1996).

Cor pulmonale and respiratory failure

Progressive airways obstruction and the resulting alveolar hypoventilation causes reflex hypoxic vasoconstriction with elevation of the blood pressure within the pulmonary circulation. Increased muscularisation of pulmonary arteries and destruction of pulmonary vascular beds leads to irreversible hypertension, right ventricular strain and cor pulmonale (secondary right heart failure).

Assessment of cor pulmonale

- Symptoms of pulmonary heart disease such as dyspnoea, syncope, chest pain and haemoptysis can also occur as a result of primary lung pathology.
- Clinical signs can be misleading but distended neck veins, parasternal heave, hepatomegaly and oedema in the absence of hypoalbuminaemia are suggestive.
- ECGs are insensitive for detecting right ventricular strain.
- Echocardiography can be technically difficult in the presence of pulmonary hyperinflation but doppler studies can successfully estimate right ventricular pressures.

Treatment

Overnight oxygen therapy can reduce pulmonary vascular resistance and provide symptom relief from the effects of chronic hypoxia (see Chapter 5).

Effects on long-term survival are not clearly established and sleep quality is not consistently improved. Some will not tolerate the inconvenience of such treatment whilst others derive useful qualitative benefits from continuous therapy. Nasal obstruction should be excluded as an exacerbating cause of nocturnal hypoxaemia. Transcutaneous or end-tidal CO_2 monitoring should be performed to detect the possible complication of worsening hypercapnia as a result of treatment.

Diuretics (for example frusemide 1 mg/kg plus potassium supplements) might be of short-term benefit to treat signs of cardiac failure or unexplained weight gain, but the prognosis is poor under such circumstances.

Theophylline is of potential benefit although increased ventilation perfusion mismatch can occur. Its effects as a respiratory stimulant and a bronchodilator might also prove useful for those with hypercapnic respiratory failure. There might be increased clearance of theophyllines. Clearance is decreased by concomitant medications such as macrolides and ciprofloxacin. Baseline measurement of plasma levels is essential and these should be repeated whenever there are significant changes in clinical status or intercurrent therapies. Intravenous Beta-2-agonists can be used to similar effect.

Ventilatory support (for example using nasal Bi-PAP or NIPPV, see Chapter 5) might be appropriate in managing those with acute reversible complications causing respiratory failure and in those with a realistic option of receiving an organ transplant.

ADJUNCT THERAPIES
rhDNase

rhDNase digests extracellular DNA released during cellular destruction and has been shown to improve the visco-elastic properties of CF sputum (Figure 4.3).

Short term benefits

Studies suggest that at least 30% will demonstrate an improvement in FEV1 of >10% within 2–4 weeks of initiating treatment (Conway 1997). However there are large inter-individual differences with some showing deterioration in FEV1 after treatment.

Subjective improvements are more common and it is sometimes difficult to differentiate true benefits from placebo effects.

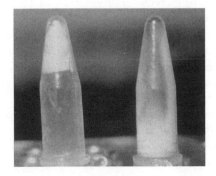

Figure 4.3 In vitro demonstration of effect of rhDNase on visco-elastic properties of sputum. Sample on the right has been treated.

Long term benefits

Phase three clinical studies demonstrated a mean improvement in FEV1 of 5.8% after 24 weeks of treatment (Fuchs et al 1994). Long-term studies have also shown modest improvements in lung function and a decreased need for treatment of infective exacerbations in mild disease (Jones & Wallis 2003).

Indications for use

It is not possible to predict who will benefit from treatment. Individual trials of treatment are warranted in those with evidence of disease progression despite the optimal use of antibiotic therapies and adequate compliance to prescribed physiotherapy regimes.

Lung function improvements are likely to be minimal in the severely affected with FVC < 40% although prolonged treatment might result in decreased need for IV therapies in this group.

Treatment protocols

Objective and subjective measures should be used over an initial trial period according to standardised protocols to accurately identify those who benefit and for whom more long-term treatment is indicated.

The standard dose is 2.5 mg once daily using a recommended nebuliser system and compressor (see Chapter 5 for practical issues).

Some benefit most from treatment last thing at night, which improves the following morning's physiotherapy session. In some this approach worsens night-time coughing.

Side effects are uncommon; voice alteration, pharyngitis and dyspepsia have been reported.

Hypertonic saline

Inhaled hypertonic saline in concentrations of up to 6% cause a transient increase in mucociliary clearance making this a potentially useful adjunct treatment prior to physiotherapy (see Chapter 24).

The intraluminal osmotic gradient draws water into the airway thus increasing sputum production.

Bronchospasm can be prevented by prior inhalation of a beta-2-agonist.

Paroxysmal coughing and oro-pharyngeal discomfort can occur after prolonged daily usage.

FUTURE THERAPIES

- Aminoglycosides have been shown to restore transcription of CFTR stop mutations, suggesting they might have novel benefits for those with this type of gene mutation. Other drugs are being developed to repair or increase expression of CFTR.
- Passive and active immunisation strategies are under evaluation. These include the use of hyperimmune globulin containing opsonising antibodies against *Ps. aeruginosa* and a variety of candidate vaccines to prevent *Ps. aeruginosa* infection. The use of vaccines to prevent chronic infection with *Ps. aeruginosa* offers great promise for the future (Keogan & Johansen 2003).
- Recombinant forms of secretory leukoprotease inhibitors and plasma purified Alpha 1 antitrypsin have been used in limited clinical trials. Transgenic animals using recombinant DNA technology might make these proteins more easily available in the future.

- Blocking increased sodium reabsorption with nebulised amiloride can improve mucociliary clearance but effects are self-limiting within 4–5 hours, necessitating frequent dosing.
- Nebulised UTP has been used to stimulate alternative chloride channels in CF epithelia but the duration of action is limited to a few hours after each dosage. Studies are determining whether limited benefits can be enhanced by its use in combination with amiloride.
- Viral and liposomal vectors have the potential for transferring the gene for CFTR to respiratory epithelia and correcting the gene defect in the CF lung. Trials are currently underway to determine the effectiveness of this exciting potential treatment.

References

Balfour-Lynn I M, Mohan U, Bush A, Rosenthal M 2004 Intravenous immunoglobulin for cystic fibrosis lung disease: a case series of 16 children. Archives of Diseases in Childhood 89:315–319

Breen L, Aswani N 2003 Elective versus symptomatic intravenous antibiotic therapy for cystic fibrosis (Cochrane Review). In: The Cochrane Library 3. Update Software, Oxford

Brett M M, Simmonds E J, Gronheim A T M et al 1992 The value of serum IgG titres against Pseudomonas aeruginosa in the management of early infection in cystic fibrosis. Archives of Diseases in Childhood 67:1086–1088

Conway S P 1997 Recombinant human DNase (rhDNase) in cystic fibrosis: is it cost effective? Archives of Diseases in Childhood 77:1–3

Dezateux C, Crighton A 2003 Oral non-steroidal anti-inflammatory drug treatment for cystic fibrosis (Cochrane Review). In: The Cochrane Library 3. Update Software, Oxford

Dezateux C, Walters S, Balfour-Lynn I M 2003 Inhaled corticosteroids for cystic fibrosis (Cochrane Review). In: The Cochrane Library 3. Update Software, Oxford

Edenborough F P, Hussain I, Stableforth D E 1994 Use of a Heimlich flutter valve for pneumothorax in cystic fibrosis. Thorax 49:1178–1179

Eigen H, Rosenstein B J, Fitzsimmons S et al 1995 A multi-centre study of alternate day prednisolone therapy in patients with cystic fibrosis. Journal of Pediatrics 126:515–523

Frederiksen B, Koch C, Hoiby N 1997 Antibiotic treatment of initial colonization with Pseudomonas aeruginosa postpones chronic infection and prevents deterioration of pulmonary function in cystic fibrosis. Pediatric Pulmonology 23:330–335

Fuchs H J, Borowitz D S, Christiansen D H et al 1994 Effect of aerosolised recombinant human DNase on exacerbations of respiratory symptoms and on pulmonary function in patients with cystic fibrosis. The New England Journal of Medicine 331:367–642

Jones A P, Wallis C E 2003 Recombinant human deoxyribonuclease for cystic fibrosis (Cochrane Review). In: The Cochrane Library 3. Update Software, Oxford

Keogan M T, Johansen H K 2003 Vaccines for preventing infection with pseudomonas aeruginosa in people with cystic fibrosis (Cochrane Review). In: The Cochrane Library 3. Update Software, Oxford

Lucas J, Connett G J, Lea R et al 1996 Lung resection in cystic fibrosis patients with localised pulmonary disease. Archives of Diseases in Childhood 74:449–451

Marchant J L, Warner, J O, Bush A 1994 Rise in total IgE as an indicator of allergic bronchopulmonary aspergillosis in cystic fibrosis. Thorax 49:1002–1005

Ryan G, Mukhopadhyay S, Singh M 2003 Nebulised anti-pseudomonal antibiotics for cystic fibrosis (Cochrane Review). In: The Cochrane Library 3. Update Software, Oxford

Ryan P J, Stableforth D E, Reynolds J et al 1995 Treatment of pulmonary aspergilloma in cystic fibrosis by percutaneous instillation of amphotericin via an indwelling catheter. Thorax 50:809–810

Smyth A, Walters S 2002 Prophylactic antibiotics for cystic fibrosis (Cochrane Review). In: The Cochrane Library 3. Update Software, Oxford

Southern K W, Barker P M, Solis A 2003 Macrolide antibiotics for cystic fibrosis (Cochrane Review). In: The Cochrane Library 3. Update Software, Oxford

Stutman H R, Marks M I 1994 Antibiotic prophylaxis study group. Cephalexin prophylaxis in newly diagnosed infants with cystic fibrosis. Sixth Annual North American Cystic Fibrosis Conference. Orlando

Valerius N H, Koch C, Hoiby N 1991 Prevention of chronic pseudomonas aeruginosa infection in cystic fibrosis by early treatment. Lancet 338:725–726

Vivek Bhargava B A, Tomashefski J F, Stern R C et al 1989 The pathology of fungal infection and colonisation in patients with cystic fibrosis. Human Pathology 20(10):977–986

Wood D M, Smyth A 2003 Antibiotic strategies for eradicating pseudomonas aeruginosa in people with cystic fibrosis. In: The Cochrane Library 3. Update Software, Oxford

Chapter 5

Physiotherapy

Allison Peebles

INTRODUCTION

All individuals with CF should have a physiotherapy programme as part of their management. The techniques used and amount of treatment recommended should be individualized, but should include the following components:

Airway clearance techniques Airway clearance techniques aim to reduce airway obstruction, improve ventilation and thereby delay disease progression.

Exercise Exercise aims to increase cardiovascular and respiratory fitness and strength of upper and lower body muscle masses thereby improving endurance, lung function and general feelings of well-being.

Maintenance of thoracic mobility, general mobility and posture Specific stretching and strengthening exercises are used to maintain or restore good posture. They prevent or treat a stiff thoracic spine and costovertebral joints thus enabling efficient, pain-free rib excursion.

STANDARDS OF CARE
Diagnosis

Shortly after diagnosis everyone should be seen by the CF physiotherapist and start to learn about the anatomy and physiology of physiotherapy, treatment techniques and an appropriate regime. The family need to be taught to recognise an increase in respiratory symptoms as a time to increase the frequency and/or duration of treatment and to seek medical advice.

Education about the disease and its management should be an ongoing part of care and form a part of each review. The amount of information given at this stage will depend on each family's needs. Written information should be checked accordingly.

It is important to introduce early discussion about exercise being part of their lifestyle. Encourage the family to think about activities they could do together. Children from active families are more likely to take up sports.

During this initial period it is important to build up a good relationship with the family to enable one to be supportive and to obtain a good understanding about how family members are coping with the diagnosis and burden of care. Good levels of rapport are essential to achieving an acceptable and effective treatment plan.

Outpatient care

Each patient should have the opportunity to be reviewed every two months by a physiotherapist with an interest in cystic fibrosis and have an annual review with a physiotherapist at a specialist centre.

Regular review

- Assessment of respiratory status and sputum production
- Review of airway clearance techniques (ACT)
- Discussion of exercise tolerance and advice on general fitness
- Assessment and advice on posture and thoracic mobility.

Annual review

In addition to the above, all patients should have a more detailed annual review to include the following:

- Full demonstration and discussion of ACT including any necessary modifications
- Measurement of exercise tolerance using a validated exercise test
- Assessment of inhaler/nebuliser techniques, timing and use of drugs and care of equipment
- Assessment of the suitability of home equipment.

Inpatient care

All patients should be assessed and treated by a physiotherapist within 24 hours of admission. Treatment should continue at an appropriate level with regular reassessment of progress. Whenever possible families should not be left to perform treatment alone. Admission to hospital is an opportunity to relieve them of this responsibility. Treatment might include the use of adjuncts with which they are unfamiliar. Everyone should have the opportunity and be encouraged to carry out daily exercise as soon as medically stable. Their programme should include a combination of cardiovascular, upper and lower body strength training (Webb & Dodd 2000). Where resources are limited, or if there are cross infection issues, exercise in their room or using hospital staircases and corridors can be as effective.

Domiciliary care

Reviews at home provide useful information about how treatment is fitted into daily routines, the space available, the degree of privacy and the level of support from the rest of the family. Whenever possible, visits should coincide with scheduled treatment times. Other benefits include:

- Children are more at ease in their own home and meeting them here can promote better relationships.
- Parents might be more relaxed and find it easier to talk about sensitive issues.
- Regular review of equipment including its suitability, requirements for servicing, and cleanliness.
- Review during home IV therapy allows close monitoring of progress, assessments of lung function, and advice and support about airway clearance.
- Close liaison between domiciliary and hospital staff is essential.

AIRWAY CLEARANCE TECHNIQUES

This chapter is an introduction to the techniques of airway clearance. Formal training including practical experience is essential.

The range of techniques include:

- Postural drainage and percussion (PD + PERC) (see page 61)
- The active cycle of breathing techniques (ACBT) (see page 66)
- Positive expiratory pressure (PEP) (see page 68)
- Oscillatory positive expiratory pressure – Flutter Cornet (see page 72)
- Autogenic drainage (AD) (see page 73)
- Modified Autogenic Drainage (see page 74)
- High frequency chest wall oscillation (HFCWO) (see page 75)
- Intra pulmonary percussive ventilation (IPV) (see page 75).

Choice depends on:

- Age
- Clinical status
- The experience of the physiotherapist
- Personal preference of the individual with CF
- Social issues, including level of support, space available, etc.

Postural drainage and percussion (Porter & Young 1991)

Postural drainage and percussion alone is generally only used in infants and young children. Treatment requires assistance and equipment for posturing in the older child.

Postural drainage

Positioning to allow gravity to assist drainage of secretions based on bronchial tree anatomy.

Everyone should have an individual regime of positions to manage their airway clearance. This might be altered because of disease progression or changing symptoms. Positions will need modifying if poorly tolerated, inconvenient or if gastro-oesophageal reflux has been demonstrated (see Modifications).

Figure 5.1 Apical segments: upper lobes. Patient is supported leaning back at 45°. Apply manual technique over collar bones.

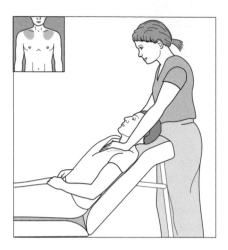

Figure 5.2 Anterior segments: upper lobes. Bed flat. Patient lying on back with pillow under their knees. Apply manual technique above nipple line on both sides.

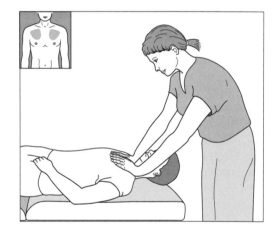

Figure 5.3 Postero-lateral segment: left upper lobe. Patient lying on right side at an inclination of 45°, head up. Trunk rotated 3/4 turn to front. Apply manual techniques over left shoulder blade.

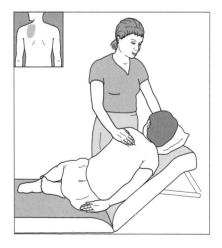

Figure 5.4 Postero-lateral segment: right upper lobe. Bed flat. Patient lying on left hand side turned 3/4 turn onto their front, supported by pillow from chest to hips. Apply manual techniques over right shoulder blade.

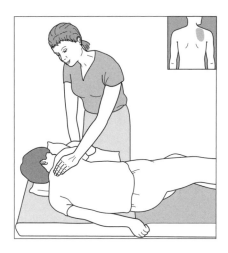

Figure 5.5 Lingula segment: left upper lobe. Patient lying on right side with head down at 25° and trunk rotated 3/4 turn back onto a pillow. Apply manual technique below the left armpit.

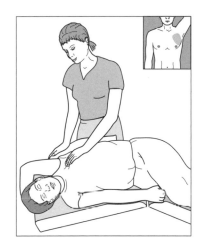

Figure 5.6 Right middle lobe. Patient lying on left side with head down at 25° and trunk rotated 3/4 turn back onto the pillow. Apply manual technique below the right armpit.

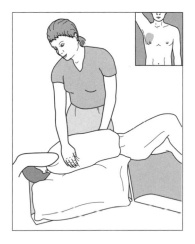

Figure 5.7   Superior segments: lower lobes. Bed flat. Patient lying flat on abdomen. Apply manual technique over mid-chest on both sides of the spine.

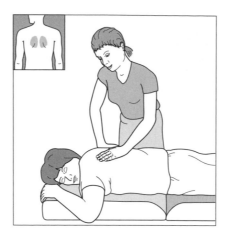

Figure 5.8   Anterior basal segments: lower lobes. Patient lying on back with head down at angle of 45° and knees bent. Apply manual technique over front of middle ribs, below nipple line on both sides.

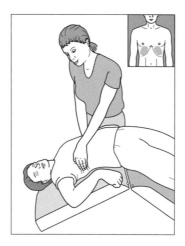

Figure 5.9   Posterior basal segments: lower lobes. Patient lying on front. Head down at an angle of 45°. Apply manual technique over the back of lower ribs.

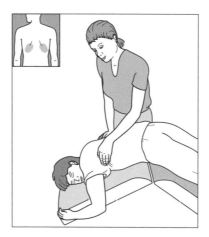

Figure 5.10 Lateral basal segment: the left lower lobe. Patient lying on right side with head down at an angle of 45°. Apply manual technique over left lower ribs.

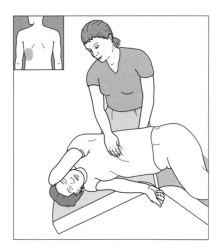

Figure 5.11 Lateral basal segment: right lower lobe. Patient lying on the left side with head down at an angle of 45°. Apply manual technique over right lower ribs.

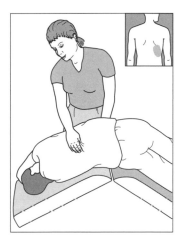

Percussion

- Performed with a cupped hand(s) over the area being drained. For an infant use 2–3 fingers.
- Can be performed independently with one hand by an older child or adult.
- Should not be so hard as to disrupt breathing – this would be counter-productive.
- Should be carried out over a layer of clothing or towel. If many layers are needed the clapping is probably too firm!
- Percussion should be used for approximately 15–20 second periods with pauses for 5 seconds or longer to minimize risks of hypoxia (Pryor, Webber & Hodson 1990).
- The rate of percussion should be comfortable for both. There is no evidence that different rates have different effects (see Modifications), although slower percussion might be better tolerated by those with increased bronchial reactivity.
- Manual percussors do not increase sputum clearance or lung function (Pryor, Parker & Webber 1981).

Figure 5.12 Mother treating infant's anterior segments of upper lobes in supine.

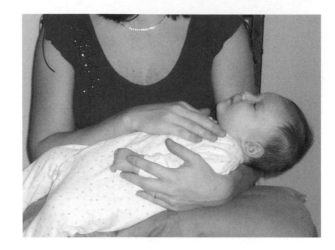

Figure 5.13 Mother treating infant's apical segments of upper lobes in sitting.

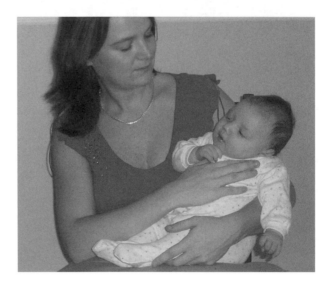

A typical regime consists of approximately 4–5 minutes of intermittent percussion in each of 2–3 postural drainage positions. If productive, the treatment time or frequency should be extended in an attempt to maximize clearance as tolerated.

Figure 5.14   Mother treating infant's apical segments of upper lobes in alternative position.

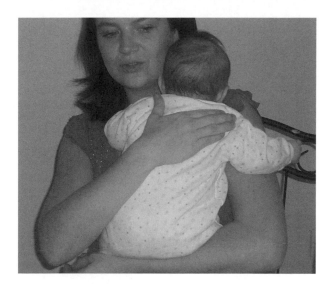

Example

Common basic postural drainage regime for a non-ambulant infant.

am   Apical segments of upper lobes, lateral segment right lower lobe, right middle lobe

pm   Anterior segments of upper lobes, lateral segment left lower lobe, lingula

When ambulant, treatment of the apical segments of the upper lobes becomes less important.

The active cycle of breathing techniques (Pryor & Webber 1979, Webber 1986, Pryor & Webber 1990, Webber & Pryor 1993)

This consists of three breathing techniques:

- Breathing control
- Thoracic expansion exercises
- The forced expiration technique.

Breathing control

Normal gentle breathing at tidal volume with shoulders and upper chest relaxed.

- Used to prevent increase in airflow obstruction and to allow patients to rest.

Thoracic expansion exercises

Deep breaths with emphasis on the breath in and a gentle breathe out. Can be used with an inspiratory hold especially if the patient has atelectasis. Can be combined with percussion or shaking/vibrations if helpful.

- Uses the principal of collateral ventilation to move air behind secretions encouraging their mobilisation (Menkes & Traystman 1977).
- Uses the phenomenon of interdependence to assist in airway expansion (Mead, Takishima & Leith 1970).

Figure 5.15 The active cycle of breathing techniques.

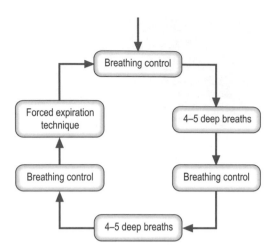

The forced expiration technique

One or two huffs with breathing control.

A huff is a forced breath out, not a blow, usually from mid to low lung volume. If correctly performed the abdominal muscles will contract. The huff is often performed too short. If this happens secretions will not be mobilised from the small airways.

- Causes an increase in intrathoracic pressure, moving the equal pressure point downstream and so mobilising secretions from smaller to larger airways.
- Secretions can be cleared from larger airways with either a high lung volume huff or cough.
- Commonly used with postural drainage but also effective in the sitting position.
- It is recommended that the number of postural drainage positions used in each treatment session is limited to two or three.

The length of each phase of the cycle can be varied and should be altered to suit each patient e.g. a very productive patient may only need one set of deep breaths in each cycle in order to cut down the treatment time, whereas a wheezy patient may need longer periods of breathing control.

Positive expiratory pressure (PEP) (Falk 1984, Groth 1985, Hofmeyr, Webber & Hodson 1990, Zach & Oberwaldner 1992, Christensen 1995)

Positive expiratory pressure can be applied via a face-mask or mouthpiece and can employ flow dependent resistors (orifice resistors) or threshold resistors.

The flow dependent resistors commonly used are the Pari-PEP and Astra-tech PEP mask. They produce pressure by imposing an adjustable orifice resistance to the exhaled flow. The pressure varies directly with resistance and flow. The threshold resistors commonly used are the Medic-Aid Threshold PEP and Vital Signs PEEP valves. These provide pressure independent of the expiratory flow. Devices of this type exert pressure as a force over surface area e.g. by compression of springs. Theoretically,

Figure 5.16   Standard PEP cycle.

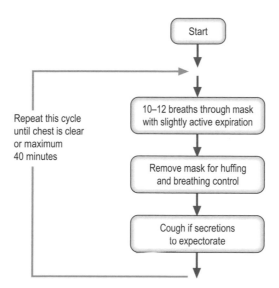

Start

10–12 breaths through mask with slightly active expiration

Remove mask for huffing and breathing control

Cough if secretions to expectorate

Repeat this cycle until chest is clear or maximum 40 minutes

threshold devices give better control over the expiratory pressure level, reducing the risk of trauma with sudden increases in airway pressure and increases in expiratory flow rates. However, all devices demonstrate flow-dependent characteristics to a variable extent especially at high flow rates (>90 L/min). Clinical studies are lacking, but long-term use of high pressure PEP in Denmark has not showed any increase in the risk of pneumothorax or haemoptysis after the significant pressures generated by coughing through the mask (see High Pressure PEP). In clinical use, the *actual* pressures should be measured to ensure agreement with the *intended* pressure. The effect of the intended pressure of 10–20 cm H_2O is to splint open central and peripheral airways to allow air to flow behind the secretions either directly or via collateral channels. The secretions are then cleared using the forced expiration technique (huffing with breathing control).

Recommendation:

Clean equipment with soap and water every day.

Flow dependent PEP

Individual initial assessment (using a PEP-Mask) is required before starting treatment. The following is recommended:

1. Position sitting upright with elbows supported on the table.
2. Allow the individual to breathe through the mouthpiece using the largest hole to become comfortable and familiar with its use.
3. Instruct them to breathe through the mouthpiece with each resistor in turn from the largest to the smallest hole. Allow at least 30 seconds with each resistor to establish a breathing pattern. Inspiration should be slightly deeper than tidal volume and expiration should be slightly active. As the resistance increases, expiration will become longer.

Encourage more active expiration if this becomes too prolonged. Conceal the manometer readings during this process as most people can and will alter their breathing (i.e. increase their flow rate) to reach the required pressures with all the resistors.

4. The correct resistor allows a good breathing pattern (maintainable for 2 minutes continuously) and gives a pressure through mid expiration of 10–20 cm H_2O. Some will find it difficult to sustain a pressure >10 cm H_2O. This is acceptable as long as the breathing pattern is good.

5. Having chosen the correct resistor, showing the manometer might help to achieve a smooth, steady breathing pattern. With correct technique the manometer dial moves smoothly up to the desired pressure, remains there during mid expiration and falls smoothly at end expiration.

6. Once established, a manometer is not essential, but most maintain a better technique with the feedback.

Review

Technique and pressures should be checked regularly and particularly during an infection to ensure the flow rate has not altered thereby changing the pressure achieved. Full assessment with all resistors is not required but as a minimum pressures with resistors above and below the one currently used should be assessed.

Threshold devices

These are very simple to use because the pressure required can be preset. However, it is difficult to check the actual pressure achieved because threshold PEP products are not designed to allow this.

Having preset the pressure individuals should be taught to achieve a good breathing pattern with a slightly extended expiration.

A simple adaptation for young children can be made (Figure 5.17).

PEP is achieved by blowing down the tube against the pressure of the water. The number of centimetres of water equates to the amount of PEP (i.e. 15 cm of water will provide 15 cm of water pressure).

High Pressure PEP (Oberwaldner 1991, Pfflegor 1992, Zack & Oberwaldner 1992)

This technique differs from the previously described PEP technique in that the *entire* treatment is performed through the PEP-mask. This is only removed to expectorate. By performing forced expiration against

Figure 5.17 Bubble PEP. Simple adaptation of threshold PEP. Cheap and popular with young children.

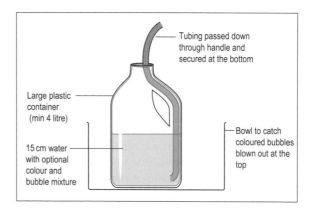

Tubing passed down through handle and secured at the bottom

Large plastic container (min 4 litre)

15 cm water with optional colour and bubble mixture

Bowl to catch coloured bubbles blown out at the top

resistance, unstable airways continue to be splinted open allowing clearance of the more peripheral secretions. This technique is useful for bronchomalacia.

Initial assessment

1. Seat with mask positioned as for low pressure PEP with the outlet of the PEP mask connected to a spirometer.
2. Perform a baseline flow volume loop.
3. Repeat flow volume loops through the mask using the full series of resistors in turn.

The resistor of choice is that which produces a graph showing maximal FVC, good plateau and no curvilinearity (i.e. no airway obstruction).

Figure 5.18 Graphs to show full series of flow volume loops.

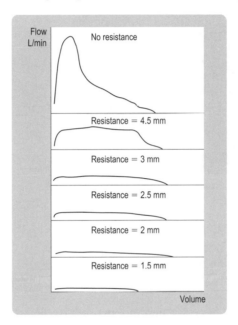

Figure 5.19 Standard high pressure PEP cycle.

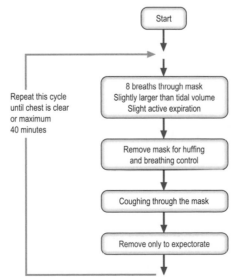

Precautions   Despite achieving pressures of 40–100 cmH$_2$O this technique has not been shown to increase the risk of pneumothorax or haemoptysis (Zach & Oberwaldner 1992). It should not be used in the presence of a large undrained pneumothorax or frank haemoptysis.

Figure 5.20 a, b Picture and drawing of the flutter.

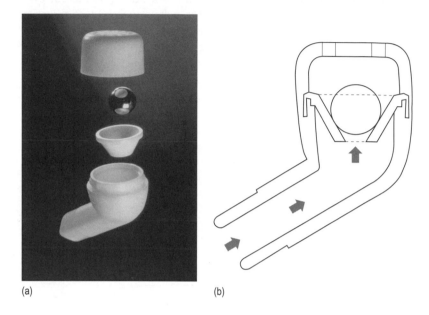

(a)   (b)

Oscillatory positive expiratory pressure

- The Flutter
- The RC Cornet
- The Acapulco.

Flutter (Konstan, Stern & Doershuk 1994, Pryor 1994, Lyons 1992, McIlwaine 1997, Schibler, Casulta & Kraemer 1992, App et al 1995)

This is performed independently, usually in the sitting position, but can also be used with gravity assisted positioning. Treatment commonly follows the cycle below but can also be used in combination with autogenic drainage.

During exhalation through the device the steel ball is raised by the air pressure behind it. This head of pressure is repeatedly released resulting in the ball oscillating back into place through gravity. This causes internal vibrations through the respiratory system resulting in an oscillating positive expiratory pressure. The oscillating frequency can be varied (usually between 6 and 26 cycles per second), by altering the inclination of the flutter device from the horizontal to achieve maximum chest vibrations. The positive expiratory pressure is 10–15 cmH$_2$O.

The RC-Cornet   Unlike the flutter, the RC-Cornet is position independent and allows fixed adjustment of the pressure and frequency.

The apparatus consists of a mouthpiece, a flattened valve tube, a pipe and a silencer. A kink in the pipe causes the valve tube to bend at a specific point. As the patient blows into the valve tube, the air-flow is

Figure 5.21   Flutter cycle.

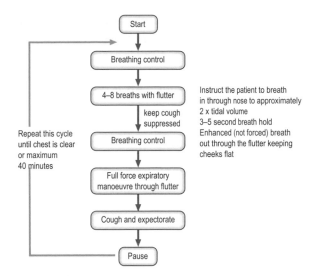

Start

Breathing control

4–8 breaths with flutter

keep cough
suppressed

Breathing control

Full force expiratory
manoeuvre through flutter

Cough and expectorate

Pause

Instruct the patient to breath
in through nose to approximately
2 x tidal volume
3–5 second breath hold
Enhanced (not forced) breath
out through the flutter keeping
cheeks flat

Repeat this cycle
until chest is clear
or maximum
40 minutes

obstructed at the bend until a critical pressure is reached which causes the bent tube to straighten. As the air escapes, this is repeated at the end of the tube causing the same build up and release of pressure. In this way a flutter action occurs with defined fluctuations in pressure and flow. By drawing out and rotating the mouthpiece, the pressure can be varied between 10 and 50 cm H_2O and the frequency between 9 and 50 Hz.

To use:

- Breathe in through the nose and out through the Cornet.
- Start by breathing at normal rate and depth.
- Intersperse normal breathing with a few deeper breaths.
- As secretions loosen they can be cleared with huffing or coughing.
- The pressure and flow can be altered by twisting the mouthpiece until an optimal effect is achieved. This may vary, but positions 3 and 4 are recommended for cystic fibrosis.
- Breathing control is used between the more active breathing manoeuvres.

Autogenic drainage (Schoni 1989, David 1991, Dab & Alexander 1979, Millar 1995, McIlwaine 1988, Gremmo 1992)

Autogenic drainage is a breathing technique performed at varying lung volumes using accelerated expiratory flows to mobilise secretions from throughout the bronchial tree. It avoids any airway compression and thus is particularly useful in individuals with increased bronchial reactivity. It is commonly performed in the sitting or supine position, but can be performed in any position found useful. This technique is often used in conjunction with the Flutter or PEP.

Instructions

Each breath comprises:

- Inspiration: Slow gentle breath in to low, mid or high lung volume (depending on the phase – see below) keeping the upper airways open.
- Breath hold: Hold breath for approximately 3 seconds keeping glottis open to allow equal filling of all lung units.

- Expiration: Breathe out as quickly as possible without causing airway obstruction. In practice this is a blow with the mouth half open or through the nose.

Initially patients rely on the physiotherapist to provide auditory and tactile guidance but with experience they use their own proprioception to detect the level of their secretions and the depth of breathing required.

Modified autogenic drainage

Each breath is performed as for autogenic drainage but there is less emphasis on the three separate phases of breathing. The length of expiration depends on the level of the secretions in the bronchial tree (i.e. high volume, shorter expiration for proximal secretions and low volume, longer expiration for distal secretions).

Figure 5.22 a, b The stages of autogenic drainage.

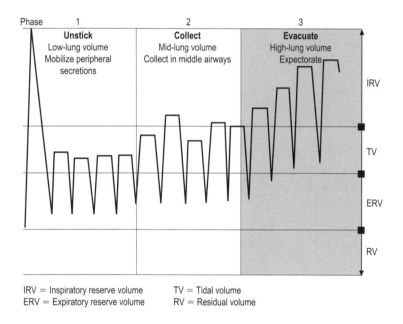

IRV = Inspiratory reserve volume   TV = Tidal volume
ERV = Expiratory reserve volume   RV = Residual volume

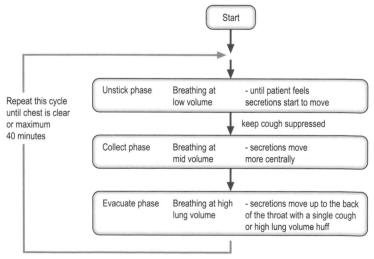

High frequency chest wall oscillation (HFCWO) (Scherer 1998)

This is a mechanical device that fits like a jacket around the patient and provides external chest wall oscillation. It has a dual pump system that generates positive and negative pressures. By electronic control of the pump the I:E ratios, frequencies, pressures and effective functional residual capacities can be altered.

There is little experience of HFCWO in the UK.

Intra pulmonary percussive ventilation (IPV) (Scherer 1998)

This device provides high frequency internal oscillations via a mouthpiece using rapid bursts of air. Devices usually allow adjustment of the I:E ratio, frequency, and drive power. As with HFCWO there is little experience in the UK. Research has only compared this treatment with postural drainage and percussion.

MODIFICATIONS TO PHYSIOTHERAPY PROGRAMME

When there are difficulties tolerating treatment because of breathlessness, wheeze, haemoptysis, pain, nausea or fatigue, modifications must be made to ensure that physiotherapy continues to be effective.

General recommendations

- Slow down treatment and increase the amount of breathing control between more active parts of the technique.
- Avoid head down tip with postural drainage positions. A very breathless patient might prefer high side lying or forward lean sitting for treatment.
- Minimise or stop chest clapping and shaking.
- Consider use of adjuncts.

Remember

- Give bronchodilators prior to treatment.
- Give medication for pain or nausea prior to treatment.
- Monitor vital signs and O_2 saturations before, during and after treatment.

Contraindications and precautions

All techniques should be stopped or used with caution in the presence of an undrained pneumothorax or recent large haemoptysis. Mechanical adjuncts such as percussion or HFCWO should be limited in those with musculoskeletal problems such as severe osteoporosis, rib fractures or uncontrolled pain. Modifications to postural drainage positioning should be considered with breathlessness, gastro-oesophageal reflux and late pregnancy. For further details refer to specific complications later in this chapter.

Adjuncts

These are used to assist with airway clearance when a patient's existing treatment is less effective or poorly tolerated. Common causes include thick secretions, dyspnoea and fatigue.

Common adjuncts include:

- Non invasive positive pressure ventilation (NIPPV)
- Periodic continuous positive airway pressure (PCPAP)
- Intermittent positive pressure breathing (IPPB)
- Humidification
- Inhalants.

> ### Remember
>
> Patients should always be encouraged to maintain their fluid intake to prevent dehydration and drying of their secretions.

Non invasive positive pressure ventilation (NIPPV)

Non invasive ventilation is used in CF as an aid to ventilation and as an adjunct to physiotherapy. It can be delivered via full face mask, nasal mask or mouthpiece. There are many different machines on the market and new models are being developed. Machines are either volume cycled or pressure cycled. Pressure cycled machines usually have positive end expiratory pressure (PEEP) which is often of benefit in moderate or severe CF. Different machines will have different variables and you will need to identify individual needs to choose the correct machine.

It is beyond the remit of this chapter to explain how to use different types of NIPPV. It should only be instigated at specialist centres. Individual companies can provide useful information and training about their products.

> ### Useful companies:
>
> Deva Medical – Breas
> Respironics (Medic-aid) – BIPAP

Figure 5.23 BIPAP with Fisher–Paykel humidification and supplemental oxygen.

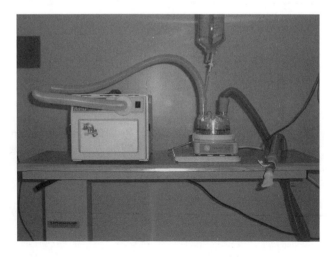

Continuous positive airway pressure (CPAP)   Provides continuous positive pressure throughout inspiration and expiration. Can be humidified if required with a Fisher Paykel heated humidifier. It has been shown to be effective in increasing functional residual capacity (Gherim, Peters & Virgilis 1979, Lindner, Lotz & Ahnefield 1987) and reducing the work of breathing (Gherim, Peters & Virgilis 1979). It is a cheaper option than NIPPV machines.

Uses
- Atelectasis, segmental or lobar collapse
- For ventilatory support in the acutely hypoxic patient where NIPPV is thought to be inappropriate.

Patient treatment
- Position patient depending on aim of treatment
- Use CPAP for 10–15 minutes (no clapping/shaking)
- Follow with airway clearance techniques (no clapping/shaking)
- Repeat as necessary.

Intermittent positive pressure breathing (IPPB)   IPPB is less commonly used in many centres with the advent of NIPPV, but it is still a useful adjunct especially where PEEP is not required.

It can be used to reduce the work of breathing (Ayers, Kozam & Lucas 1963) and augment tidal volumes (Sukumalchantra, Park & Williams 1965) during exacerbations in adults and cooperative children.

- Provides positive pressure throughout inspiration
- Can only be used with spontaneously breathing patients
- Can be used in conjunction with ACBT.

Use of equipment
Sensitivity   Sets the inspiratory pressure required to trigger the machine. This should be kept low in most cases for minimal effect.

Flow control   Sets the flow rate of the inspired gas delivered. The initial setting should match the patient's own pattern of breathing. The flow rate will probably need altering throughout treatment.

Pressure control   Sets the maximum inspiratory pressure at the mouth. If the patient's technique is good this will be indicative of the airway pressure. If the patient is allowed to blow back into the mouthpiece or holds a lot of gas in their mouth this will cut off the breath too early. Blowing back onto the machine can be identified by a sharp rise of the pressure gauge.

Air mix control   If driven by oxygen, the air mix should usually be pulled out giving a concentration of 45% (Porter & Young 1991).

Nebuliser   Normal saline administered through the nebuliser component should be used to humidify the inspired gases. For the severely dyspnoeic, the delivery of a bronchodilator through this system might result in improved airway deposition although there is little evidence for benefit compared with conventional nebuliser systems (Webber, Shenfield & Paterson 1974).

Oxygen or air?   Most should use oxygen with IPPB. Despite delivering concentrations of 45%, hypercapnic patients are not at risk because treatment times are short, their ventilation is assisted and resultant airway clearance should improve arterial blood gas concentrations (Gormezano & Branthwaite 1972, Starke, Webber & Branthwaite 1979).

For a breathless patient, a positive end expiratory pressure (PEEP) valve can be placed on the outlet valve.

Treatment
- Connect ventilator to gas source.
- Assemble circuit and fill nebuliser with appropriate solution.
- Use mouthpiece, flange or mask as appropriate.
- Set sensitivity low at 5–7 cmsH$_2$O and flow at 7 l/min.
- Set pressure at 10 cmsH$_2$O for an adult; lower for a child.
- Position and explain the procedure.
- Instruct to keep a tight lip seal around the mouthpiece during inspiration; allow the breath in until the machine stops before gently breathing out. Relaxation is important to enable the ventilator to provide the work of breathing.
- The initial flow setting should reflect the patient's own pattern of breathing; for example, a breathless patient may need a faster flow rate initially which can be reduced once they are familiar with the equipment. Lower flow rates will result in more beneficial slower inspiratory times.
- The pressure can be altered to change the size of breath as treatment progresses.

Can be used with ACBT

- To augment thoracic expansion exercises and minimise effort
- After expectoration to provide support during recovery.

Contraindications to positive pressure
- Undrained pneumothorax or a history of recurrent pneumothoraces
- Large bullae
- Severe haemoptysis
- Lung abscess.

Humidification Although there is little evidence that inspired saline or water vapour improves mucous transport or changes the rheological properties of mucous, all inspired wall gasses should be humidified to minimize the dehydration of secretions.

Inhalants
- rhDNase – Has been shown to reduce the visco-elasticity of sputum. It can be inhaled daily or on alternate days and should be taken within 6 hours of physiotherapy due to the drug's short half-life. It should not be inhaled within 1 hour of nebulised colistin (see Chapter 4).
- Hypertonic saline (4.5% is commonly used in clinical practice) – Has been shown to increase the effectiveness of physiotherapy and

improve mucocilliary clearance compared with 0.9% normal saline. Some patients will require a bronchodilator prior to its use to prevent bronchospasm.

EXERCISE (Cooper 1995)

Although children are naturally active, it is important to educate parents and children about the benefits of exercise as an essential part of treatment. Exercise should be fun and introduced from a young age with trampolines or a simple circuit in the garden with hoops, skipping ropes and bikes.

School age children partake in variable amounts of formal physical training but parents should encourage any sporting activity and try to find something of interest for those not naturally inclined to exercise.

As school progresses, academic work may take priority and many adolescents no longer have exercise in their timetables. Teenage years are often characterised by decreased adherence to treatment and so it is an important time to maintain general fitness. Some local gyms have started 'teenzones' where under 16 year olds can use gym equipment under supervision. This is a good social way of exercising and can set a routine for later life.

An exercise programme should include aerobic training to enhance VO_2 and general fitness, resistance training to improve FEV1, weight gain and strength, and stretching to maintain thoracic and general mobility.

Exercise will augment airway clearance. Occasionally, healthy patients with normal lung function and no respiratory symptoms can use a reduced airway clearance programme *provided* they maintain high levels of daily exercise. In general, exercise should *not* be considered as a substitute for airway clearance techniques (Salh 1989).

Everyone should be encouraged to exercise during hospital admissions. Whenever possible this should be in the gym thereby offering them a break from the ward. If this is impractical because of infection control and staffing issues, exercise in a side room should be part of the treatment plan. Dance mats, trumpets, skipping ropes, hand weights and hoops can be used to make exercise varied. These are more portable and less expensive than static bikes.

Those with severe disease requiring oxygen or even ventilatory support, should still be encouraged to exercise. Their programme should include aerobic, resistance and mobility training but may need to be performed in situ.

A generous intake of salt and water is important when exercising, especially in warm climates.

Diabetics should check their BM prior to vigorous exercise. If it is less than 5 mmol/l they should eat extra carbohydrate before exercising.

Contraindications to specific sports
- Contact sports should be avoided by patients with severe osteoporosis and splenomegaly.
- Scuba diving should be avoided by patients with air trapping or symptomatic sinus disease.
- Exercise at altitude should be avoided by hypoxic patients.

> **Remember**
>
> It is easier to maintain then rehabilitate.

Exercise testing

An exercise test will:

- Assess functional ability
- Measure oxygenation during exercise and subsequent recovery
- Raise the profile of exercise and provide reassurance about the safety and ability to exercise
- Help formulate an exercise programme
- Assess response to intervention.

Exercise testing should be a routine part of the annual assessment and in some it should be carried out more regularly. It is essential for establishing a baseline exercise capacity before prescribing an appropriate exercise programme.

> Undertaking exercise testing in the community, where emergency medical assistance is unavailable, is not recommended.

Desaturation with exercise is rare in patients with an FEV1 $>$ 60% predicted (Marcotte 1986). A fall $>$4% in O_2 saturation with exercise is significant.

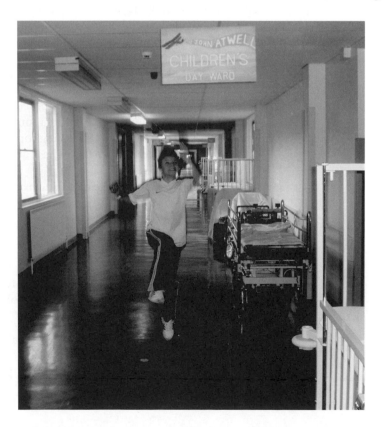

Figure 5.24   Exercise should be fun and wherever possible.

Practical considerations

- Testing should not be carried out immediately after eating.
- Do not perform during acute illness.
- Most tests require a quiet corridor or gym.
- Give a full explanation and an opportunity to practice the method of testing.
- Ideally oxygen saturations should be measured throughout the test with a portable monitor or at the beginning and end of testing as a minimum.
- Borg or VAS scores of breathlessness can be used to measure perceived shortness of breath and muscle fatigue.

Methods of testing

There are a number of suitable exercise tests.

Incremental tests (progressive maximal tests)

Cycle ergonometry   Uses a static exercise bicycle. Speed set at 60 rpm throughout test. Start at 10, 15 or 20 watts (resistance) and increase by the same amount each minute until unable to continue. The choice of starting resistance is determined by size, sex and general level of fitness e.g. a fit man who did regular exercise would start at 20 watts and increase to 40 for minute 2, 60 for minute 3 etc. A child would start at 10 watts, and a fit female 15 watts. Being a static test, it is easy to get accurate saturation readings throughout.

Modified shuttle test   An externally paced progressive test where the pace is set by an audio cassette.

This has recently been modified and is proving to be a maximal test for all but the fittest of patients. The patient walks between two points 10 m apart (a shuttle). The cassette bleeps when they should be at each end and starting the next shuttle. Each minute the bleeps are closer together thereby increasing the number of shuttles and therefore the pace. The patient starts to run when needed, to keep up with the bleeps and continues until they cannot maintain the speed.

20 m shuttle test (Bleep test)   This test differs from the modified shuttle test in that the individual runs between two points 20 m apart. This test starts at a gentle jog for an adult and is only suitable for very fit adolescents and adults. It gives a predicted VO_2 max.

Non incremental tests

Timed walks (2, 6, 12 minute)   Measures the maximum distance walked in a set time.

Individuals set their own pace and should achieve maximum exertion by the end of the test. They are allowed to stop if necessary with any rests noted by the tester. It requires two practices to provide a reasonably accurate and reproducible result. It is important to allow sufficient time to recover between tests.

- Can be performed in any quiet corridor
- No special equipment required
- Very dependent on patient motivation.

Figure 5.25 Modified shuttle test.

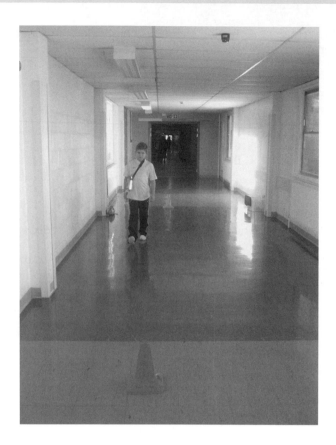

Figure 5.26 Illustration of modified shuttle test.

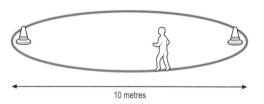

10 metres

Step test (Balfour-Lynn) A simple, quick, reproducible test using a 6-inch step. The individual is asked to step up and down at a set rate of 30 steps/minute for 3 minutes. The rate is set using a metronome.

Spontaneous and vigorous exercise is more common in children. Studies have shown that children tend to engage in short bursts of high intensity physical activity with intervening periods of low and moderate intensity. Most of the exercise tests are progressive and focus on VO_2 max, but these do not necessarily mimic real life. The step test is closer to the exercise pattern of children and so an abnormal physiologic response to this is more likely to indicate impairment in their lives.

Once the exercise test has been performed, recommendations can be made to help formulate an exercise plan. The reasons for stopping tests are important. A surprising number will be limited by lack of fitness rather than the respiratory symptoms they expected. Recommendations for improving fitness are the same as generally advised:

- Start work at 50% of peak work capacity (this is easily worked out if using the cycle ergometry test)
- Work at 70–80% of peak heart rate (as achieved during exercise test)
- There should be shortness of breath without distress
- Training should take place 3–4 times per week for 20–30 minutes.

Thoracic mobility and posture

Postural abnormalities and reduced thoracic mobility are common in CF. There is usually a postural component but in some it becomes fixed. A stiff thoracic spine can be associated with stiff costovertebral joints. These problems reduce rib excursion and the ability to develop normal transpleural pressure for lung expansion. Shortening of some muscle groups might also occur. This is most apparent in the anterior muscles of the neck, the trapezei, the anterior muscles of the hip and the hamstrings. This alteration of muscle length will alter the length tension curves of these muscles and can result in less efficient muscle action.

Tight muscles and a stiff chest wall cause a restrictive impairment in addition to a primarily obstructive lung condition and increase the work of breathing.

Chest pain is common. Musculoskeletal pain can be referred around the chest wall mimicking pleuritic pain. The physiotherapist has a role in determining the cause of symptoms. Most treatments rely on the reproduction of signs and symptoms and using an appropriate treatment rationale. The use of forward lean sitting for palpation may be a more suitable position than prone. The possibility of osteoporosis must be considered.

> ### Remember
>
> The physiotherapist's role includes assessment of posture and teaching exercises to mobilise and strengthen the thoracic cage to prevent future complications.

SPECIAL SITUATIONS

Pneumothorax

Small pneumothorax

Continue physiotherapy but avoid the use of positive pressure. Watch for signs of increased breathlessness indicative of extension. Give analgesia if required. Avoid prolonged or frequent forced expiratory manoeuvres. Humidify supplemental oxygen. Encourage mobility but avoid strenuous exercise.

Large pneumothorax

Withhold physiotherapy until drain inserted then recommence normal physiotherapy. Ensure adequate analgesia. Humidify supplemental oxygen. Encourage mobility, particularly shoulder range of movement and correct posture, but avoid strenuous exercise.

Pneumothorax requiring surgery

Withhold physiotherapy until the post-operative period then recommence with adequate analgesia. Humidify supplemental oxygen. Encourage early mobilisation as above.

Gastro–oesophageal reflux (GOR) (Phillips 1998, Button 1997a, Button 1997b, Button 1998)

- Management depends on the results of 24-hour pH monitoring (see Chapter 6).
- Those who *only* reflux whilst in a head down position should modify their postural drainage routine.
- Those who reflux intermittently in *all* positions will not benefit from modifying their postural drainage routine.

Haemoptysis

Mild haemoptysis (Blood streaked sputum)

Continue normal airway clearance.

Moderate haemoptysis (less than 250 mls)

Modify airway clearance until bleeding stops:

- Avoid head down tilt
- Minimise coughing
- Stop percussion and shaking
- Avoid PEP, flutter or any other devices which will increase intrathoracic pressure
- Continue gentle exercise avoiding any tachycardia.

Severe haemoptysis

Treatment should be stopped until bleeding has settled or arterial embolisation has been carried out. Treatment should continue as for moderate haemoptysis.

Stress incontinence

Stress incontinence is well recognized. Identification needs careful, sensitive questioning.

Pregnancy

Airway clearance should be continued throughout pregnancy. Head down tipped positions will need modifying as uterine size increases and pushes against the diaphragm. The lower lobes will need careful attention with the resultant reduction in FRC and early closing volumes causing gas trapping in these lung areas. PEP devices or adjuncts such as NIPPV can be useful for some patients.

Exercise should be continued but care should be taken with weight training due to ligament laxity.

The need for pelvic floor exercises must be emphasised.

Surgery

General anaesthesia and surgery will affect lung function by altering both lung mechanics and gas exchange (see Chapter 18).

Preoperative work up might include IV antibiotics but should include optimal physiotherapy treatment to ensure the patient goes for surgery with as clear a chest as possible.

There is an ideal opportunity to clear secretions whilst the patient is intubated. This can be done using manual hyperinflation, chest shaking and suction or lavage.

In the postoperative period pain control should be optimal and timed to cover physiotherapy sessions. Supplemental oxygen should be humidified. Physiotherapy might need modifying initially. Early mobilization is advised.

At discharge, ensure the patient has appropriate advice about returning to normal physiotherapy and activity.

Transplant

Pre-transplant

Ensure optimal airway clearance. Encourage and design an exercise programme to fulfill criteria described in the exercise section.

Post-transplant

The initial management will be undertaken at the transplant centre and close liaison with the referring centre is essential. The patient will continue with airway clearance as necessary to assess and clear their chest. They will monitor daily lung function to detect early signs of infection and continue with an exercise programme.

Terminal care

During the final phase of an individual's life, the role of the physiotherapist changes. It is important to be involved in symptom control with the use of humidified oxygen therapy, nebuliser systems, physiotherapy adjuncts and support. It is important not to withdraw, simply because airway clearance is less effective or appears inappropriate. Help can still be given clearing upper airway secretions, positioning, facilitating relaxation with massage, breathing control and support. Those who prefer to die at home should be supported with domiciliary physiotherapy (see Chapter 23).

TREATMENT ADHERENCE

Most individuals will have times when they do not adhere to physiotherapy. It is commonly rejected because it is time consuming and the effects of omission might not be immediately felt.

The physiotherapist needs to be sympathetic and work to re-establish an achievable regime.

Young children

- Keep treatment fun. Make games out of breathing exercises. Use a trampoline or tickling games to induce cough.
- Try to keep some routine going even if it is not effective treatment.
- Spread the responsibility for treatment throughout the family.
- Distract during treatment with stories or videos (this can be a problem if you want the child to concentrate on breathing exercises).
- Use star charts and positive reinforcement as an incentive for cooperation.

Older children and adults

- Identify reasons for stopping physiotherapy.
- Discuss and re-negotiate a new routine that you both think is adequate and achievable (be sure to set a minimum).
- Re-educate about how physiotherapy works.
- Try alternative airway clearance techniques.
- Encourage exercise to supplement physiotherapy.
- Offer professional counselling if there are issues that need discussing.

Figure 5.27 Venturi mask and humidity cap with entrained humidified air.

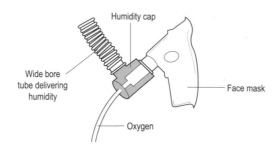

Humidity cap

Wide bore tube delivering humidity

Face mask

Oxygen

OXYGEN THERAPY
(Dodd & Haworth 1998)

Oxygen is given to correct hypoxaemia and minimize work of breathing.

Delivery systems

Venturi mask and valve – fixed concentration masks

Flow rates are recommended for each concentration based on estimated peak inspiratory flow rates of 40–50 L/min during tidal breathing.

- They provide a reliable Fraction of inspired Oxygen (FiO_2). The flow delivered is greater than the patient's inspiratory flow rate. However, with severe breathlessness, the inspiratory flow rate can rise above 40–50 L/min and an increased flow of oxygen will be needed to deliver the same concentration.
- A low FiO_2 does not require humidification because a high proportion of room air is entrained.
- A higher FiO_2 needs humidifying because of the higher proportion of inspired dry walled gas.
- Humidity caps should always be used to humidify this system.

> **Warning**
>
> Never try to humidify narrow bore tubing leading to the venturi valve.

Venturi humidity systems

- Reliable FiO_2 because the flow delivered is greater than inspiratory flow rate.
- Humidified (not always necessary).
- Can be set up to provide >60% oxygen using two nebulised Venturi systems in parallel connected with a Y connector. An oxygen analyser can be placed in the system. The Venturis are closed or nearly closed and the flow rate turned up until the required oxygen level is reached. With this system 98% oxygen can be provided (note the two 10 cm lengths of wide bore tubing attached to the holes in the face mask in Figure 5.28).

Nasal specs

- Unreliable concentration as the 1–4 L/min O_2 delivered is diluted by the patient's inspiratory flow rate.
- Can be used with bubble-through system but no objective benefits have been shown.

Simple face mask

- Less reliable as inspired FiO_2 percentage will depend on patient's inspiratory flow rate.

Figure 5.28 Shows face mask with two 10 cm wide bore tubes attached.

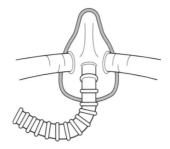

Monitoring

Modern pulse oximeters accurately estimate arterial oxygen saturation and should be used to titrate inspired oxygen concentrations. Oxygen supplementation will mask hypoxaemic respiratory failure and patients with ongoing respiratory difficulties despite oxygen therapy should have a capillary or arterial blood gas to detect CO_2 retention. Transcutaneous or end tidal CO_2 monitoring can be used to detect trends towards worsening hypercarbia.

HOME OXYGEN THERAPY

Daytime sleepiness and morning headaches with poor ability to concentrate might be due to nocturnal hypoxaemia in those with advanced lung disease.

Assessing the patient

The need for oxygen can be assessed by overnight pulse oximetry. Those with prolonged desaturations <92% are most likely to benefit symptomatically. Flow rates can be adjusted following treatment according to repeat measurements and symptomatic responses.

Types of equipment available and prescribing

The prescribing of home oxygen is due to change in 2005. At present it is prescribed by the GP and allows only the prescription of large cylinders or concentrators. The new arrangements transfer prescribing to the hospital consultant and allows the contractor to decide, with the patient, the best and most up-to-date method of delivery. This will include the prescription of liquid and lightweight oxygen.

The GP will continue to be able to prescribe oxygen for patients who need small amounts.

Concentrators

Concentrators are the most commonly used method of providing supplemental oxygen. They run off mains electricity so a cylinder is provided in case of power failure. They can be ordered with variable flow rates depending on requirements.

Disadvantages include size (they are approximately the size of a bed-side cabinet) and the tendency to 'hum' when in use. They are not portable. Mobile patients require long lengths of tubing.

Cylinders

Cylinders are available in a variety of sizes and are generally used as back up to concentrators. Small cylinders tend to last for only a short period and require frequent refilling. This is discouraged by the manu-facturers. They can be portable but if they are taken into a car a warning label must be displayed.

Tubing, masks or nasal cannula

Most people prefer a less obtrusive nasal cannula. However, the choice of face mask or cannula should be individualised.

If mobile individuals require a considerable length of tubing to enable them to move around, it is important to check that oxygen delivery remains adequate.

Tubing should be changed regularly, as should the nasal cannula or face mask.

> **Remember**
>
> Families must inform their house and/or car insurance companies if supplemental oxygen is in use and display a sign in the back of their car (see Chapter 21).

Introducing therapy

Currently, equipment is installed by the companies providing it. Their installation representative will provide teaching.

A CF team member should check that equipment has been installed and that the family know how to operate it. Individuals can have diffi-culties adjusting to a nasal cannula or an oxygen mask but this usually ceases to be a problem after continued use.

Once therapy has begun it is important to re-monitor oxygen satur-ations to ensure that an appropriate amount of oxygen is delivered.

INHALATION THERAPY

Inhalers (Gregson & Warner 1995)

There are three methods for delivering drugs directly to the airways:

- Metered dose inhaler (MDI)
- Dry powder inhaler (DPI)
- Nebuliser (compressed gas or ultrasonic).

An MDI via a spacer is a simple and effective drug delivery system for mild to moderate CF-related lung disease. Children under the age of 3 years will not be able to coordinate breathing through a mouthpiece and so spacer devices should be adapted with a face-mask attachment. Increased compliance with inhalation therapy in older children and adults might be achieved by the use of smaller DPI devices. Inhaled antibiotics are currently given via nebulisers although formulations for dry powder delivery will become available. Nebulisers are best used for all medications when symptoms are severe.

Optimal inhaler technique for MDI and spacer

- Shake the MDI (necessary for most devices).
- Stand or sit upright to allow good diaphragmatic excursion.
- Place device in mouth and make a firm seal with lips.
- Activate the device and immediately start inhalations.
- Takes 5 steady tidal breaths after each actuation without breath holding.

Common faults

- Tongue and or teeth block inhalation
- Lip seal inadequate
- Head bent forward
- Inhaler device inserted too far into the mouth, blocking inspiratory holes
- Inspiration too short.

Nebulisers (Association of Chartered Physiotherapists with an Interest in CF 1996)

Compliance with nebulisation is a problem. Individuals are less likely to persevere with time-consuming therapies if there are no perceived benefits. Careful discussion and education is needed to ensure that the family understand the reasons for treatment. They should be able to admit to the team if they are not managing to take prescribed treatment. The time taken to nebulise drugs varies with different equipment and between individuals. Generally, they should be advised to stop after 10 minutes.

Exerpts from *Practical Guidelines for the use of Nebulisers in Cystic Fibrosis* – Reprinted with kind permission of Association of Chartered Physiotherapists with an Interest in Cystic Fibrosis.

Factors affecting success

- Incorrect equipment for the type of drug used
- Nebulisation time too long for patient leading to poor compliance
- Incorrect particle size (optimal size 1–5 microns)
- Inadequate volume of drug (be aware of residual volume of equipment used)
- Patient education.

Factors affecting aerosol deposition

Increased

- Slowing of raised respiratory rates
- Correct use of mouthpiece
- Comfortable supported sitting position
- Nebulisation of aerosols at appropriate time in relation to airway clearance techniques (see below)
- Minute volumes between 10–15 L/min
- Tidal volume interspersed with slow deep breaths may improve deposition.

Decreased

- Airways obstruction
- Fast mean inspiratory flow rate
- Use of mask
- Poor technique
- Small tidal volume.

Compressors

The compressor is an electrically powered machine driving air flow. The output is measured in L/min. There are many on the market and constantly updated models. It is important that the correct compressor and nebuliser are used for each type of drug (see Table 5.1).

When using a compressor:

- It must conform to BS5724 (or European standard equivalent).
- It must be serviced according to the manufacturer's instructions and checked before issue.
- Written instructions for use, including cleaning and maintenance, what to do in emergency, and on holidays, must be provided.

Maintenance of nebuliser equipment

- Note manufacturer's guidelines for duration of use of nebuliser and cleaning methods.
- Change mouthpiece, mask and tubing every three months.
- Change discoloured valves/filters.

Table 5.1 Choice of nebulisers and compressors for drugs.

Compressor	Nebuliser	Fill volume	Special note
Bronchodilators			
Flow rate 6–8 L/min	Jet nebuliser	2 ml	• Use before physiotherapy • If wishing to mix with other medication, check compatibility with pharmacist
Antibiotics			
Do not use with ultrasonic nebuliser			
Flow rate 6–8 L/min	Active venturi	2–4 ml	• Give after physiotherapy
Flow rate 8–10 L/min	Active venturi	2–4 ml	• Pre-prescription challenging with spirometry to exclude bronchoconstriction
Flow rate 8–10 L/min	Venturi	4 ml	
Steroids			
Do not use with ultrasonic nebuliser			
Flow rate 6–8 L/min	Active venturi	2 ml respules	• Give after physiotherapy
Flow rate 6–8 L/min	Venturi	2 ml respules	• Rinse mouth out thoroughly after use • Ideally use a mouthpiece or self-sealing mask • Vaseline can be used around the mouth
Mucolytics			
Same as bronchodilators	Same as bronchodilators	2–4 ml	• Give before physiotherapy • Pre-prescription challenging with spirometry
DNase			
6–8 L/min	Giving respiratory fraction 40–60% of particle size 3.5 μm	2.5 ml	• Do not combine • Do not give within an hour of nebulised antibiotic

Preparation of drugs and equipment

- Collect drugs, additives and equipment together on a clean surface.
- Wash hands thoroughly with warm soapy water and dry thoroughly.
- Prepare needle and syringe (if required) or nebule. Check drug and additive for expiry date. It should be noted that manufacturers recommend a new needle and syringe each time.
- Mix contents thoroughly; some antibiotics need gentle agitation. Wait for any foaming to subside – a suggestion would be to prepare an antibiotic drug before doing physiotherapy ready for inhalation after treatment.
- Put the solution into the chamber.
- Use the appropriate driving force (cylinder or air compressor) taking care not to occlude the ventilation of the machine. We would recommend not putting it on the floor by the bed because of the possibility of drawing in cold and dusty air.
- Nebulise the solution in the chamber (see breathing pattern and patient technique in next section).

Table 5.2 Trouble shooting.

Problem	Solution
Nebulisers	
Frothing	Leave longer to settle, do not shake
Spitting/no mist	Clean thoroughly; if unsuccessful change nebuliser
Leaking	Hold upright, check that connections are well-fitted
Dirty	Change reusable/durable annually, and disposable 3-monthly
Taking a long time	(1) Clean or (2) Replace with new (also see below for compressors)
Compressors	
Difficult to transport	Seek advice about portable type
Taking a long time	(1) Change filter or (2) service compressor
When to change inlet or outlet filter, if appropriate	3-monthly or when discoloured
Servicing/electrical check	Annually or according to manufacturers' instructions
Broken case	Service or replace
Too noisy	Service or newer model needed
Narrow bore tubing	
Blows off compressor	Use high pressure tubing
Dirty	Change 3 monthly
Mouthpieces	
Nose breathing	Use nose clip
Cleaning	After each use
Changing	Disposable; 3-monthly. Durable; annually
Masks	
Antibiotic usage	Sealing mask required
Child objects to mask	Persevere!
Uncomfortable	Try different size or mouthpiece

Table 5.3   Side effects.

Problem	Solution
Light-headedness	Adjust breathing pattern to control hyperventilation
Wheeziness	Check temperature (? solution too cold); breathing pattern; pre-prescription drug challenge with spirometry is recommended
Wheeziness with antibiotic	Check tonicity (solution should not be hypertonic); administer bronchodilator first
Irritation around face/eyes	Mouthpiece if appropriate; wash face after treatment; protect with Vaseline
Sore mouth	Rinse mouth or brush teeth after use
Tachycardia and shaking	Seek medical advice

- When nebulisation is complete, separate the components of the pot and wash and dry thoroughly after each use.
- Dispose of all sharps in a safe manner (i.e. sharps Box).
- Keep all equipment (used or unused) safely out of the reach of children.
- All solutions when prepared should be used immediately or kept in a refrigerator according to the manufacturer's recommendations. Refrigerated solutions should be brought to room temperature prior to inhaling.

Advice for inhalation

- Sit comfortably in an upright position.
- Preferably use a mouthpiece. Seal lips around it and breathe through mouth. A nose clip will help with this.
- Breathe at a comfortable rate.
- Intersperse normal breathing with occasional slower deeper breaths.
- Do not talk whilst using nebuliser.
- Have technique checked regularly by a member of the cystic fibrosis team.

> **Note**
>
> Children too young to use a mouthpiece should be encouraged to use a close fitting mask either held or strapped on.

Recommendations following use

- Disconnect the nebuliser from the tubing.
- Turn on the compressor for a short time to clear moisture from the narrow bore tubing.
- Disassemble the nebuliser circuit completely after each use.
- Wash each component in warm soapy water.
- Rinse and dry thoroughly.
- Hang up the wide bore tubing to dry.
- Certain equipment may be boiled, autoclaved or dishwashed.
- Check manufacturer's guidelines.

References

App E M, Danzl G, Schweiger K et al 1995 Sputum rheology changes in cystic fibrosis lung disease following two different types of physiotherapy VRP1 (flutter) versus autogenic drainage. Respiratory and Critical Care Medicine 151:4

Association of Chartered Physiotherapists with an interest in CF and CF Nurse Specialists Group 1996 Nebulisation. Practical guidelines for the use of nebulisers in cystic fibrosis.

Ayres S M, Kozam R L, Lukas D S 1963 The effects of intermittent positive pressure breathing on intra thoracic pressure, pulmonary mechanics and the work of breathing. American Review of Respiratory Disease 87:370–379

Balfour-Lynn I M, Prasad S A, Laverty A et al Step test versus 6 minute walk: assessing exercise tolerance in children with CF. Paediatric Pulmonology Tenth Northern American CF Conference. Abstract 347

Button B M, Heine R G et al 1997a Postural drainage and gastro-eosophageal reflux in infants with cystic fibrosis. Archives of Diseases in Childhood 76:148–150

Button B M, Heine R G et al 1997b A twelve month comparison of standard versus modified chest physiotherapy in twenty infants with cystic fibrosis. Paediatric Pulmonology 14:A338

Button B M, Heine R G, Calto-Smith A G et al 1997 Postural drainage and gastro-oesophageal reflux in infants with CF. Archives of Diseases in Childhood 76(2):148–150

Button B M, Heine R G et al 1998 Postural drainage in cystic fibrosis: is there a link with gastro-oesophageal reflux? Journal of Paediatric Child Health 34:330–334

Christensen E F, Jensen R H et al 1995 Flow dependent properties of positive expiratory pressure devices. Monaldi Archives of Chest Disease 50:2

Cooper D 1995 Rethinking exercise testing in children: a challenge. American Journal of Respiratory and Critical Care Medicine 152:1154–1157

Dab I, Alexander F 1979 The mechanism of autogenic drainage studied with flow volume curves. Monographs of Paediatrics 10:50–53

David A 1991 Autogenic drainage – the German approach. Respiratory Care (ed JA Pryor). Churchill Livingstone, London, p 65–78

Dodd M E, Haworth C, Webb A K. 1998 A practical approach to oxygen therapy in cystic fibrosis. Journal of the Royal Society of Medicine 34:91

Falk M, Kelstrup M, Anderson J B et al 1984 Improving the ketchup bottle method with positive expiratory pressure, PEP, in CF. European Journal of Respiratory Disease 65:423–432

Gherim S, Peters R M, Virgilis R W 1979 Mechanical work on the lungs and work of breathing with positive end expiratory pressure and continuous positive airway pressure. Chest 76:251–256

Gormezano J, Branthwaite M A 1972 Pulmonary physiotherapy with assisted ventilation. Anaesthesia 27:249–257

Gregson R K, Warner J O 1995 Asthma inhalers – developments or distractions? A guide to progression of inhaler devices. Maternal and Child Health Dec:383–389

Gremmo M, Cerioni E, Guenza M C et al 1992 Association of oscillating PEP (flutter) and controlled ventilation in patients with CF. 11th International CF Congress, Dublin

Groth S, Statangel G, Dirksen H et al 1985 Positive expiratory pressure (PEP mask) physiotherapy improves ventilation and reduces volume of trapped gas in cystic fibrosis. Bulletin of European Physiopathology and Respiration 339–343

Hofmeyr J L, Webber B A, Hodson M E 1986 Evaluation of positive expiratory pressure as an adjunct to chest physiotherapy in the treatment of cystic fibrosis. Thorax 41(12):951–954

Konstan M S, Stern R C, Doershuk C 1994 Efficacy of the flutter device for airway mucous clearance in patients with CF. Journal of Pediatrics 124(5):689–693

Lindner K H, Lotz P, Ahnefeld F W 1987 Continuous positive airway pressure effect on functional residual capacity, vital capacity and its subdivisions. Chest 92:66–70

Lyons E, Chatham K, Campbell I A et al 1992 Evaluation of the flutter VRPI device in young adults with cystic fibrosis. Thorax 47:237

Mcllwaine M, Davidson A G F, Wong L T K et al 1988 Comparison of positive expiratory pressure and autogenic drainage with conventional percussion and drainage therapy in the treatment of CF. 10th International CF Congress, Sydney, Australia, Excerpta Medica, Asia Pacific Congress Series p 120

Mcllwaine P M, Wong L T K, Peacock D et al 1997 Flutter versus PEP. A long term comparative trial of positive expiratory pressure (PEP) versus oscillating positive expiratory pressure (flutter) physiotherapy techniques. Paediatric Pulmonology 14:339

Marcotte J E, Grisdale R K, Levison H et al 1986 Multiple factors limit exercise capacity in cystic fibrosis. Paediatric Pulmonology 2(5):274–281

Mead J, Takishima T, Leith D 1970 Stress distribution in lungs: a model of pulmonary elasticity. Journal of Applied Physiology 28:596–608

Menkes H A, Traystman R J 1977 Collateral ventilation. American Review of Respiratory Diseases 116:287–309

Millar S, Hall D O, Clayton C B, Nelson R 1995 Chest physiotherapy in cystic fibrosis: a comparative study of autogenic drainage and the active cycle of breathing techniques with postural drainage. Thorax 50:165–169

Oberwaldner B, Theissl B, Rucker A et al 1991 Chest physiotherapy in hospitalised patients with CF: a study of lung function effects and sputum clearance. European Respiratory Journal 4:152–158

Pfflegor A, Theissl B, Oberwaldner B, Zach M S 1992 Self-administered chest physiotherapy in cystic fibrosis: a comparative study of high pressure PEP and autogenic drainage. Lung 170:323–330

Phillips G, Pike S et al 1998 Holding the baby:head downwards positioning does not cause gastro-eosophageal reflux. European Respiratory Journal 12:954–957

Porter A E, Young C S 1991 The physiotherapy management of cystic fibrosis in children. Physiotherapy 75:193–194

Pryor J A, Webber B A 1979 An evaluation of the forced expiratory technique as an adjunct to postural drainage. Physiotherapy 65:304

Pryor J A, Parker R A, Webber B A 1981 A comparison of mechanical and manual percussion as adjuncts to postural drainage in the treatment of cystic fibrosis in adolescents and adults. Physiotherapy 67:140–141

Pryor J A, Webber B A, Hodson M E 1990 Effect of chest physiotherapy on oxygen saturation in patients with cystic fibrosis. Thorax 45:77

Pryor J A, Webber B A, Hodson M E 1994 The flutter VRPI as an adjunct to chest physiotherapy in cystic fibrosis. Respiratory Medicine 88:677–681

Salh W, Bilton D, Dodd M et al 1989 Effect of exercise and physiotherapy in aiding sputum expectoration in adults with cystic fibrosis. Thorax 44:1006–1008

Scherer T, Barandun J et al 1998 Effect of High-frequency oral airway and chest wall oscillation and conventional chest physical therapy on expectoration in patients with stable cystic fibrosis. Chest 113:1019–1027

Schibler A, Casulta C, Kraemer R 1992 Rational of oscillatory breathing as chest physiotherapy performed by the flutter in patients with cystic fibrosis (CF). Paediatric Pulmonology 8:301

Schoni M H 1989 Autogenic drainage: a modern approach to chest physiotherapy in CF. Journal of Royal Society of Medicine 82(16):32–37

Starke I D, Webber B A, Branthwaite M A 1979 IPPB and hypercapnia in respiratory failure: the effect of different concentrations of inspired oxygen on arterial blood gas tensions. Anaesthesia 34:283–287

Sukumalchantra Y, Park S S, Williams M H 1965 The effect of intermittent positive pressure breathing (IPPB) in acute ventilatory failure. American Review of Respiratory Disease 92:885–893

Webb A K, Dodd M E 2000 Exercise and training for adults with cystic fibrosis. In: Hodson M E, Geddes D M (eds) Cystic Fibrosis, 2nd edn. Arnold, London, p 433–448

Webber B A, Shenfield G M, Paterson J W 1974 A comparison of three different techniques for giving nebulised albuterol to asthmatic patients. American Review of Respiratory Disease 109:293–295

Webber B A, Hotmeyr J L, Morgan M D L et al 1986 Effects of postural drainage incorporating the forced expiration technique on pulmonary function in CF. British Journal of Diseases of the Chest 80:353–359

Webber B A, Pryor J A 1993 Physiotherapy for respiratory and cardiac problems. Churchill Livingstone, Edinburgh

Zach M S, Oberwaldner B 1992 Effect of positive expiratory breathing in patients with cystic fibrosis. Thorax 47:66

Further reading

Paediatric Respiratory Care – A Guide for Physiotherapists and Health Professionals. Chapman and Hall, London. Prasad SA, Hussey J.

Physiotherapy for Respiratory and Cardiac Problems. Churchill Livingstone. Webber BA, Pryor JA.

Chapter **6**

Gastrointestinal problems

June Abay, Mark Beattie

CHAPTER CONTENTS

INTRODUCTION

The differential diagnosis of gastrointestinal symptoms in children with CF includes the following (Littlewood 1992):

- CF-related complications
- Gastrointestinal (GI) pathology unrelated to CF
- Non-organic abdominal pain.

PATHOLOGY

Pancreas

There is marked variability in the functional consequences of exocrine pancreatic damage. Non-functioning CFTR results in dehydration of zymogen granules, thickened pancreatic secretions and low bicarbonate excretion. Pathological changes include proximal ductular obstruction, acinar cell destruction, fibrosis, fatty change, calcification and cyst formation. Increased circulating immune reactive trypsin (IRT) as detected in the newborn period is a result of leakage of enzymes that cannot flow through

Figure 6.1   Malabsorption can result in malnutrition as demonstrated in this child at late presentation.

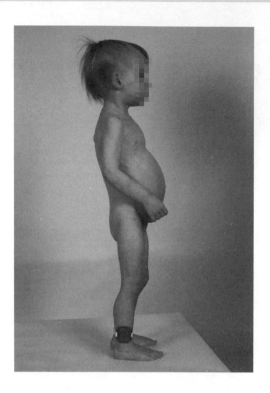

Figure 6.2   Nutritional status is intimately related to respiratory status; the most important factor determining long term survival.

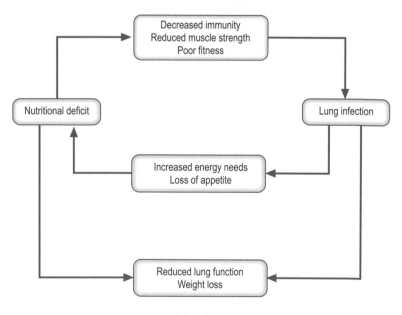

blocked ductules. Levels decrease in most cases as a result of local tissue destruction – autodigestion.

GI tract

CFTR is expressed on the apical membrane of epithelia throughout the GI tract. Functional consequences include the dehydration of intestinal fluid resulting in thick, viscid intestinal secretions. This can lead to the clinical problem of distal intestinal obstruction syndrome (DIOS). Secondary changes in intestinal gut hormones might explain some of the abnormalities of gut transit that are encountered (see below).

NUTRITIONAL ISSUES

Good nutrition is vital for successful CF care and is addressed in detail in Chapter 7.

Nutritional deficiencies occur as a result of one or more of the following:

- Inadequate intake or excessive losses
- Increased metabolic demand without increased intake
- Maldigestion and malabsorption (see Figure 6.1).

Nutritional status is intimately related to respiratory health (see Figure 6.2).

DIARRHOEA

It is essential to confirm stools are loose by objective assessment. Fatty stools are characteristic of maldigestion due to pancreatic insufficiency and have a characteristic smell.

CF-related causes of diarrhoea

- Insufficient pancreatic enzyme replacement therapy (PERT)
- Adherence issues
  - Toddler refusal
  - Chaotic household with multiple meal givers
  - Frustration or desire to be 'normal', omitting PERT with school lunch
  - Desire to be slim in adolescence
  - Perception that enzymes are not needed with milk or snacks
- Inappropriate timing of enzymes or prolonged meal times
- Poor enzyme activity as a result of:
  - Approaching the end of shelf life
  - Accelerated 'natural decay' in lipase strength by exposure to sunlight, heat or high humidity
  - Gastric acid hypersecretion and deficiency of pancreatic bicarbonate reducing the pH within the proximal small bowel below that for dissolution of the enteric coating
  - Increased small bowel transit
- Disorders of bile acid metabolism resulting in increased faecal loss of bile salts, increased glycine conjugated and decreased taurine conjugated bile salts
- Short gut syndrome following resection for meconium ileus in infancy
- Bacterial overgrowth either secondary to antibiotic usage or post bowel resection (this can be a late complication)
- Use of energy-dense high osmolality enteral feeds
- Side effects of concurrent medication

Diarrhoea unrelated to CF

- Toddler diarrhoea: Food residues, such as peas, carrots and sweet corn are typically present. Adjustment to enzyme dose does not improve loose stools but symptoms can improve after toilet training. The child should be otherwise well and thriving.
- Chronic infections such as giardiasis should be excluded by stool culture

- High laxative diet, e.g. blackcurrant drinks and excessive bran
- Laxative abuse
- Constipation presenting with overflow diarrhoea
- Other causes of malabsorption can occur concurrently with CF including:
  - Lactose intolerance
  - Cow's milk protein intolerance
  - Coeliac disease (increased incidence in CF)
- Colitis, e.g. inflammatory bowel disease, pseudomembranous colitis.

Investigation and management

A careful history and stool examination might provide clues to the cause of symptoms. Features suggesting fat malabsorption as the cause of diarrhoea include:

- Abdominal distension
- Abdominal discomfort relieved by defecation
- Pale, bulky, loose stools with a rancid smell
- Orange oil around the stool, visible fat globules, or an oily sheen on the surface of the toilet pan. Pistachio green coloured stools suggest protein malabsorption.
- Faecal incontinence.

Persisting symptoms should be investigated. Consider the following:

- Arrange expert dietetic input to ensure accurate titration of enzyme dose (see Chapter 7). Consider stock rotation, timing and brand of enzymes and a trial of treatment with a proton pump inhibitor.
- Consider a period of inpatient observation to facilitate the above.
- Arrange stool collection to obtain objective measures of fat malabsorption (see Chapter 8).
- Arrange stool examination, microscopy and culture including tests for *Clostridium difficile*.
- Further investigations might include
  - Coeliac antibody screen
  - Inflammatory markers
  - Skin prick tests
  - A trial of milk-free diet
  - Abdominal ultrasound including measurements of bowel wall thickness in those who have received Eudragit coated enzymes
  - Small and large bowel imaging
  - Upper and lower gastrointestinal endoscopy.

ABDOMINAL PAIN

Always consider a medical cause for abdominal pain but remember that, even in children with underlying organic pathology, functional causes are common. Abdominal surgical emergencies are dealt with in Chapter 17.

CF-related causes of abdominal pain

The following should be considered:

- Persistent malabsorption (see Chapter 8)
- Distal intestinal obstruction syndrome
- Constipation

- Splenic pain in individuals with massive splenomegaly
- Oesophagitis secondary to chronic gastro-oesophageal reflux
- Surgical problems: acute or sub-acute intestinal obstruction should be considered, particularly in individuals who have had surgery for meconium ileus or appendicitis (see Chapter 17)
- Fibrosing colonopathy
- Pain can occur as a result of poorly understood abnormalities of small and large bowel motility (dysmotility).

Abdominal pain unrelated to CF

- Recurrent abdominal pain of childhood is common
- Psycho-social causes such as bullying, school phobia, sexual abuse and depression
- Urinary tract pathology
- Acute appendicitis (see Chapter 17)
- Mesenteric adenitis
- Inflammatory bowel disease
- Gynaecological causes
- Acute cholecystitis (see Chapter 12)

DISTAL INTESTINAL OBSTRUCTION SYNDROME

Distal intestinal obstruction syndrome (DIOS), previously called meconium ileus equivalent, is a relatively common problem although there are wide variations in the extent to which it is reported between centres. This might reflect differences in recommendations for PERT dosing. There is an increased incidence of DIOS in adolescence and adult life but it can occur at any age. Abnormally viscid mucofeculent material causes gradual narrowing of the terminal ileum, partial and occasionally complete obstruction. The caecum and ascending colon can also be involved. Episodes can be precipitated by dehydration and intercurrent infections but often occur spontaneously. Some cases are chronic and/or relapsing. The differential diagnosis of DIOS includes acute appendicitis, intussusception, and volvulus (see Chapter 17).

Abdominal pain:

- Is of gradual onset, with occasional symptoms becoming more frequent
- Is colicky and usually referred to the right lower quadrant
- Occurs at any time and may wake individuals from sleep
- Fever is unusual but can occur and there may be leucocytosis
- There may be abdominal distension, vomiting, anorexia and decreased defecation
- Typically there is a diffuse right lower quadrant tenderness with a palpable mass
- Abdominal X-ray characteristically shows a 'foamy' gas pattern in the right flank.

Management

- Correct dehydration using intravenous fluids if necessary
- Consider surgical review by an experienced paediatric surgeon
- Mild cases might respond to oral lactulose

- More severe cases can be relieved with oral Gastrograffin (see Chapter 24)
- If there is no response to the above use a balanced intestinal lavage solution (GoLytely) (see Chapter 24). This usually requires a nasogastric tube for administration
- Those unable to tolerate oral intake because of vomiting will require a Gastrograffin enema under X-ray screening and/or irrigation via colonoscopy.

Recurrences of DIOS are common. Advise:

- Adequate hydration
- Adequate PERT
- Laxatives such as senna and lactulose can be helpful for chronic cases
- Consider daily oral N-acetylcysteine for relapsing cases (see Chapter 24)
- Proton pump inhibitors can be of benefit in some cases.

CONSTIPATION

Recurrent abdominal pain despite adequate PERT to correct malabsorption is often due to constipation. In one retrospective case notes review (Rubinstein, Moss & Lewiston 1986) 32% had experienced at least one episode of constipation. DIOS occurred in 9% of individuals and was more common in those with a history of constipation.

Relevant factors

- Energy-dense diets tend to have a low fibre content (Gavin & Connett 1997)
- Inadequately controlled steatorrhoea
- Poor fluid intake
- Viscid intestinal secretions
- Large bowel dysmotility
- Peri-anal pathology.

Assessment

Particular note should be made of stool frequency, pain (location, duration and severity) and stool consistency. Stools are often soft and abdominal symptoms are relieved by defecation. Faecal masses are usually impalpable. Abdominal X-rays often reveal colonic faecal loading in unaffected CF individuals but this can be gross when constipated. Constipation can occur even with a daily bowel action if there is incomplete emptying of the colon.

Consider the possibility that peri-anal pathology has triggered initial stool withholding (e.g. prolapse, local inflammation secondary to antibiotic induced diarrhoea, or excessive enzyme usage, peri-anal Group A streptococcal infection, anal fissures and threadworm infection).

Management

- Get the diagnosis right. In difficult cases transit studies can be helpful.
- Address identifiable risk factors.
- Encourage generous fluids, fibre and regular toileting.
- Keep laxative regimes simple. Lactulose as a softener and senna to promote emptying are usually effective either separately or together.

It is important, if the regime is effective, to continue for several weeks or months.

- Consider co-existing DIOS necessitating more intensive treatment (see above).

GASTRO-OESOPHAGEAL REFLUX (Beattie 2001)

Gastro-oesophageal reflux represents a considerable disease spectrum ranging from mild to life-threatening disease. Gastro-oesophageal reflux disease (GERD) implies significant morbidity. Individuals with reflux symptoms require investigation and consideration of the differential diagnosis. Individuals with CF are particularly prone to reflux and in particular during early childhood (Heine 1998). Severe complications can occur with few or no obvious symptoms. Although it is often difficult to confirm reflux aspiration, it is now widely accepted that GERD can contribute significantly to progressive lung damage.

Mechanisms include

- High volume feeds
- Delayed gastric emptying
- Inappropriate relaxation of the lower oesophageal sphincter
- A flattened diaphragm altering the gastro-oesophageal junction
- Increased acid production and possibly abnormal stomach motility
- Respiratory exacerbations: raised intra-abdominal pressure during coughing bouts
- Physiotherapy: postural drainage positions may exacerbate reflux in some children.

Indications for investigation

Mild reflux is common. It rarely requires specific investigation and is a clinical diagnosis.

Children who require further investigation include those with:

- Symptoms attributable to reflux not responsive to simple treatment strategies
- Poorly controlled respiratory disease where reflux may be a factor.

Investigations

No test directly connects pulmonary disease to reflux. A therapeutic trial of acid suppression with proton pump inhibitors over a period of 2–3 months can be useful.

Barium radiology

This is not sensitive or specific for reflux but will rule out an anatomical cause for vomiting such as a large hiatus hernia, oesophageal stricture or web, atypical pyloric stenosis, gastric web, duodenal web, malrotation and volvulus.

pH study

The pH study is considered by many to be the gold standard. Its advantages are the ability to quantify reflux over a period of time and establish temporal relationships with atypical symptoms and events such as apnoea. There is a standard protocol for the methodology and interpretation of pH

Figure 6.3 pH study showing severe post prandial reflux in a 6-month-old infant with CF – arrows indicate feed times.

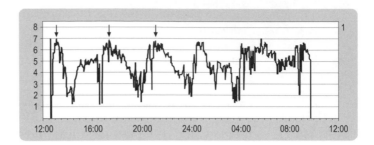

studies (Vandenplas et al 1992). Anti-reflux medication must be stopped four days prior to the procedure. An event marker can be used for position, sleep, feeds and symptoms. Reflux episodes occur when the pH falls below 4.

The reflux index is the time pH is less than 4(%):

- 5–10% = mild reflux
- 10–20% = moderate reflux which is usually controlled by medical therapy
- 30% plus = severe and often requires surgical intervention.

Indications for a pH study:

- Gastro-oesphageal reflux where there is diagnostic uncertainty or no response to treatment
- If surgery is being considered
- Suspicion of occult reflux
- Unexplained or difficult to control respiratory disease
- Unexplained apnoea.

Children with simple reflux do not require a pH study.

Reproducibility is a concern. If the result is not as expected, the study may need to be repeated.

Nuclear medicine: milk scan

This uses continuous evaluation after a radiolabeled meal. It is independent of pH and can detect alkaline reflux. It is performed over a period of up to an hour with a delayed (24-hour) film to look for aspiration. The technique is particularly useful to diagnose non-acid reflux. It also assesses gastric emptying.

Oesophagoscopy and oesophageal biopsy

When oesophagitis is suspected, upper GI endoscopy is a useful investigation and is mandatory for severe symptomatic reflux. There is poor correlation between endoscopic appearances and histology and so biopsies should always be taken.

Management

General measures

- Explanation and reassurance
- Positioning
- Avoid large meals and food 1–2 hours before going to bed
- Avoid tea, coffee and gaseous drinks
- Elevate head of bed
- Avoid head down positioning during physiotherapy.

Some cases of reflux can occur as a result of cow's milk protein intolerance. A trial of cow's milk avoidance over a defined period and under dietetic supervision should be considered.

Medication (Cucchiara et al 2000, Mazur et al 2000)

Antacids   Antacids such as Gaviscon are effective treatment of symptomatic GERD. In infants Gaviscon can be added to feeds and the liquid suspension or tablets used in older children.

Acid suppression
- Proton pump inhibitors e.g. omeprazole, lansoprazole
- H2 blockers e.g. ranitidine.

Children with proven oesophagitis or severe symptomatic GER confirmed by investigation are more effectively treated with proton pump inhibitors. Omeprazole is most frequently used in children. It is available in tablet or capsule formulations that can be crushed or broken. Lansoprazole can also be used and is available as a suspension.

H2 receptor antagonists can be used to treat mild symptomatic reflux. Ranitidine is safe and well tolerated.

Prokinetics   These increase lower oesophageal sphincter pressure, improve oesophageal clearance and aid gastric emptying. Metoclopramide is an effective dopamine antagonist but not widely used because of concerns about extrapyramidal side effects. Domperidone has a much better side effect profile but is also a dopamine antagonist.

Cisapride is an effective treatment but has been withdrawn because of concerns about cardiotoxicity. It can be obtained on a named patient basis.

Surgery   This is rarely required although carefully selected patients may benefit. Significant post-operative complications include bloating, abdominal pain, dysphagia and retching. Ongoing respiratory disease can exacerbate these problems.

RECURRENT ABDOMINAL PAIN

Recurrent abdominal pain is common and affects up to 10% of school-aged children. It occurs more frequently in those with chronic diseases including CF. It is more common in girls and there is often a family history. Pain is usually peri-umbilical and rarely associated with other GI symptoms such as diarrhoea, rectal bleeding or weight loss.

Non-organic or 'functional' abdominal pain usually occurs in children aged older than 5 years with peaks at 8–9 years and around senior school entry. Pain is usually of gradual onset, variable severity (with symptom-free periods), peri-umbilical (although not always), lasts 1–3 hours and unclear in nature so that children find it difficult to describe. The pain rarely causes a child to wake from sleep; this would suggest more sinister pathology. It is not usually related to meals, activity or bowel movement. Loose diagnostic criteria are 3 or more significant episodes that impact on a child's functioning during 3 months. The pain can become a very significant issue, particularly if it interferes with school attendance.

Extra-intestinal symptoms such as headaches are common. There is often a positive family illness history. The child is often offered positive reinforcement for symptoms. Examination and investigations are all normal.

Functional abdominal pain is associated with:

- Timid, nervous, anxious characters
- Perfectionists – over-achievers
- Increased number of stresses and more likely to internalize problems than other children
- School absence
- Positive family history.

Management

- Remember that the pain is real to the child, not psychogenic or imaginary.
- The child should be supported with avoidance of environmental reinforcement.
- The goal of management cannot be total freedom from pain.
- Associated symptoms should be reviewed and dietary triggers avoided.
- Lifestyle issues such as school attendance and exercise should be addressed.
- A diary of symptoms is occasionally useful in severe cases enabling the child to focus on more severe episodes of pain and how to deal with them.

There are many social and psychological factors impacting on children with chronic disease and a reduced life expectancy. There are likely to be difficult issues during adolescence when the normal transition from dependency to full autonomy will be inhibited by CF complications and their management. A number of children with recurrent abdominal pain will develop migraine or recurrent tension headaches as adults.

Abdominal migraine

A small group of children with abdominal pain have a clustering of symptoms often associated with nausea, headache, photophobia and tiredness. Some will be helped by migraine prophylaxis.

Functional dyspepsia

This phenotype is increasingly recognized in adults who have epigastric discomfort after meals with no underlying disease process. Functional dyspepsia is often associated with poor diet and inactivity. Lifestyle measures and antacid treatment usually suffice.

Irritable bowel syndrome

This is an umbrella term relevant to all of the above. Irritable bowel syndrome is common in adults and increasingly recognised in children. It can be associated with diarrhoea or constipation. Laxatives can alleviate constipation. Antispasmodics are not generally helpful and lifestyle measures such as diet and exercise are usually the most helpful.

SHORT BOWEL SYNDROME

This is intestinal failure secondary to massive resection for conditions such as necrotising enterocolitis, volvulus and gut atresia. Management should be in conjunction with a paediatric gastroenterologist.

Management

- Maintain normal growth and development
- Promote intestinal adaptation
- Prevent complications
- Establish enteral nutrition
- Total parenteral nutrition.

Factors that influence outcome

- Ileum adapts better than jejunum
- Better prognosis if ileo-caecal valve present
- Better outcome if colon present
- Co-existent disease e.g. enteropathy
- Presence of liver disease is an adverse risk factor.

Outcome

Less than 40 cm of small bowel is usually associated with the need for long term nutritional support. Bowel lengthening procedures and small bowel transplantation are options to consider with an appropriate specialist unit.

BACTERIAL OVERGROWTH

This diagnosis should be considered in individuals with risk factors such as previous gastrointestinal surgery and short bowel syndrome. Repeated courses of antibiotics are also a risk factor. Stasis causes bacterial proliferation and the emergence of resistant strains causing fat and fat-soluble vitamin malabsorption.

Hydrogen breath testing might be useful. Radioisotope labelled breath testing may also have a role. Barium studies are indicated if obstruction is suspected.

Treatment involves appropriate management of the underlying cause. Metronidazole is effective orally. Probiotics have also been used.

GIARDIASIS

Giardia is a protozoal parasite found in contaminated food and water. Clinical manifestations vary. Individuals may be asymptomatic, have acute diarrhoeal disease or chronic diarrhoea. Partial villous atrophy is occasionally seen. Diagnosis is made by stool examination for cysts or examination of the duodenal aspirate at small bowel biopsy. Treatment is with metronidazole and is often given empirically in suspicious cases.

CLOSTRIDIUM DIFFICILE INFECTION

Clostridium difficile and/or clostridium toxin is commonly found in the stools of well CF individuals. Pseudomembranous colitis with fever and bloody diarrhoea is rare despite intense antibiotic exposure. Treatment of symptomatic disease is with oral vancomycin and oral or intravenous metronidazole.

PEPTIC ULCERATION

This is uncommon despite a low duodenal pH. The routine use of oral antibiotics, H2 antagonists and proton pump inhibitors might result in lower rates of infection with *Helicobacter pylori* in individuals with CF.

If there are symptoms of dyspepsia, question the family about the use of non-steroidal anti-inflammatory drugs (NSAIDs). Some individuals might self medicate with NSAIDs because of data suggesting they have useful anti-inflammatory properties to treat CF-related lung disease.

COELIAC DISEASE

Due to the increased prevalence of coeliac disease in the general population any individual with poor growth or persistent gastrointestinal symptoms should have their coeliac serology checked.

INTUSSUSCEPTION
(See Chapter 17)

This occurs more frequently in CF and later than in the general population. It is usually ileo-colonic. The lead point is usually the terminal ileum or proximal caecum. Intussusception can mimic the findings of DIOS (Holmes 1991). Occasionally surgery will be required particularly if diagnosis is delayed, but conservative treatment using either air or gastro-graffin enema under radiological control is usually successful.

APPENDICITIS
(See Chapter 17)

Appendicitis can mimic DIOS. Symptoms of appendicitis may be masked or modified (Coughlin 1990).

FIBROSING COLONOPATHY

Fibrosing colonopathy (FC) was first described in 1994. Five children with strictures of the ascending colon were reported from Liverpool (Smyth 1994). All had presented with symptoms suggesting DIOS but had not responded to conventional treatment. Strictures were characterised by marked sub-mucosal fibrosis, intraluminal narrowing and little or no inflammation. Subsequent epidemiological data suggested that FC was related to the ingested dose of methacrylic acid copolymer coating (Eudragit) used in pancreatic enzymes given to children at that time (Smyth 1995, Prescott & Bakowski 1999). Fibrosing colonopathy was particularly associated with the recent ingestion of large doses of high strength enzymes coated with Eudragit.

No FC cases have been reported in individuals receiving non-Eudragit-containing PERT including the high strength enzyme preparations Creon 25,00 and Creon 40,000 despite these accounting for over 97% of the UK market (Bakowski 1999).

There are two reports of FC in adults; a 25-year old female with CF (Hausler 1998) and a 66-year-old female without CF (Bansi 2000). The latter patient had received high doses of methacrylic acid copolymer-coated enzymes following a pancreatoduodenectomy and tested negative for the CF gene. Although new cases of fibrosing colonopathy are now exceedingly rare in the UK there have been 42 cases reported worldwide between 1994–2000; one in Germany, four in the UK, and 37 in the US. All four UK cases had been treated with low-strength methacrylic acid copolymer-coated enzymes. Any suspected cases of FC should be referred to the specialist centre.

ORAL PATHOLOGY
Salivary glands – sialolithiasis

Rare cases of salivary gland stones are probably caused by the high calcium content of saliva. The salivary glands are slightly enlarged in most CF individuals. This usually causes no problems. Salivary amylase and lipase might usefully contribute to digestion.

Aphthous ulcers

Aphthous ulcers can result from chewing enzyme granules, disrupting the enteric coating and thus releasing active enzymes.

Oral candidiasis

Use of inhaled corticosteroids and disruption of the normal oral flora with antibiotics can result in overgrowth of candida. Asking individuals to rinse their mouth after corticosteroid inhalation and judicious use of topical antifungals can help to prevent this.

Dental decay

A high sugar diet and syrup formulations containing sugar can increase the risk of tooth decay. Good dental hygiene and fluoride supplements (in areas where the water supply is not supplemented) are recommended.

References

Bakowski M 1999 Pancreatic enzymes and fibrosing colonopathy. Letter. Lancet 354:249

Bansi D S, Price A, Russell C et al 2000 Fibrosing colonopathy in an adult owing to over use of pancreatic enzyme supplements. Gut 46:283–285

Beattie R M 2001 Diagnosis and management of gastro-oesophageal reflux. Current Paediatrics 11(4):269–275

Coughlin J P, Gaurderer M W, Stern R C et al 1990 The spectrum of appendiceal disease in CF. Journal Paediatric Surgery 25(8):835–839

Cucchiara S, Franco M T, Terrin G et al 2000 Role of drug therapy in the treatment of gastro-oesophageal reflux disorder in children. Paediatric Drugs 2(4):265–272

Gavin J, Connett G J 1997 Dietary fibre and the occurrence of gut symptoms. Archives of Diseases in Childhood 76:35–37

Hausler M, Meilicke R, Biesterfeld S et al 1998 Brief case reports. First adult patient with fibrosing colonopathy. American Journal of Gastroenterology 93:1171–1172

Heine R G, Button B M, Olinsky A et al 1998 Gastro-oesophageal reflux in infants under 6 months with CF. Archives of Diseases in Childhood 78(1):44–48

Holmes M, Murphy V, Taylor M et al 1991 Intussusception in CF. Archives of Diseases in Childhood 66(6):726–727

Littlewood J 1992 CF: gastrointestinal complications. British Medical Bulletin 48(4):847–859

Mazur L J, Baker R D, Boyle J T et al 2000 Gastro-oesophageal reflux. In: Moyer V A (ed) Evidence based child health. BMJ books

Prescott P, Bakowski M T 1999 Pathogenesis of fibrosing colonopathy: the role of methacrylic acid copolymer. Pharmacoepidemiol Drug Safety 8:377–384

Rubinstein S, Moss R, Lewiston N 1986 Constipation and meconium ileus equivalent in patients with CF. Pediatrics 78(3):473–479

Smyth R L, van Velzen D, Smyth A R et al 1994 Strictures of ascending colon in CF and high-strength pancreatic enzymes. Lancet 343:85–86

Smyth R, Ashby D, O'Hea U et al 1995 Fibrosing colonopathy in CF: results of a case controlled study. Lancet 346:1247–1251

Vandenplas Y, Belli D, Boige N et al 1992 A standardized protocol for the methodology of esophageal pH monitoring and interpretation of the data for the diagnosis of gastro-oesophageal reflux. ESPGHAN society statement. Journal of Pediatric Gastroenterology and Nutrition 14:467–471

Recommended reading

Wyllie R, Hyams J S (eds) 1999 Paediatric gastrointestinal disease, 2nd edn. W B Saunders

Rothbaum R J 1999 Gastrointestinal and hepatobiliary problems in CF. Recent Advances in Paediatrics David TJ (editor) 17th edn

Chapter 7

Nutritional care

Joan Gavin

INTRODUCTION

Nutritional requirements in CF depend on

- Age
- Sex
- Efficacy of digestion and absorption
- Respiratory status
- Activity levels.

Improved nutrition benefits growth, respiratory muscle strength and immunological status. There is good evidence that poor nutrition is associated with more frequent exacerbations of respiratory illness (Durie & Pencharz 1989).

The main objectives of nutritional care are:

- Monitor nutritional status at each clinic visit
- Encourage a regular intake of energy dense meals and snacks with a generous salt intake to meet estimated requirements
- Advise on vitamin and mineral supplements
- Advise on the titration of pancreatic enzyme replacement therapy to minimise stool energy losses
- Encourage a positive attitude to eating and mealtimes
- Advise on nutritional supplements or enteral tube feeding when normal foods cannot meet estimated energy requirements.

Table 7.1 Estimated average requirement (EAR) for energy (Department of Health 1992).

Age	EAR Kcal/d (MJ/d)			
	Males		Females	
0–3 months	545	(2.28)	515	(2.16)
4–6 months	690	(2.89)	645	(2.69)
7–9 months	825	(3.44)	765	(3.20)
10–12 months	920	(3.85)	865	(3.61)
1–3 years	1,230	(5.15)	1,165	(4.86)
4–6 years	1,715	(7.16)	1,545	(6.46)
7–10 years	1,970	(8.24)	1,740	(7.28)
11–14 years	2,220	(9.27)	1,845	(7.92)
15–18 years	2,755	(11.51)	2,110	(8.83)
19–50 years	2,550	(10.60)	1,940	(8.10)
51–59 years	2,550	(10.60)	1,900	(8.00)
60–64 years	2,380	(9.93)	1,900	(7.99)
65–74 years	2,330	(9.71)	1,900	(7.96)
75+ years	2,100	(8.77)	1,810	(7.16)

NUTRITIONAL REQUIREMENTS

Energy

The energy requirements of individuals with CF can be increased by uncontrolled maldigestion and malabsorption despite optimal pancreatic enzyme replacement therapy (PERT). Stool losses can be up to three times the upper limit of normal and cause sufficient energy loss to limit growth (Murphy 1991). Catabolic lung inflammation caused by infection and the increased work of breathing to overcome airways obstruction can increase the basal metabolic rate by 30% (Levison & Cherniak 1968). As a result the energy requirements can be up to 120–150% of Estimated Average Requirement (EAR) for energy although many children will grow normally by consuming just 100% of their energy requirements (Table 7.1). An equation has been developed incorporating these factors to estimate energy requirements specifically for CF (Ramsey 1992) (see Chapter 8).

Estimates of actual energy intake can be made using a five-day weighed or non-weighed food diary and analysing the data using a nutritional computer package such as 'Compeat' (Nutritional Systems Ltd, London, UK) or 'Microdiet' (Salford University, UK).

The most practical way to assess the adequacy of energy intake at routine clinic visits is to monitor weight gain and growth.

Ways to implement a higher energy intake from food

- Increase the intake of full fat milk, cheese and yoghurts; cheese can be added to savoury dishes such as casseroles, stews, baked beans and mashed potatoes.
- Increase intake of full fat polyunsaturated or monounsaturated margarines by adding to a variety of savoury foods such as mash and vegetables.
- Increase the use of polyunsaturated and monounsaturated oils; fry foods such as sausages, bacon, eggs, and fry foods more frequently than grilling.

- Increase intake of higher calorie puddings such as crumble, custard and ice cream.
- Restrict consumption of squash (including fizzy) especially before mealtimes as sugar laden drinks can reduce appetite for whole foods.
- Eat regularly and include high energy snacks such as biscuits and cake provided they do not compromise intake at mealtimes.

Recommendation

It is recommended that the high energy CF diet contains:

- 35–40% calories from fat
- 10–15% calories from protein
- 45–50% calories from carbohydrate.

Fat

Due to the increasing life expectancy of individuals with CF, it is important to consider the type of fat recommended. Monounsaturated and polyunsaturated fats such as sunflower, olive oil and margarines are not only more efficiently absorbed (Jones, Pencharz & Clandinin 1985) but are also advised for prevention of heart disease in the general population. It therefore seems prudent to encourage these types of fat in the CF diet.

The fat soluble vitamins

Due to fat maldigestion and malabsorption, individuals are at risk of deficiency of these vitamins. Low vitamin levels have been associated with compromised clinical status (Rayner 1989) and reduced lung function (Carr & Dinwiddie 1996). Routine supplementation of Vitamins A, D and E in the amounts recommended below should help prevent these problems. Fat soluble vitamin supplements should be taken with PERT to maximise digestion and absorption. A convenient time is often at breakfast.

Vitamin A

Vitamin A deficiency

This is associated with night blindness (Rayner 1989), xerophthalmia, and dry thickened skin but these symptoms are now rarely seen in the UK. Plasma Vitamin A (retinol) is reduced during acute infection (Duggan 1996) and should be measured when individuals are clinically stable. Unfortunately plasma retinol concentrations are now regarded as insensitive indicators of Vitamin A status. Low levels might occur despite high body stores as a result of liver accumulation (Eid, Shoemaker & Samiec 1990). Low plasma Vitamin A levels might reflect low retinol binding protein levels or poor mobilisation from liver stores, especially in malnourished individuals. In the absence of a reliable indicator of status, plasma Vitamin A results should be interpreted with caution.

Excess vitamin A

Prolonged excessive Vitamin A intake has been associated with hepatic damage (Eid, Shoemaker & Samiec 1990). Whilst currently recommended doses might be in excess of body requirements further evidence is necessary before changes to current practice can be recommended.

Table 7.2 Vitamin A supplementation (current UK recommendations).

Age	Dose
<6 weeks	600 ug (2000 iu)
6 weeks to 6 months	1200 ug (4000 iu)
>6 months-adult	2400 ug (8000 iu)

Note: Recommendations might change in the future.

Table 7.3 Recommended formulations of Vitamin A supplementation.

Vitamin A+D BPC capsules	1 capsule = 4,000 iu
Halibut Cold Liver Oil capsules	1 capsule = 4,000 iu
Dalivit	1.2 ml = 8,000 iu

Note: Ketovite and Abidec do not contain an appropriate dose of Vitamin A.

Normal plasma levels of Vitamin A are 1–4.2 μmol/litre. Table 7.2 shows current UK recommendations for supplementation, and Table 7.3 shows recommended formulations of Vitamin A supplements.

Dietary sources of Vitamin A to be encouraged

- Dairy products
- Butter
- Margarine
- Egg yolk
- Liver
- Oily fish
- Oranges
- Yellow coloured fruit and vegetables.

Vitamin D

Vitamin D deficiency

The majority of Vitamin D is synthesised in the skin through sunlight but reduced plasma levels of 25-hydroxyvitamin D have been described in some studies (Congden 1981, Durie & Pencharz 1989). Osteopenia and osteoporosis have been increasingly recognised in children and adults with CF (Bachrach, Loutit & Moss 1994, Haworth 1999). Reduced bone mineralisation appears to correlate with poor nutritional status, chronic lung infection, poor calcium intake, corticosteroid use and limited exercise. See Chapter 14 for investigations and treatment of individuals at risk of deficiency. Plasma 25-hydroxyvitamin D gives a good indication of status but there are seasonal variations in levels and these should be taken into consideration when interpreting results (Reiter 1985, Wolfe, Conway & Brownlee 2001).

Excess Vitamin D

Excess Vitamin D intake can cause hypercalcaemia in infancy (Martin, Snodgrass & Cohen 1984) and nephrocalcinosis in adults but toxicity has not been reported in CF.

Normal plasma levels of Vitamin D are 4–40 μmol/litre. Aim to achieve levels at the high end of the normal range. Table 7.4 shows current UK

Table 7.4 Vitamin D supplementation (current UK recommendation).

Age	Dose
<6 weeks	5 ug (200 iu)
6 weeks to 6 months	10 ug (400 iu)
>6 months to adult	20 ug (800 iu)

Table 7.5 Available formulations of Vitamin D.

Vitamin A+D BPC capsules	1 capsule = 400 iu
Halibut Cold Liver Oil capsules	1 capsule = 400 iu
Dalivit	1.2 ml = 800 iu

Table 7.6 Vitamin E supplementation (current UK recommendation).

Age	Dose
<12 months	50 mg
1–10 years	100 mg
>10 years	200 mg

Table 7.7 Available formulations of Vitamin E.

Alpha-tocopherol acetate chewable tablets	100 mg tablets
Alpha-tocopherol acetate capsules	50 mg/200 mg
Vitamin E suspension	5 ml = 500 mg

recommendations for supplementation, and Table 7.5 shows recommended formulations of Vitamin D supplements.

Dietary sources of Vitamin D to be encouraged

- Egg
- Margarine
- Evaporated milk
- Oily fish
- Liver.

Vitamin E

Vitamin E deficiency

Vitamin E deficiency is associated with neurological impairment. A variety of clinical features have been described including loss of reflexes (Bye 1985), tremor, ataxia and ophthalmoplegia. Plasma levels of Vitamin E represent only a small proportion of the vitamin in the body and might not accurately reflect status. Red blood cell Vitamin E levels are more indicative of long-term treatment and thus adherence to prescribed doses (Peters & Rolles 1993).

Excess Vitamin E

There is no clear evidence that Vitamin E is toxic even when taken in doses far in excess of physiological requirements.

Normal red blood cell levels of Vitamin E are 4.41–8.13 μmols/litre. Normal plasma levels of Vitamin E are 11.6–37.1 μmols/litre. Table 7.6 shows current UK recommendations for supplementation, and Table 7.7 shows recommended formulations of Vitamin E supplements.

Water miscible preparations of Vitamin E are more efficiently absorbed than fat soluble Vitamin E preparations, but are less readily available (Peters & Kelly 1996).

Dietary sources of Vitamin E to be encouraged

- Margarine
- Butter
- Vegetable oils
- Wheat products.

Vitamin K

Vitamin K deficiency

Vitamin K is necessary for the manufacture of clotting factors in the liver. Marked deficiency is manifest by a bleeding tendency and prolonged pro-thrombin time (INR). However the INR is rarely abnormal in CF (Durie 1994, Rashid 1999). Recent studies suggest that a sub-clinical deficiency exists in the majority of pancreatic insufficient individuals. This is even more likely in those with liver disease, see Chapter 12 (Wilson 2001). Vitamin K might also be of importance in preventing osteoporosis, see Chapter 14. Further studies are needed to establish a suitable dose of Vitamin K to correct deficiency.

Vitamin K supplementation

The water soluble preparation (Phytomenadione) is recommended at a standard dose of 10 mg daily (for children and adults). One tablet of mena-diol phosphate provides this.

Water soluble vitamins

Deficiency of water soluble vitamins is rare (Peters & Kelly 1993) although riboflavin deficiency has recently been described (McCabe 2001). Regular dietary assessment should prevent deficiencies.

Trace elements

High energy diets should not be recommended without considering the intake of other food groups such as fruit and vegetables. Micronutrients from a wide range of foods are important to ensure efficient metabolism of high fat foods, and play a role in stimulating appetite. Monitoring of nutritional status should include measurements of trace element plasma levels. Suitable multivitamin and mineral supplements should be used when deficiencies are detected (e.g. Forceval Junior or Sanatogen Gold).

Fibre

Individuals with CF consume less than half the fibre intake of non-CF age-matched controls (Gavin, Ellis & Dewar 1997) and those with the lowest fibre intake tend to have the lowest energy intake. Increasing dietary fibre might further compromise total energy intake whilst having no significant benefit to colonic function. This is because the role of dietary fibre appears to be partly simulated by large quantities of maldigested and malabsorbed nutrients, despite PERT, that pass through to the CF colon (Gavin 2000). Stool softeners and stimulant laxatives should be used to treat constipation rather than increasing fibre intake beyond normal amounts.

Table 7.8 Recommendation for sodium supplementation.

Age	Dose
0 to 1 year	2 mmol/kg (NaCl solution)
1 to 5 years	600 mg od (10 mmol Na) tablets
6 to 10 years	600 mg bd (20 mmol Na) tablets
11 years +	600 mg tds-qds (30–40 mmol Na) tablets

Sodium

Urinary sodium measurements usefully indicate salt balance. Salt loss in sweat is excessive in CF but UK individuals do not require routine sodium supplements. In infants with faltering growth, a sodium supplement of 1–2 mmol/kg/day added to breast or formula feed has been shown to improve weight gain without the addition of energy supplements (MacDonald 1996). During hot weather, increased sweating and therefore increased salt loss can result in negative salt balance with associated leg cramps, anorexia and vomiting. In such circumstances supplements should be given according to the doses shown in Table 7.8 (MacDonald 1996). Many people use low salt substitutes in cooking and at the table but as these contain potassium rather than sodium chloride. Individuals with CF should be advised to avoid these and to use regular table salt.

One tablet of Slow Sodium contains 600 mg of sodium.

PANCREATIC ENZYME REPLACEMENT THERAPY (PERT)

Enteric coated microsphere enzyme preparations have revolutionised nutritional management in CF and supplanted their non enteric coated predecessors. The enteric coated microspheres or minimicrospheres are contained within a gelatine capsule. When swallowed whole the gelatine capsule dissolves in the stomach. The enteric coating remains intact until the intraluminal pH is alkaline within the small bowel and the enzymes are then released. Children should be encouraged to swallow enzyme capsules whole so that the gelatine capsule is of benefit. This can be achieved by learning to swallow an empty capsule first. With encouragement many children can do this by 2–3 years of age. If infants or younger children cannot swallow whole capsules they can be opened and the enteric coated contents taken directly into the mouth or mixed with yoghurt or fruit puree. They must not be chewed. Enzymes should never be sprinkled onto food. They might be activated before ingestion and thus be less effective in the duodenum. Enzymes should generally be taken throughout a meal for maximum effect but taking them before food is often more practical.

Indication

Pancreatic enzyme replacement therapy should only be introduced when there is growth failure and symptoms of pancreatic insufficiency confirmed by direct microscopy for fat globules (Walters 1990) and measurement of faecal elastase. Concentrations of less than 200 mcg elastase per gram of stool are indicative of pancreatic insufficiency (Cade 2000). All pancreatic insufficient individuals should be commenced on low strength enzyme preparations. High strength preparations should only be considered as an

Table 7.9 Types of pancreatic enzyme replacement therapy available.

Product (Manufacturer)	Composition (Per Capsule/Tablet/) BP Units		
	Lipase	Protease	Amylase
Enteric coated microspheres			
Pancrease (Janssen Cilag)	5000	350	3000
Nutrizym GR (Merck)	10000	650	10000
Enteric coated minimicrospheres			
Creon 5000 (Solvay) #	5000	3600	200
Creon 10000 (Solvay)	10000	600	8000
Creon 25000 (Solvay)	25000	1000	18000
Creon 40000 (Solvay)	40000	25000	1600
Enteric coated microtablets			
Pancrease HL (Cilag)	25000	1250	22500
Nutrizym 10 (Merck)	10000	500	9000
Nutrizym 22 (Merck)	25000	1100	19800
Cotazym S (Organo)	8000	30000	30000

* There is a powdered enzyme preparation available i.e. Pancrex V but it is thought to be less effective due to lack of protection from the acidic environment in the stomach and are therefore not generally recommended.
# Creon 5000 presentation is in a tub with scoop attached: 1 scoop = 5000 lipase units.

alternative when large numbers of capsules are necessary to correct malabsorption. Enzymes should be taken with all food and drink except:

- Fruit juice
- Fruit cordials
- Water
- Boiled sweets
- Fresh fruit
- Fizzy drinks.

Remember

A small percentage of CF individuals are pancreatic sufficient and some have a gradual decline in pancreatic function after birth. Enzyme preparations should only be introduced after obtaining evidence for pancreatic failure.

Table 7.9 shows the types of pancreatic enzyme replacement therapy available.

Dosage As dietary fat is almost completely dependent on pancreatic lipase for its digestion, it is sensible to educate the individual and their families about the quantity of enzyme capsules that might be required to digest low, medium and high fat foods. Although studies suggest that on average 2000 units lipase are required to digest every 1g fat (Constantini 1998) (Borrowitz 1995), such prescriptive practice is unjustified because of the large inter-individual variability in digestion and absorption of fat (Murphy 1991). Such practices might result in individuals becoming obsessed with food intake whilst achieving no difference in stool fat output compared to more liberal methods. It is preferable for people to learn to monitor stool output and self titrate enzyme dose as a result of personal experience, within sensible limits set by the dietitian. To encourage self reporting of bowel symptoms and stool output accurately a symptom diary or questionnaire can be used.

The use of high doses of Eudragit containing lipase preparations has been associated with the development of colonic strictures (Smyth 1995, Freiman & Fitzsimmons 1996). As a result, the Committee on Safety of Medicines recommends that 'Pancrease HL and Nutrizym 22 should not be given to children aged <15 years'. Because of the confounding association with high strength preparations it was recommended that 'the total dose of pancreatic enzymes should not usually exceed 10,000 units lipase/kg body weight daily'.

Most children require less than 10,000 units lipase/kg/day to correct pancreatic insufficiency. In practice it is impossible to accurately estimate an individual's lipase intake because the stated capsule dose is actually a minimum of capsule content at the end of shelf life. This is because capsules are overfilled to compensate for enzyme degradation during storage (e.g. Creon 25,000 capsule contains 40,000 lipase units at manufacture and 25,000 at end of shelf life). The amount of overfill is different between enzyme preparations making it difficult to compare lipase doses when changing from one product to another.

Containing enzyme dosage is impractical in a small number of children requiring more than 10,000 units lipase/kg/day to correct pancreatic insufficiency. Attempting to do this will result in enzyme driven diets whereby daily energy intake is constrained to the total number of enzymes allowed or displacement of normal diet with elemental supplements not requiring pancreatic enzymes. A less prescriptive policy of using 'the smallest enzyme dose to control steatorrhoea and achieve a normal pattern of growth and weight gain' (Littlewood & Wolfe 2000) without the strict imposition of an absolute dose limit is far more appropriate.

Because of enzyme degradation it is important that emergency supplies of enzyme capsules kept in the car or at a neighbour's house are regularly checked for use-by date. Enzymes consumed after this date or kept in hot temperatures are less effective and can result in maldigestion when consumed. Always advise that pancreatic enzyme capsules are kept at room temperature.

SPECIAL SITUATIONS

Nutritional requirements vary throughout life and each age group presents new challenges to the dietitian.

Feeding infants

Breast feeding

This should be encouraged. Breast milk contains lipase and essential fatty acids.

Formula feeding

Standard infant formulae are recommended unless there has been significant small bowel resection when hydrolysed formulae may be required.

Feeding should aim to achieve 150–200 ml/kg/day or 100–130 Kcal/kg/day. These can be increased to 150–200 Kcal/kg/day if the baby is not gaining weight.

Administration of enzymes to infants

Enteric coated mini-microspheres should be recommended for all infants with clinical findings and biochemical evidence of pancreatic insufficiency.

An initial dose of 1/4 low strength capsule (or 1/2 scoop of Creon 5000) per feed should be offered to infants and increased until maldigestion and malabsorption are controlled e.g. no fat globules on stool microscopy. Increases should be by 1/4–1/2 capsule at a time.

Enzymes should be given irrespective of whether infants use standard or hydrolysed feeds. They should be given directly before a feed and not mixed in the infant's bottle.

After giving enzymes a parent should feel around the gums with their finger to ensure no mini-microspheres are present; they can cause gum irritation.

If infants are receiving continuous feeds give enzymes orally 3–4 hourly. Decrease the dosage if there is peri-anal excoriation.

If stools are persistently fatty (i.e. pale and bulky) despite several increases in enzyme dose, antacid therapy or a proton pump inhibitor should be considered. This should make the duodenum more alkaline and thus maximise enzyme activity at the appropriate place in the GI tract.

If the infant is 'nil by mouth', on TPN or recovering from surgery, it is prudent to give a small dose of enzymes 4 hourly to digest gastro-intestinal mucus secretions thus preventing intestinal obstruction.

High energy supplements might be required if there is poor weight gain. These can be added to the infant formula in proportions recommended by the dietitian (see supplement section).

Weaning

This should follow standard practice for all infants, aiming to wean children at 4–6 months of age (Department of Health 1994). Packaged weaning foods can be reconstituted with infant formula instead of water for extra calories. Fresh pasteurised cows milk should not be introduced until the infant is one year old. It might require a slight increase in enzyme dosage.

Food refusal

Parents should be reassured that food refusal or 'faddy eating' is typical in this age group and not symptomatic of CF. Such behaviour can cause extra stress to parents who are struggling to maintain a high energy intake for their child. Early referral to a psychologist at the specialist CF centre might avoid long-term behavioural feeding problems. The booklet 'Help: my child won't eat' by The Children's Society and Paediatric Group of the BDA provides useful practical advice. The following advice can be helpful:

- The child should be offered small portions of their favourite food and rewarded with praise for cooperation.
- A time limit of 30 minutes should be set for completing each course and any uneaten food removed without comment.
- The family should be encouraged to eat together to provide role models of good eating habits.
- Distractions such as television should be avoided during mealtimes.
- Serve small easily consumable portions – they can always ask for more.
- Avoid excessive fluids before mealtimes.
- Sweet foods should not be used as rewards; this will encourage the child to believe that sweet foods are nicer than savoury.
- Discourage discussion of poor eating behaviour in the presence of the child.

Enzyme refusal   Enzyme doses can be split throughout the meal to ease administration.

If the child is hungry they will be inclined to be irritable and resist enzymes so allow them to eat a few mouthfuls of food before giving enzymes.

Mixing enzymes in honey, syrup, or jam makes them sticky and more difficult to spit out. Stage 1 baby food can also be used to administer enzymes more easily.

The use of positive reinforcement such as a star chart to reward the child for compliance and conversely avoiding anger or signs of stress when the child will not comply is recommended.

Toddlers to teens

Eating disorders are of more concern in older children, especially if the behaviour has become established over several years. It is useful to discuss the problem with parents and the child as he/she might be using food as a form of control over the family. Food diaries can be used to clarify the problem by depicting eating patterns, food likes and dislikes.

Teenagers

Non-compliance in this age group should be anticipated. The adoption of 'healthy eating' trends can be a rebellion against CF and a result of peer pressure. Self consciousness is common and many teenagers resent being different from their peers. They will be aware that it is possible to lose weight through enzyme dose manipulation. In most cases open discussion with parents and teenager about these issues will be sufficient to overcome any problems. True anorexia is a real risk and it is important to detect signs of persistent non-compliance early. Poor nutrition in adolescence can result in irreversible deteriorations in health. Early aggressive nutritional intervention is essential if there is a poor response to simple measures.

Nutritional intervention for the anorexic

- If rapid weight loss has occurred (weight for height <85% or BMI <19) the individual will need admission for overnight tube feeding and eating behaviour therapy from a psychiatric team. Overnight feeds should initially provide half the nutritional requirements gradually increasing to meet all requirements as needed. A gradual increase will prevent oedema from rapid re-feeding.

- Bed rest or exercise restriction should only be implemented when rapid weight loss has occurred.
- Individuals should initially be offered quarter-sized portions at mealtimes.
- The meal should be left with the individual for 30 minutes and then removed without comment.
- Nursing staff and family can offer encouragement to eat at mealtimes but no pressure or force should be used.
- Aims of psychological therapy and target body weight should be discussed with the individual, psychiatrist, dietician and doctor.

Diabetes

See Chapter 11.

Pregnancy

See Chapter 16.

Persistent faltering growth

There are four strategies to pursue when managing continued poor weight gain:

- Ensure maldigestion and malabsorption are controlled (see 'dosage of pancreatic enzymes')
- Maximise calories from the diet
- Provide oral high energy supplements
- Commence enteral feeding via nasogastric or gastrostomy routes.

> **Remember**
>
> - Poor weight gain can also be a result of deterioration in respiratory status. Aggressive treatment of chest disease can improve nutrition.
> - Always consider diabetes as a cause of poor weight gain (see Chapter 11).

SUPPLEMENTS

Table 7.10 shows criteria for different levels of nutritional intervention.

> **Remember**
>
> Irrespective of the reason for admission, never overlook nutrition when patients are hospitalised.

Types of oral high energy supplements

- Calorie powders and emulsions
- Nutritionally fortified high calorie milk shakes and fruit juices
- Glucose drinks.

Calorie powders and emulsions

Calorie powders and emulsions are ideal for mixing with infant formula feeds. There are three types, (see Table 7.11).

Table 7.10 Criteria for different levels of nutritional intervention (UK CF Trust Nutrition Working Group 2002).

	<5 years	5–18 years	>18 years
Normal nutritional state	Weight/height 90–110%	Weight/height 90–110%	BMI 19–25 +/or no recent weight loss
Consider supplements	Weight/height 85–89% OR weight loss over 4 months OR plateau in weight over 6 months	Weight/height 85–89% OR weight loss over 4 months OR plateau in weight over 6 months	BMI <19 OR 5% weight loss over >2 months
Growth failure – aggressive nutritional support	Supplements tried and either weight/height <85% OR weight falling 2 centile positions	Supplements tried and either weight/height <85% OR weight falling 2 centile positions	Supplements tried and either BMI <19 OR >5% weight loss over >2 months

N.B. For all age categories special attention must be given where stunting is evident (defined as height centile <0.4th centile).

Figure 7.1 Oral high energy supplements. A variety of products are available to suit individual preferences.

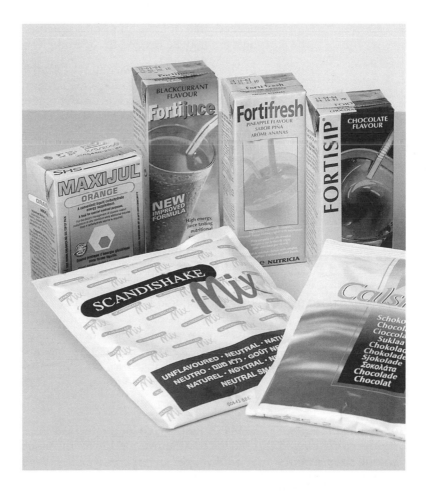

Table 7.11   Calorie powders and emulsions.

Glucose polymers	Maxijul – Scientific Hospital Supplies (SHS)	(380 Kcal/100 g)	132 g/200 g/2.5 kg
	Caloreen – Nestle Clinical Nutrition	(390 Kcal/100 g)	500 g
	Polycal – Nutricia Clinical Care	(380 Kcal/100 g)	400 g
	Polycose – Abbott Nutrition	(376 Kcal/100 g)	350 g
	Vitajoule – Vitaflo	(380 Kcal/100 g)	125 g/200 g/500 g/2.5 kg
Fat and glucose polymer	Duocal – SHS	(492 Kcal/100 g)	400 g
	MCT Duocal – SHS	(497 Kcal/100 g)	400 g
Fat emulsions	Calogen (SHS)	(450 Kcal/100 ml)	250 ml/1 litre
	Liquigen (SHS)	(450 Kcal/100 ml)	250 ml/1 litre
	MCT oil (SHS)	(855 Kcal/100 ml)	500 ml

Recommended dose of calorie powders

Glucose polymer powder should be introduced at 1 g per 100 ml feed and increased in 1 g portions on alternate days (to reduce the risk of osmotic diarrhoea) to a maximum of 5 g per 100 ml feed or to a maximum of 8 g per 100 ml feed for fat and glucose polymers. No extra PERT should be needed after the addition of a glucose polymer to a feed but a slight increase may be needed for fat and glucose polymers.

- The addition of 5 g Maxijul to 100 ml milk equates to 86 Kcal/100 ml.
- The addition of 8 g Duocal to 100 ml milk equates to 100 Kcal/100 ml.
- Normal infants receive on average 67 Kcals/100 ml (depending on formula).

All supplements are prescribable, 'ACBS' listed and the calorie powders are available in 132 g sachets, 200 g tubs, 400 g tubs and 2.5 kg tubs.

High energy infant formulae are now available to provide additional calories in a ready prepared form and are 'ACBS' listed.

- SMA High Energy (SMA Nutrition) – 91 Kcals/100 ml (available in 100 ml bottles/250 ml cartons)
- Infatrini (Nutricia Clinical Care) – 100 Kcals/100 ml (available in 100 ml bottles).

Recommended dosage of fat emulsions

The liquid should be introduced at 1 ml per 100 ml feed and increased by 1 ml on alternate days to a maximum of 3 ml per 100 ml feed. The maximum dose is often used in conjunction with 5 g glucose polymer per 100 ml feed to provide a 1 Kcal/ml feed. Enzymes are required to digest the fat emulsion (commence an extra 1/4–1/2 capsule per 100 ml feed) whether it be Calogen (LCT fat) or Liquigen (MCT) fat.

Monitoring weight gain in infants commencing calorie supplements

- In hospital: weigh alternate days
- In the community: weekly for the first month, fortnightly, then monthly until weight gain is consistent.

Table 7.12   Liquid high energy supplements.

Milkshakes	Fortisip (Nutricia Clinical Care)	(150 Kcal/100 ml) – 200 ml carton
	Fortimel (Nutricia Clinical Care)	(100 Kcal/100 ml) – 200 ml carton
	Ensure/Ensure Plus (Abbott Nutrition)	(100 Kcal/150 Kcal/100 ml) – 250 ml/220 ml carton
	Scandishake (Scientific Hospital Supplies)	(240 Kcal/100 ml) – 85 g sachet (made with milk)
	Calshake (Fresenius Kabi Ltd)	(240 Kcal/100 ml) – 87 g sachet (made with milk)
	Fresubin/Fresubin Energy (Fresenius Kabi Ltd)	(100 Kcal/150 Kcal/100 ml) – 200 ml carton
	Resource Shake (Novartis) Clinutren Iso/	(174 Kcal/100 ml) – 175 ml carton
	Clinutren 1.5	(100 Kcal/150 Kcal/100 ml) – 200 ml (Nestle Nutrition) carton
Paediatric Milkshakes (8–20 kg body weight)	Paediasure/Paediasure Plus (Abbott Nutrition)	(100 Kcal/150 Kcal/100 ml) – 200 ml carton
	Fortini (Nutricia Clinical Care)	(150 Kcal/100 ml) – 200 ml carton
	Frebini Energy (Fresenius Kabi Ltd)	(150 Kcal/100 ml) – 200 ml carton
Yogurt-style drinks	Fortifresh (Nutricia Clinical Care)	(150 Kcal/100 ml) – 200 ml carton
	Ensure Plus yogurt style (Abbott Nutrition)	(150 Kcal/100 ml) – 220 ml carton
Fortified fruit juices	Fortijuice (Nutricia Clinical Care)	(150 Kcal/100 ml) – 200 ml carton
	Provide Xtra (Fresenius Kabi Ltd)	(125 Kcal/100 ml) – 200 ml carton
	Enlive (Abbott Nutrition)	(125 Kcal/100 ml) – 240 ml carton
Glucose drinks	Liquid Maxijul (Scientific Hospital Supplies)	(200 Kcal/100 ml) – 200 ml carton
	Liquid Polycal (Nutricia Clinical Care)	(247 Kcal/100 ml) – 200 ml bottle
	Liquid Duocal (Scientific Hospital Supplies)	(158 Kcal/100 ml) – 250 ml/1 litre
Nutritional powders	Pro-cal (Vitaflo)	(667 Kcal/100 g) – 15 g/510 g/1.5 kg
	Quickcal (Vitaflo)	(780 Kcal/100 g) – 13 g/520 g/1.5 kg

Table 7.13   Recommended dosage of supplements (Macdonald 1996).

1 to 2 years	200 Kcals per day
3 to 5 years	400 Kcals per day
6 to 11 years	600 Kcals per day
>12 years	800 Kcals per day

Nutritionally fortified high calorie milk shakes and fruit juices

These are used to supplement a high energy diet. Products currently available in the UK are listed in Table 7.12. Recommended dosages (MacDonald 1996) are shown in Table 7.13.

Restricting energy contribution from supplements to 1/3–1/4 of total energy requirement helps to ensure individuals with CF do not become dependent on supplements as their main source of calories.

Use of liquid high energy supplements

- Supplements should only be given after meals or before bedtime.
- Supplements must not be used to replace meals.
- Fat-based emulsions e.g. Calogen/Liquigen when given in large quantities e.g. 100 ml per day, might require additional vitamin and mineral supplements such as Sanatogen Gold or Forceval Junior to ensure efficient metabolism of fat.
- Enzymes should be taken with milk-based supplements and other fat containing supplements.

- The dose of enzymes required is generally equivalent to that required for the same volume of full cream milk or foods with a similar fat and protein content.

> **Remember**
>
> High energy liquid supplements are best used as a temporary calorie boost and should be discontinued when appetite returns to prevent dependence on supplements and 'taste fatigue'. Professional dietary advice is required to ensure maximum energy intake from food before supplements are discontinued.

ENTERAL FEEDING

Enteral feeding can be introduced at any age but is most often needed around puberty when diet and supplements alone are insufficient to meet the increased energy requirements that occur at this time. Respiratory status can also deteriorate as a result of poor adherence and this puts an additional stress on the body's ability to gain weight. Correctly used, long-term enteral feeding should achieve good catch-up growth and improvements in lung function (Boland 1986, Steinkamp & Von der Hardt 1994). Indications for starting enteral feeds are listed in Table 7.10.

> **Remember**
>
> Long-term enteral feeding is invasive and places considerable demands on the family. They should be fully informed and assessed as to their ability to meet these demands. Necessary equipment should be obtained and community support arranged. We recommend that feeding is initiated in a hospital setting and the individual only discharged home when confident.

Types of enteral feed available

- Whole protein
- Semi-elemental
- Elemental.

Whole protein

This is the preferred choice. A variety of products are available (Table 7.14).

Advantages of a whole protein feed are its ready-to-feed composition, the fact that it is inexpensive, and its low osmolality. It can be rapidly introduced without risking osmotic diarrhoea. However, intolerance can occur after gastrointestinal surgery and in individuals with milk allergy.

Peptide semi-elemental feed

Peptide semi-elemental feed is a semi-hydrolysed protein formula used in cases of whole protein feed intolerance, e.g. secondary milk protein intolerance or short gut syndrome.

Table 7.14 Whole protein feeds.

Nutrison/Nutrison Energy*	Nutricia Clinical Care	500 ml/1 litre/1500 ml
Fresubin/Fresubin Energy*	Fresenius Kabi Ltd	200 ml/500 ml/1 litre
Osmolite/Osmolite Plus*	Abbott Nutrition	250 ml/500 ml/1 litre/1500 ml
Jevity/Jevity Plus*	Abbott Nutrition	500 ml/1 litre/1500 ml
#Nutrini/Nutrini Energy*	Nutricia Clinical Care	200 ml/500 ml/1000 ml
#Tentrini/Tentrini Energy*	Nutricia Clinical Care	500 ml
#Paediasure/Paediasure Plus*	Abbott Nutrition	250 ml/500 ml
#Frebini/Frebini Energy*	Fresenius Kabi Ltd	200 ml/500 ml

Available as standard 1 Kcal/ml solutions or as *higher energy 1.5 Kcal/ml products.
Paediatric enteral feeds (1 Kcal and 1.5 Kcal/ml) should be used for ages 1–6 yrs (8–20 kg) except for Tentrini designed for children aged 7–12 years (21–45 kg).

Table 7.15 Peptide semi-elemental feeds.

Peptisorb	Nutricia Clinical Care	500 ml/1 litre
Perative	Abbott Nutrition	237 ml/500 ml/1 litre
Peptamen	Nestle Nutrition	200 ml/375 ml/500 ml/1 litre
MCT Pepdite/MCT Pepdite 1+	Scientific Hospital Supplies	400 g
Pepdite/Pepdite 1+	Scientific Hospital Supplies	400 g

Table 7.16 Elemental feeds.

Products	Energy content	Type of fat	Presentation
Elemental E028 (Scientific Hospital Supplies)	388 Kcal/100 g	5% MCT	100 g
Elemental E028 Extra (Scientific Hospital Supplies)	443 Kcal/100 g	65% MCT	100 g
Emsogen (Scientific Hospital Supplies)	438 Kcal/100 g	83% MCT	100 g

The advantages of peptide semi-elemental feeds are their ready-to-feed composition, and the fact that a proportion of fat is MCT so enzyme dose can usually be reduced by 30–50% with close monitoring of gut symptoms and stool output.

Semi-elemental feeds must be introduced slowly. These feeds have a higher osmolality and risk causing osmotic diarrhoea.

Elemental feed   Elemental feeds are a completely hydrolysed formula for use in patients with short gut syndrome or intolerance of semi-elemental feed. Up to 83% of fat is present as MCT. Only half the enzyme dose is usually required although bowel symptoms and stool output should be monitored closely. Feeds can be concentrated up to 2.5 Kcal/ml but tolerance problems may develop at this concentration because of high osmolality.

Elemental feeds are only available in powdered form, thus reconstitution of feed will increase care load at home. There is a risk of bacterial contamination. Elemental feeds are expensive – although the cost may be partly offset by some reduction in enzyme dosage.

Figure 7.2   Child with long–term NG tube in situ.

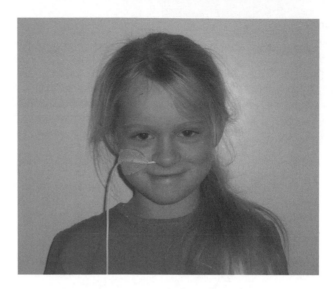

Pulmocare
(Abbott Nutrition)

Pulmocare is a 1.5 Kcal/ml whole protein feed with a high fat, low carbohy-drate content. It is advocated for moderate to severe chest disease to reduce CO_2 production and thus energy expenditure through respiration although these theoretical advantages have not been substantiated (Kane & Hobbs 1991). It is available in 250 ml cans or 500 ml ready-to-hang containers.

Home Delivery of Enteral Feeds (UK)

General Practitioners prescribe enteral feeds. However, transporting bulky feed bottles from the pharmacist to home can be difficult. The following companies will deliver feed and consumable equipment to the home.

Nutricia Clinical Care Homeward
Tel: 01225 711531 – Information Hotline

Fresenius Home Care
Tel: 01928 579333 – Patient Services

Abbott Nutrition Hospital to Home
Tel: 0800 0183799 – Patient Services

Nasogastric feeding

Choice of enteral feeding route depends on individual preference and likely duration.

Nasogastric feeding is often the precursor to gastrostomy feeding. Some individuals opt to continue with nasogastric feeding and pass the tube themselves every night. Most change to a gastrostomy for aesthetic reasons. Six French gauge paediatric incubator (22 or 36 inch) or 8 French gauge fine bore (22 or 36 inch) feeding tubes are the most suitable for pump feeding. These can stay in situ for three months (Figure 7.2). Weighted tubes are ideal because they are less likely to be regurgitated with coughing.

Starting nasogastric feeding

Home NG feeding needs careful teaching and preparation. Before discharge from hospital families must have information about:

- Care of the tube (for example flushing) and how often it requires changing
- How to pass a tube, including measuring for the correct length
- How to check the tube is correctly positioned using an aspiration technique (use 30–50 ml syringes for this technique as a lower pressure is exerted)
- Skin care, with particular reference to changing tape
- The importance of hygiene when dealing with the tube and feed
- How to use the feeding pump, giving sets, etc.
- How to obtain further supplies of feed and equipment.

Insertion of NG tube: practical tips

- Always measure and cut the tape before passing the tube and have it close at hand, ready to use.
- Some tubes have lubricants that are activated by water, so flush the tube with 10 mls of water prior to insertion – it makes it much easier to pass and more comfortable.
- If the tube does not have a lubricant, a lubricating gel can be used instead.
- Passing tubes is easier if the individual can swallow at the appropriate moment. Getting them to drink water can help.
- Once inserted, flush the tube to enable easy removal of the guide wire.
- Blocked tubes can be unblocked using flat cola (not Pepsi), meat tenderiser or cranberry juice.
- The procedure for unblocking tubes is as follows:
  - Insert a small amount of liquid, stopping as soon as resistance is felt. Leave it for a few minutes and repeat.
  - Gently try to insert a few more mls of liquid and allow this to stand for a few more minutes.
  - Gently pull back to see if you can remove any of the blockage.
  - Repeat this process until the line is clear.
  - Never use the wire introducer to try and clear a blockage.

If, after a new tube has been passed, it is not possible to aspirate any liquid from the stomach, give the individual a drink, wait for a few minutes and then try to aspirate again.

Gastrostomy feeding

In general we recommend gastrostomy insertion for individuals requiring long-term enteral feeding. For further details about gastrostomy choice and management see Chapter 17.

Administering the feed

Rotary peristaltic pumps are recommended to regulate the flow of feed. The rate and quantity of feed required depends on:

- Age and weight
- Additional oral intake prior to enteral feeding

Table 7.17 Problems with enteral feeding.

Problem	Possible cause	Solution
Diarrhoea	Over rapid infusion of feed	Reduce rate
	Cold feed	Deliver feed at room temperature
	Contaminated feed	Check microbiology of equipment used for feeding
	Intolerance	Ensure adequate enzymes being taken before changing feed to semi-elemental or elemental feed
	Pharmaceutical e.g. antibiotics, laxatives antacids	Review drugs
	Hypoalbuminaemia, e.g. liver failure	Seek medical/dietetic advice to correct albumin levels.
Gastrostomy tube blockage	Insufficient flushing	Flush with carbonated mineral water, fruit juice or flat cola (not Pepsi) If still blocked recommend a small dose of powdered enzymes – leave in tube for 15 minutes then flush.
	Drug precipitation	Ensure flushing before, after and between each drug.
Gastro-oesophageal reflux		Keep elevated at 45 degrees whilst feeding and for 30 minutes after. Consider use of prokinetics
Nausea/Vomiting	Over rapid infusion rate	Reduce rate of infusion
	Contaminated feed	Check microbiology of equipment used for feeding
	Electrolyte imbalance	Review blood profile and correct levels.
	Delayed gastric emptying	Consider use of gut motility drugs
	Cows milk protein intolerance	Change feeds
	Over-rapid infusion rate	Reduce rate
Abdominal distention	Over rapid infusion rate	Reduce rate of infusion
	Delayed gastric emptying	Consider use of gut motility drugs

- The presence of other fluid infusions, for example concurrent intravenous infusions
- Total fluid requirement.

Feeds should be started at full strength and the rate of infusion gradually increased as tolerated. Initially the feed should aim to provide 30% of

---

Example

Total energy requirement for 19 kg, 7-year-old child (Department of Health 1992)	= 1740 Kcals
Energy from overnight enteral feed	= 600 Kcals

Using a 1.5 Kcal/ml feed we would recommend an incremental rate increase over three nights as follows:

Night 1	30 ml per hour for 12 hours = 360 ml = 540 Kcal
Night 2	40 ml per hour for 10 hours = 400 ml = 600 Kcal
Night 3	50 ml per hour for 8 hours = 400 ml = 600 Kcal

---

estimated energy requirement building up to approximately 1000 Kcals provided by the overnight feed in children more than 20 kg. The feed should aim to provide only a third of the energy requirements in those less than 20 kg although this might need adjusting according to subsequent weight gain.

Administering enzymes with enteral feeds

- Overnight feeds should ideally be given over an 8–10 hour period starting early enough so that the feed can be completed by approximately 6.00 am, to try and give the individual an appetite for breakfast.
- The feed should be stopped at least 1 hour before physiotherapy to avoid vomiting.
- The total number of enzymes given should be based on the number required for a similar quantity of full cream milk with adjustment according to bowel symptoms, stool output and weight gain. Enzyme doses are generally split with one dose taken pre-feed and another before sleep. If an individual habitually wakes just as the feed finishes, a dose of enzymes could be taken at this time rather than before sleep.

References

Bachrach L K, Loutit C W, Moss R B 1994 Osteopenia in adults with CF. American Journal of Medicine 96:27–34

Boland M P, Stocki D S, McDonald N E et al 1986 Chronic jejunostomy feeding with a non-elemental formula in undernourished CF patients. Lancet ii:232–234

Borrowitz D S, Grand R J, Durie P R and Consensus Committee 1995 Use of pancreatic enzyme supplements for patients with CF. Journal of Pediatrics 127:681–684

Bye A M E, Muller D P R, Wilson J et al 1985 Symptomatic Vitamin E deficiency in CF. Archives of Diseases in Childhood 60:162–164

Cade A, Walters M P, McGinley N et al Evaluation of faecal pancreatic elastase-1 as a measure of pancreatic exocrine function in children with CF. Pediatric Pulmonology 29:172–176

Carr S B, Dinwiddie R 1996 Vitamin A as a predictor for poor lung function in CF. Paediatric Pulmonology 13(suppl):317

Congden P J, Bruce G, Rothburn M M et al 1981 Vitamin status in treated patients with CF. Archives of Diseases in Childhood 56:708–740

Constantini D, Padoan R, Curcio L et al 1988 The management of enzymatic therapy in CF patients by an individualised approach. Journal of Pediatric Gastroenterology and Nutrition 7:(Suppl) 1, 1–14

Department of Health 1992 Dietary reference values for food energy and nutrients for the UK. Report No 41. HMSO, London

Department of Health 1994 Weaning and the weaning diet. Report No 45. HMSO, London

Duggan C, Collin A A, Agil A et al 1996 Vitamin A status in acute exacerbation of CF. American Journal of Clinical Nutrition 64:635–639

Durie P R, Pencharz P B 1989 A rational approach to the nutritional care of patients with CF. Journal of Royal Society of Medicine 82:11–20

Durie P R 1994 Vitamin K and the management of patients with CF. Canadian Medical Association Journal 151:933–936

Eid N S, Shoemaker L R, Samiec T D 1990 Vitamin A in CF: case report and review of the literature. Journal of Paediatric Gastroenterology and Nutrition 48:655–656

Freiman J P, Fitzsimmons S C 1996 Colonic strictures in patients with CF: results of a survey of 114 CF care centres in the US. Journal of Paediatric Gastroenterology and Nutrition 22:153–156

Gavin J 2000 MPhil Thesis. Influence of nutrient intake on colonic function and stool composition in enterally fed CF patients. Institute of Human Nutrition, University of Southampton

Gavin J, Ellis J, Dewar A L 1997 Dietary fibre and the occurrence of gut symptoms in CF. Archives of Diseases in Childhood 76:35–37

Haworth C S, Selby P L, Webb A K et al 1999 Low bone mineral density in adults with CF. Thorax 54:961–967

Jones P J H, Pencharz P B, Clandinin M T 1985 Absorption of 13C-labelled stearic, oleic and linoleic acids in humans: application to breath tests. Journal of Laboratory and Clinical Medicine 105:647–652

Kane R E, Hobbs P 1991 Energy and respiratory metabolism in CF. The influence of carbohydrate content of nutritional supplements. Journal of Pediatric Gastroenterology and Nutrition 12:217–223

Levison H, Cherniak R 1968 Ventilatory cost of exercise in chronic obstructive pulmonary disease. Journal of Applied Physiology 25:21–27

Littlewood J P, Wolfe S P 2000 Control of malabsorption in CF. Paediatric Drugs 2:205–222

McCay P B, Pfeifer P M, Stide W H 1972 Vitamin E protection of membrane lipids during electron transport function. Ann NY Acad Sci 203:62–73

MacDonald A 1996 Nutritional management of CF. Archives of Disease in Childhood 74:81–87

Martin N D T, Snodgrass G J, Cohen R D 1984 Idiopathic infantile hypercalcaemia – a continuing enigma. Archives of Diseases in Childhood 59:605–613

Murphy J 1991 PhD thesis. Influence of diet and disease on human intestinal microflora, colonic function and faecal energy. Institute of Human Nutrition, University of Southampton

Murphy J L, Wootton S A, Bond S A et al 1991 Energy content of stool in healthy controls and patients with CF patients. Archives of Diseases in Childhood 66:495–500

Peters S A, Rolles C J 1993 Vitamin Therapy in CF – a review and rationale. Journal of Clinical Pharmacy and Therapeutics 18:33–38

Peters S A, Kelly F J 1993 Vitamin E supplementation in CF. Journal of Pediatric Gastroenterology and Nutrition 22:341–345

Ramsey B W, Farrell P M, Pencharz P and the Consensus Committee 1992 Nutritional assessment and management in CF: a consensus report. American Journal of Clinical Nutrition 55:108–116

Rashid M, Durie P R, Andrew M et al 1999 Prevalence of Vitamin K deficiency in CF. American Journal of Clinical Nutrition 70:378–382

Rayner R J, Tyrell J C, Hiller E J et al 1989 Night blindness and conjunctival xerosis caused by vitamin deficiency in patients with CF. Archives of Disease in Childhood 64:1151–1156

Reiter E O, Brugman S M, Pike J W et al 1985 Vitamin D metabolites in adolescents and young adults with CF: effects of sun and season. Journal of pediatrics 106:21–25

Smyth R L, Ashby D, O'Hea U et al 1995 Fibrosing colonopathy in CF: results of a case-control study. Lancet 346:1247–1251

Steinkamp G, von der Hardt H 1994 Improvement of nutritional status and lung function after long term nocturnal gastrostomy feeding in CF. Journal of Pediatrics 124:244–249

UK CF Trust Working Group 2002 Nutritional management of CF: CF Trust. Bromley

Walters M P, Kelleher J, Gilbert J et al 1990 Clinical monitoring of steatorrhoea in CF. Archives of Diseases in Childhood 63:99–102

Wilson D C, Rashid M, Durie P R et al 2001 Treatment of Vitamin K deficiency in CF. Effectiveness of a daily fat soluble vitamin combination. Journal of Pediatrics 138:851–855

Wolfe S P, Conway S P, Brownlee K G 2001 Seasonal variation in Vitamin D levels in children with CF in the United Kingdom. 14th European CF Conference. Vienna. Journal of Cystic Fibrosis P115

Chapter 8

Monitoring and investigations

Joan Gavin, Graeme Jones, Valerie Walker, Gary Connett

CHAPTER CONTENTS

INTRODUCTION

Regular follow-up and the appropriate use of investigations to detect and treat any deterioration in well-being are central to CF care. Good communications with support services are vital.

SWEAT TESTS

The only acceptable diagnostic sweat test procedure is pilocarpine iontophoresis with analysis of sweat chloride (see Chapter 2). This has three steps:

- Stimulation of sweating
- Sweat collection
- Sweat analysis.

Approved NCCLS Guidelines are in use in the USA. UK Guidelines are available on the Association of Clinical Biochemists website: www.acb.org.uk.

The flexor surface of the forearm is the preferred collection site, but the thigh or back can be used in small babies. Eczematous areas and skin rashes must be avoided. Simultaneous testing of both arms guards against errors, but is not essential.

Figure 8.1   Electrodes secured in position.

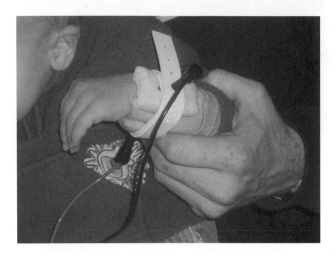

The skin is cleaned thoroughly with de-ionised water and dried. One of two procedures is then used:

The Gibson and Cooke filter paper collection procedure

Stimulation of sweating

Pads are prepared with 4–8 thicknesses of hospital lint for use as electrolyte reservoirs. These must be at least 1 cm larger than the electrode, to prevent electrode-skin contact. They may be sewn into calico pockets to contain the electrode.

The pads are saturated by soaking with the electrode solution before applying to the skin. Pilocarpine nitrate (2–5 g/L) is used for the positive electrode (anode). Pilocarpine nitrate, magnesium sulphate or other solutions are used for the negative electrode (cathode). Steel 'button' electrodes, are slipped into the calico pockets. When older style flat copper electrodes are used, the soaked pads are wrapped tightly around them, covering all bare metal.

The anode is applied to the flexor surface of the forearm and the cathode to the extensor surface. The electrodes are secured by a flexible perforated strap of soft rubber, wrapped in a crepe bandage and connected to a power supply. This must be battery driven and should include a safety cut-out.

The electrical current is increased gradually from 0.5 mA to 4 mA and maintained at 4 mA for 5 minutes. Longer times do not enhance sweating. The patient will experience a tingling sensation.

The electrodes are removed and the area beneath the anode is washed thoroughly with de-ionised water and dried.

Sweat collection

Sweat is collected onto sodium chloride-free filter paper that has been weighed dry in an air-tight container. The size should equal the stimulated area (for example, 5 cm × 5 cm). Using forceps, it is removed from the container (Figure 8.2), placed over the cleaned area, covered with a piece of polythene or parafilm, at least 1 cm larger than the paper, and taped securely in place to achieve a complete seal (Figure 8.3).

Figure 8.2   Filter paper removed from container with forceps.

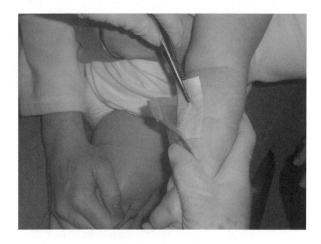

Figure 8.3   Filter paper is taped in position under plastic cover.

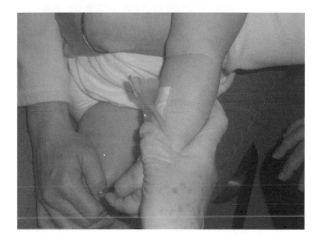

After a minimum of 20 minutes and no more than 30 minutes, the filter paper is transferred quickly, using forceps, to its container, which is immediately sealed. The paper is re-weighed in the container as quickly as possible, to obtain the accurate weight of sweat. The sweat is eluted with water and analysed for chloride +/− sodium. After weighing, the paper can be stored in the sealed container for up to 3 days at 4°C prior to analysis.

The Wescor–Macroduct® system (Wescor inc, Logan, Utah, USA)

Stimulation of sweating

Pilocarpine nitrate is impregnated into 2.8 cm diameter Pilogel® iontophoretic gel disks, supplied by the manufacturer. These are fitted into a pair of circular stainless steel electrodes, which are strapped to the flexor and extensor surfaces of the forearm as above. Usually only one arm is tested. They are connected to a battery-operated power pack, which raises the current to a maximum of 1.5 mA.

The electrodes are removed. The skin on the flexor surface of the arm is cleaned with de-ionised water and dried.

The Macroduct® collector is then attached with a strap. This is disposable. It consists of a slightly concave plastic disk with a hole in the centre. The hole connects to a small plastic tube, which is coiled over the top of the disk. As it is secreted, sweat is forced through the hole into the tubing. A tiny amount of dye is also carried into the tube with it, to allow visualisation of the sweat.

Sweat is removed with a micropipette and either analysed immediately for chloride +/− conductivity, or transferred into a small airtight tube and stored at 4°C pending analysis.

Who can have a sweat test?

Tests can be done from two weeks of age in babies over 3 kg weight, who are normally hydrated and without systemic illness. If there is urgency, tests can be attempted from 7 days of age. Tests can be carried out during treatment with intravenous fluids or diuretics, providing the individual's condition is stable.

Tests should be deferred if the patient

- is <7 days of age or <3 kg in weight
- is dehydrated, systemically unwell or oedematous
- has extensive eczema
- is receiving oral corticosteroids.

When should tests be repeated?

Tests should be repeated:

- If the sample is insufficient.
- A negative result, inconsistent with the clinical features.
- An equivocal result (40–60 mmol/L; 35–60 mmol/L if <6 weeks old).
- A previous diagnosis of CF, but not following a typical course.

Risks

Transient reddening of the skin is quite common and does not matter. Urticaria occurs very infrequently, perhaps due to hypersensitivity to pilocarpine or the electric current. Give an antihistamine if needed. Blisters and frank burns occur in fewer than 1% of tests and are avoidable. They are caused by:

- Bare metal touching the skin
- Oxidised/corroded electrodes
- Current >4 mA
- Pads covering the electrodes not moist enough.

If necessary, treatment with an antibiotic ointment is generally adequate.

Patient information

Families should understand about the test and should have written information prior to the test. Informed consent should be obtained in accordance with local policy.

Responsibility for testing and training

Sweat collection must be performed by:

- Centres undertaking at least 50 tests per year
- Individuals undertaking at least 10 tests per year.

Personnel must be fully trained. Their competence should be re-validated regularly and this should be recorded. Laboratories analysing sweat should participate in an external quality assessment scheme.

MONITORING NUTRITIONAL STATUS

Weight

- Infants should attend the clinic every 2 weeks until thriving and their weight checked at least 2 monthly thereafter.
- Beam balance scales are the most accurate, but portable scales (e.g. Salter) are more practical in the community.
- Infants should be weighed without nappies and older children in undergarments without shoes and socks.
- Weigh standing upright with hands by the side, not leaning on the scales or on the person undertaking the weighing.
- Weigh with an empty bladder if possible.
- For consistency, weighing should be by the same experienced staff using the same equipment.
- Weights should plotted on centile charts.

Length/height

- Measure at least two monthly until growth ceases and then annually. Plot on centile charts and regularly calculate the height velocity. If puberty is delayed this will result in reduced height velocity at the expected time.

Figure 8.4   Always weigh in undergarments.

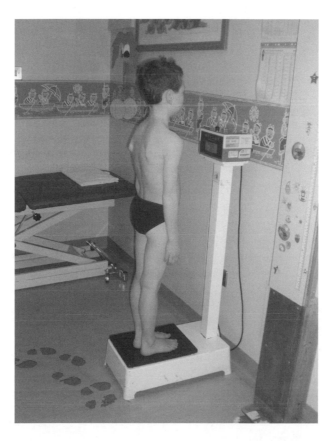

Figure 8.5   Technique for measuring height in a child.

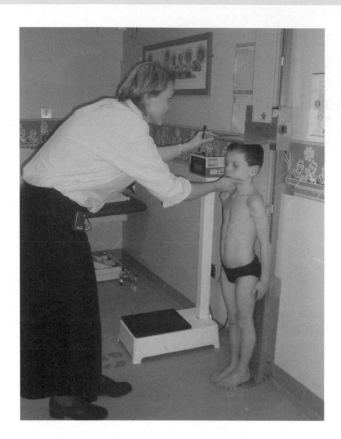

- Measure standing upright with shoes removed, shoulders straight, heels together and back to the stadiometer.
- Remove all hair accessories and ask the individual to look straight ahead.

Head circumference

This can be reduced. Measure regularly until 5 years (Ghoshal 1995).

Body Mass Index

This helps assess whether weight is in proportion to height. It can be used to assess nutrition at a particular time and documented serially. Values are age and sex standardised and should be plotted on specific BMI centile charts (Cole, Freeman & Preece 1995). Measurements need careful interpretation when height has been affected by malnutrition or delayed puberty. BMI is calculated by the formula:

$$\frac{\text{Weight (kg)}}{\text{Height}^2 \, (\text{m}^2)}$$

Percentage weight for height

This is the more traditional measure of weight in proportion to height but also does not account for stunting:

$$\frac{\text{Current weight (kg)} \times 100}{\text{Weight (kg) equivalent to current height centile}}$$

Figure 8.6 Measurement of upper arm skin fold thickness.

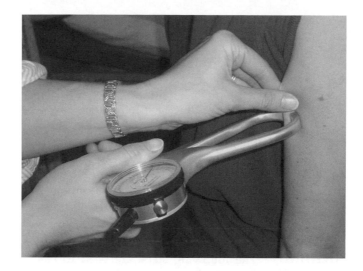

Anthropometric measures

Skinfold thickness reflects total body fat and is measured using skin callipers at the mid-point of the upper arm. An average of three measures can be plotted on specific centile charts (Frisancho 1981) (Figure 8.6).

Mid arm circumference reflects lean body mass. An average of three measures taken by the same person should be plotted on specific centile charts (Frisancho 1981).

Waist measurements can be useful to evaluate weight distribution after refeeding.

Anthropometric measures have poor reproducibility (Frisancho 1981) and are not routine.

TESTS FOR MALABSORPTION

Fat microscopy is a simple test indicating malabsorption, but is not quantitative. It can provide useful information around the time of diagnosis. Some centres use steatocrits as a semi-quantitative test for stool fat but the gold standard is the three-day faecal fat test.

Three-day faecal fat measurement

- A stool collection is made whilst consuming habitual diet.
- Carmine markers are consumed at the beginning and end of the three-day study.
- Intake is measured using a food diary.
- Findings are expressed as the coefficiency of absorption (CA):

$$CA = \frac{\text{dietary fat} - \text{faecal fat} \times 100\%}{\text{dietary fat}}$$

Table 8.1 shows normal CA ranges.

If there is excess fat individuals should undergo careful evaluation of enzyme usage (see Chapter 7).

Faecal elastase

Pancreatic function around the time of diagnosis can best be evaluated by measurements of stool faecal elastase. Pancreatic insufficient individuals

Table 8.1 Normal range for Coefficiency of Absorption.

Term infants	80–85%
10 months–3 years	85–90%
Older than 3 years	95%

requiring PERT will have very low levels (<15 mcg/g of stool). Those with higher levels might usefully be re-evaluated should there be faltering growth or symptoms suggesting malabsorption.

Other tests

Stool chymotrypsin levels are less reliable for assessing pancreatic function but might be useful for determining whether PERT doses are being given beyond the amounts needed to address symptoms. Tests of pancreatic function by duodenal intubation and PABA excretion are rarely necessary.

CALCULATING DAILY ENERGY REQUIREMENTS

The following steps are used to calculate the Daily Energy Requirement (DER).

1. Basal metabolic rate (BMR) can be calculated using a Deltatrack machine. If this method is unavailable, daily energy requirements can be calculated (Ramsey 1992) using the following World Health Organization Equations for predicting BMR (in calories) from body weight (kg).
2. Calculate daily energy expenditure (DEE) by multiplying the BMR by activity coefficient (AC) plus disease coefficient (DC):

$$DEE = BMR \times (AC + DC)$$

Activity coefficients (AC)

1.3 – confined to bed
1.5 – sedentary
1.7 – active

Disease coefficients (DC)

0 – FEV1 80% of that predicted
0.2 – FEV1 40–79% of that predicted
0.3 – FEV1 <40% of that predicted

---

3. Calculate DER from DEE taking into account the presence of steatorrhoea.

   DER = DEE where fat absorption >93% of intake
   DER = DEE × 0.93/0.85 if fat stool collection unavailable.

MONITORING OF RESPIRATORY STATUS

Microbiology

The major pathogens associated with pulmonary infection in CF are:
- *Staphylococcus aureus* (Gram positive cocci)
- *Haemophilus influenzae* (small Gram negative bacilli)
- *Pseudomonas aeruginosa* (large Gram negative bacilli) – particularly mucoid strains

Table 8.2   Estimated BMR.

Age range	BMR
Females	
0–3 years	$61.0 \times$ weight (kg) $- 51$
3–10 years	$22.5 \times$ weight (kg) $+ 499$
10–18 years	$12.2 \times$ weight (kg) $+ 746$
18–30 years	$14.7 \times$ weight (kg) $+ 496$
30–60 years	$8.7 \times$ weight (kg) $+ 829$
Males	
0–3 years	$60.9 \times$ weight (kg) $- 54$
3–10 years	$22.7 \times$ weight (kg) $+ 495$
10–18 years	$17.5 \times$ weight (kg) $+ 651$
18–30 years	$15.3 \times$ weight (kg) $+ 679$
30–60 years	$11.6 \times$ weight (kg) $+ 879$

- *Burkholderia cepacia* (large Gram negative bacilli) – previously *Pseudomonas cepacia.*

Mycoplasma pneumoniae, Aspergillus fumigatus, atypical Mycobacteria species, and an increasing variety of Gram-negative bacilli, including *Stenotrophomonas maltophilia,* might be recovered and play a role in disease. Culture for these less typical organisms should be made after discussion with the laboratory to optimise recovery rates.

Microbiological examination

The recovery and recognition of respiratory pathogens from sputum samples depends on the quality of the specimen, and the use of suitable microscopical and culture techniques.

Quality of specimen

This depends on:

- The adequacy of the specimen.
- Avoidance of contamination and overgrowth by upper respiratory tract flora.
- Current antimicrobial treatment.

Sputum samples expectorated from the lower respiratory tract are preferred. The ratio of white blood cells to squamous epithelial cells in the Gram stain is indicative of specimen quality. Generally, the higher the ratio of epithelial cells to white blood cells the more likely the culture results will represent oropharyngeal flora.

Specimens should be transported and cultured as soon as possible. Sputum can be refrigerated for up to 2–3 hours without an appreciable loss of pathogens. Delay beyond this time can lead to the overgrowth of upper respiratory tract flora and a reduction in the numbers of some pathogens, particularly *Haemophilus influenzae*. Where a delay in transport is unavoidable specimens should be refrigerated. In those who have difficulty expectorating, a sputum sample sent by post might yield the hardier *Pseudomonas aeruginosa* and *Burkholderia cepacia*.

Ideally, all microbiological specimens should be taken prior to commencing antibiotics. Where this is not practical, all antimicrobial agents used in treatment should be indicated on the request.

Microscopy and cultural techniques

Microscopy on sputum specimens is usually carried out after staining using the Gram stain. Gram stains can be used for determining the quality of the specimen and for predicting the presence of likely pathogens based on their staining reaction and microscopic appearance (Flourney & Davidson 1993).

The main problem in culturing CF respiratory specimens arises from difficulties in detecting major respiratory pathogens amongst contaminating oropharyngeal flora. Most laboratories attempt to overcome this problem in one, or a combination of the following ways:

- Liquefaction and dilution of the sputum specimen to dilute out the presence of oropharyngeal flora leaving the respiratory pathogens, which are normally present in higher numbers (Dixon & Miller 1995)
- The use of highly selective differential culture media to suppress the growth of oropharyngeal flora. Suitable media are commercially available for the detection of *Pseudomonas aeruginosa*, *Burkholderia cepacia*, *Staphylococcus aureus*, and *Haemophilus influenzae*.

All pathogens should be identified to species level and be accompanied by appropriate antimicrobial susceptibility test results. These can be useful markers of organism identification as well as aiding treatment regimes (e.g. *Burkholderia cepacia* is invariably resistant to colomycin whilst *Pseudomonas aeruginosa* is generally sensitive).

Decisions about the selection of antibiotics to treat infective exacerbations should not be based solely on sensitivity test results. Standard methods to obtain such data are usually derived from a single test colony and might not reflect the considerable heterogeneity found, particularly in *Ps. aeruginosa* populations. New antibiotic sensitivity testing techniques include mixed morphotype testing and testing of antibiotic combinations with potential in-vitro synergy, but their role in management is unclear (Morlin 1994, Aaron 2000).

All isolates of *Ps. aeruginosa* should be reported as 'mucoid' or 'non mucoid' because alginate production, which leads to mucoid colonies, is an important virulence factor (Stenvang 1992) (Figure 8.7).

There are risks of cross infection with *B. cepacia*, multi-resistant *Ps. aeruginosa* and MRSA (see Chapter 1). Strict adherence to local infection control policies is essential (McCallum 2001). New isolates of these organisms should be characterised by phenotypic or genotypic typing techniques as part of surveillance for cross infection episodes. This will generally require the isolate to be sent to a regional or national reference laboratory. All other organisms with unusual or unexpected resistance patterns should also be referred to a reference laboratory. This should be arranged through the local laboratory service.

Figure 8.7   Mucoid
Pseudomonas aeruginosa.

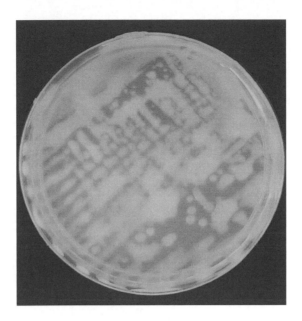

LUNG FUNCTION

Early respiratory complications occur in the small airways resulting in:

- Airways obstruction
- Hyperinflation
- Gas trapping
- Ventilation–perfusion mismatch.

This results in an increased residual volume (RV), functional residual capacity (FRC), total lung capacity (TLC) and decreased forced expiratory volume in one second (FEV1).

As disease progresses, lung destruction and fibrosis reduces TLC and restricts lung volumes. FRC and RV remain elevated. Gas dilution measurements progressively underestimate TLC because of increased gas trapping, although a lung clearance index using stable gas isotopes might prove useful for the early detection of airway complications (see Figure 8.8).

Detailed lung function assessment including body plethysmography can be a useful part of annual assessment. Some individuals maintain high FEV1 measurements at the expense of increasing lung volumes. Simple spirometry provides the most useful information for routine assessment.

Spirometry (Figure 8.9)

After some practise, the majority of children aged over 5 years can perform reproducible spirometry. All children should be taught the necessary forced respiratory manoeuvres as soon as is practical. Incentive devices usefully help young children achieve maximal flow volume loops.

Serial pulmonary function tests usefully detect changes in clinical status and should be recorded sequentially so that deteriorations are readily apparent.

Figure 8.8 Static lung volumes showing the progression of increasing hyperinflation (increasing FRC and RV) and the subsequent development of restrictive airways disease with increasing fibrosis (Levison & Godfrey 1976).

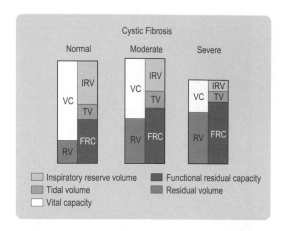

Figure 8.9 Performing lung function tests.

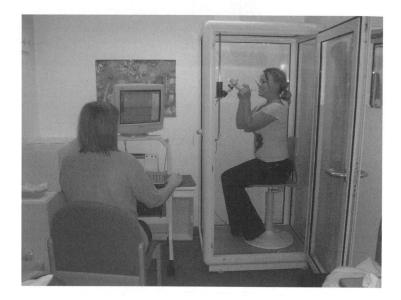

Spirometry is mandatory at all clinic visits with assessment of bronchoreversibility if there is increased airflow obstruction.

FEF 25–75% is the most sensitive indicator of early airway changes as reflected by increased convexity of the flow–volume loop but there is considerable inter and intra-subject variability in this measurement.

Significant decreases in FEV1 and FVC indicate the need for a change in treatment. Further measurements should be used to assess the efficacy of such interventions.

Within-patient variability of lung function:

- Is greater than in normals
- Is generally consistent within individuals
- Increases with worsening respiratory status.

Serial measurements of pulmonary function when well can be used to determine an individual's coefficient of variation (CV) (i.e. the standard

Figure 8.10 Spirometry in CF. Solid lines: normal values; dotted lines: expiratory flow volume curve, typical of airways obstruction and hyperinflation seen with moderately severe respiratory disease.

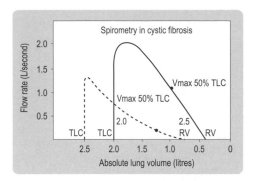

deviation of repeated measurements as a percentage of the mean of these measurements).

Example

Calculation of Coefficient of Variation: Example

Serial FEV1 measurements when well:

2.1, 2.3, 2.3, 2.4, 2.2, 2.2, 2.4, 2.1.

Mean FEV1 = 2.25

$\qquad$ SD = 0.12

Coefficient of variation $= \dfrac{0.12}{2.25} \times \dfrac{100}{1} = 5.3\%$

Pulse oximetry   Resting pulse oximetry usefully reflects oxygen uptake although hypoxaemia does not normally occur until there are moderately severe reductions in lung function. Resting oxygen saturations of less than 95% are indicative of moderately severe lung damage. Such individuals are likely to have significant hypoxaemia, particularly during acute respiratory exacerbations. In-patient treatment should include careful overnight monitoring with oxygen therapy as appropriate to achieve normal saturations.

Blood gas measurements   Capillary blood gas measurements of CO_2 should be performed in those with FVC < 40% to detect chronic hypercapnia. If detected, oxygen therapy should be used cautiously.

Bronchoscopy   The role of bronchoscopy and analysis of bronchoalveolar specimens in CF has not yet been clarified. Its value is unlikely to be scrutinised by

Figure 8.11 Bronchoscopy performed as a day case procedure.

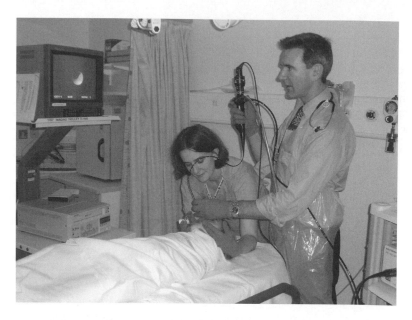

randomised controlled trials but clinical experience indicates that the procedure can identify unsuspected problems and provide useful prognostic and aetiological information to the direct benefit of the individuals studied.

Indications for bronchoscopy

Therapeutic interventions

Bronchoscopy was first used to try and clear diffuse mucoid impaction and selectively aspirate mucous plugs or secretions to resolve lobar or segmental atelectasis. Whilst manifest benefits can be achieved these are rarely sustained in those with moderate or severe lung involvement (Connett 1996). Early intervention to treat atelectasis, or persistent pneumonic consolidation despite intensive antibiotics and physiotherapy, is more likely to be of benefit. The use of rhDNase at the time of bronchoscopy might help loosen and dislodge areas of mucous plugging. Prolonged lavage and suctioning might be needed to effectively remove bronchial casts extending into the distal bronchi.

Bronchoscopy also has a role in the management of haemoptysis where it might usefully identify the site of bleeding prior to pulmonary artery embolisation (Fabian & Smitheringale 1996).

Diagnostic interventions

Antibiotic treatment when sputum is unavailable is often empirical. Whilst the use of antibiotics for increased symptoms is mandatory, significant lower respiratory infection can occur with minimal symptoms. There are limitations in the use of oro-pharyngeal cultures for detecting early infection with *Ps. aeruginosa* (Armstrong 1996). Bronchoscopy might usefully detect this and other organisms for which specific antibiotics would be needed. Additional information about gastro-oesophageal reflux (using a quantitative fat-laden macrophage index) and levels of cellular and cytokine inflammation are also potentially available (Dean 1993).

Bronchoscopy is easily performed as a day-case procedure under sedation (Connett 1996). Many centres perform bronchoscopy under general anaesthesia but this limits the extent to which individuals are able to cough and thus potentially benefit from the procedure. Slight fever on the night following lavage is the only commonly reported side effect. In experienced hands the risks are minimal.

References

Sweat testing

NCCLS 2000 Sweat testing: sample collection and quantitative analysis; approved guidelines. 2nd edn. NCCLS document C34-A2 (ISBN 1-56238-407-4) Wayne PA

Monitoring of nutritional status

Cole T J, Freeman J V, Preece M A 1995 Body mass index reference curves for the UK 1990. Archives of Diseases in Childhood 73:25–29

Frisancho A R 1981 New norms of upper limb fat and muscle areas for assessment of nutritional status. American Journal of Clinical Nutrition 34:2540–2545

Ghosal S, Taylor C J, Pickering M et al 1995 Disproportionate head growth retardation in CF. Archives of Diseases in Childhood 72:150–152

Ramsey B W, Farrell P M, Pencharz P and the Consensus Committee 1992 Nutritional assessment and management in CF: a consensus report. American Journal of Clinical Nutrition 55:108–116

Weltman E A, Stern R C, Doershuk C F et al 1990 Weight and menstrual function in patients with eating disorders and CF. Pediatrics 85:282–287

Microbiology

Aaron S D, Ferris W, Henry D A et al 2000 Multiple combination bactericidal antibiotic testing for patients with CF infected with Burkholderia cepacia. American Journal of Respiratory Critical Care Medicine 161:1206–1212

Dixon J M, Miller D C 1995 Value of dilute inocular in cultural examination of sputum. Lancet 2:1046–1048

Flourney D J, Davidson L J 1993 Sputum Quality: can you tell by looking? American Journal of Infection Control 21(2):64–69

McCallum S J, Corkill J, Gallagher M et al 2001 Superinfection with a transmissible strain of Pseudomonas aeruginosa in adults with CF chronically colonised by P. aeruginosa. Lancet 358:558–560

Morlin G L, Hedges D L, Smith A L et al 1994 Accuracy and cost of antibiotic susceptibility testing of mixed morphotypes of Pseudomonas aeruginosa. Journal of Clinical Microbiology 32:1027–1030

Stenvang S, Hoiby N, Espersenf et al 1992 Role of alginate in infection with mucoid Pseudomonas aeruginosa in CF. Thorax 47:6–13

Bronchoscopy and lung function

Armstrong D S, Grimwood K, Carlin J B et al 1996 Bronchoalveolar lavage or oropharyngeal cultures to identify lower respiratory pathogens in infants with CF. Pediatric Pulmonology 21(5):267–275

Connett G J, Doull I J, Keeping K et al 1996 Flexible fibre-optic bronchoscopy in the management of lung complications in CF. Acta Paediatrica 85(6):675–678

Dean T P, Dai Y, Shute J K et al 1993 Interleukin-8 concentrations are elevated in bronchoalveolar lavage, sputum, and sera of children with CF. Pediatric Research 34(2):159–1561

Fabian M C, Smitheringale A 1996 Haemoptysis in children: the hospital for sick children experience. Journal of Otolaryngology 25(1):44–45

Levison H, Godfrew S 1976 Pulmonary aspects of CF. In: Mangos J A, Talamo R C (eds) CF – Projections into the Future. Stratton Intercontinental Book Corp., New York

Chapter **9**

Radiology

Joanna J. Fairhurst

REGULAR CHEST X-RAY EVALUATION

Regular annual assessment should include evaluation of chest X-rays using a scoring system. Systems currently in use include:

- Chrispin and Norman Score (Chrispin & Norman 1974) – the most commonly used system in the UK*
- Brasfield Score (Brasfield 1979) – preferred in the United States of America*
- Wisconsin system (Weatherley 1993) – greater sensitivity in mild disease, but needs a computer programme to run it
- Bhalla system (Bhalla 1991) – based on chest computed tomography
- Northern score (Conway 1994) – requires only a PA chest X-ray

* Both these systems were devised in the 1970s when progression of disease was more rapid and radiographic abnormalities more pronounced. They provide poor discrimination in milder disease in infants and young children.

Chrispin and Norman score

Both postero-anterior and lateral chest X-rays are required for complete scoring. Each lung is divided into upper and lower zones by a line passing through the middle of the hilum. These four zones are assessed for

Figure 9.1 AP and lateral chest X-ray showing flattened diaphragm, kyphosis and sternal bowing.

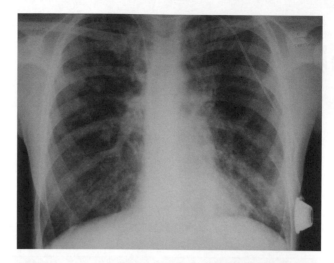

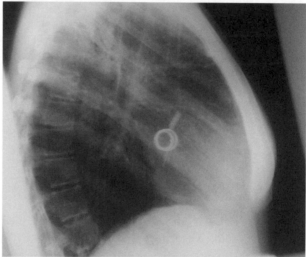

the presence and severity of the following features which may be absent (score 0), present but not marked (score 1) or marked (score 2):

Hyperinflation (Figure 9.1) – as evidenced by flattening of the diaphragm, sternal bowing and kyphosis.

- Peribronchial thickening – seen either as tramline in longitudinal section or circular shadow in cross section (Figure 9.2)
- Mottled shadows – Small, rounded shadows up to 0.5 cm diameter, representing centrilobular consolidation secondary to mucus plugging of bronchioles with super imposed infection (Figure 9.3)
- Ring shadows – Air filled bronchiolectatic cavities (Figure 9.4)
- Large shadows – Representing confluent lung collapse or consolidation. Can affect a segment or whole lobe (Figure 9.5). Involvement of a single segment scores 1, two or more segments scores 2.

The full scoring system is outlined in Table 9.1.

Figure 9.2   Coned view of the right lower lobe showing peribronchial thickening.

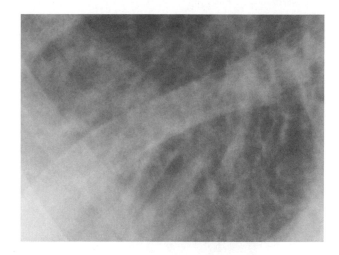

Figure 9.3   Coned view of the right mid zone showing mottled shadows.

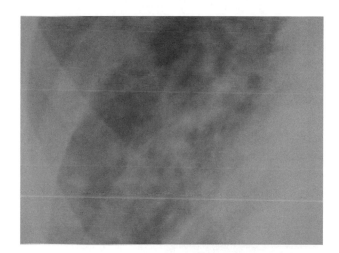

Figure 9.4   Coned view of the right upper zone showing ring shadows.

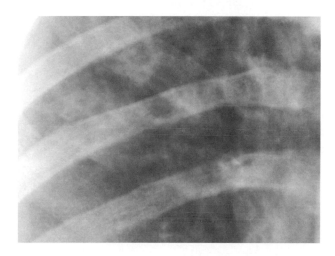

Figure 9.5 Focal consolidation in the middle lobe and lingula.

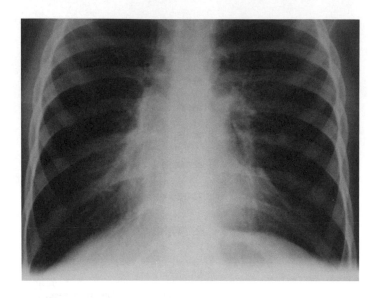

Table 9.1 Chrispin and Norman Score.

Feature	Not present	Present but not marked	Marked
Chest configuration:			
Sternal bowing	0	1	2
Diaphragmatic depression	0	1	2
Spinal kyphosis	0	1	2
Bronchial line shadows:			
Right upper zone	0	1	2
Right lower zone	0	1	2
Left upper zone	0	1	2
Left lower zone	0	1	2
Mottled shadows:			
Right upper zone	0	1	2
Right lower zone	0	1	2
Left upper zone	0	1	2
Left lower zone	0	1	2
Ring shadows:			
Right upper zone	0	1	2
Right lower zone	0	1	2
Left upper zone	0	1	2
Left lower zone	0	1	2
Large shadows:			
Right upper zone	0	1	2
Right lower zone	0	1	2
Left upper zone	0	1	2
Left lower zone	0	1	2

Brasfield score

Both postero-anterior and lateral chest X-rays are required for complete assessment. The films are assessed for the presence and severity of five features: air trapping, linear markings (peribronchial thickening), nodular-cystic lesions (the equivalent of mottled shadows), large lesions (segmental shadowing) and general severity.

Absence of any of the above features scores 0, increasing severity scores from 1 to 4.

The final score is obtained by subtracting the total points scored by the chest X-rays from 25. The full scoring system is outlined in Table 9.2.

Chest CT score

Bronchiectasis and mucous plugging are consistently underestimated on plain chest X-rays. To overcome this, and to permit more sensitive and accurate assessment, several chest CT scores have been developed.

Table 9.2 Brasfield score.

Category	Definition	Scoring	
Air trapping	Generalised pulmonary overdistention presented as sternal bowing, depression of diaphragms, and/or thoracic kyphosis	0	absent
		1	
		2	increasing
		3	severity*
		4	
Linear markings	Line densities due to prominence of bronchi; may be seen as parallel line densities, sometimes branching, or as 'end-on' circular densities with thickening of bronchial wall	0	absent
		1	
		2	increasing
		3	severity*
		4	
Nodular-cystic lesions	Multiple discrete small rounded densities, 0.5 cm in diameter or larger, with either radiopaque or radiolucent centres (does not refer to irregular linear markings); confluent nodules not classified as large lesions	0	absent
		1	
		2	increasing
		3	severity*
		4	
Large lesions	Segmental or lobar atelectasis or consolidation; includes acute pneumonia	0	absent
		3	segmental or lobar atelectasis
		5	multiple atelectasis
General severity	Impression of overall severity of changes on roentgenogram	0	absent
		1	
		2	increasing
		3	severity
		4	
		5	complications (e.g. cardiac enlargement, pneumothorax)

*Score of 4 is most severe.

Figure 9.6 Coned view of the right lung showing pneumothorax.

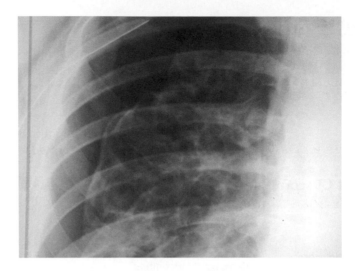

The main disadvantages to routine use of CT in regular assessment are lack of universal availability, the potential need for sedation in younger patients and the significant radiation exposure. Doses from modern, low dose, thin-section techniques are beginning to approach those acquired from two view conventional chest radiographs. The scoring system devised by Bhalla evaluates the severity of involvement by assessing the presence and extent of bronchiectasis, peribronchial thickening, mucous plugging, abscesses, bullae, emphysema and collapse/consolidation.

IMAGING RESPIRATORY COMPLICATIONS

Chest radiograph

Indications Other than as part of the annual review, indications for chest radiography include:

- Severe exacerbation of respiratory symptoms
- Chest pain
- Pyrexia.

The chest X-ray may reveal:

- Pneumothorax, particularly in older children and adults (Figure 9.6)
- Focal infection.

> **Remember**
>
> **Atypical organisms (for example, mycobacteria/mycoplasma) particularly in patients on immunotherapy.**
>
> Although hilar enlargement, whether due to lymphadenopathy, pulmonary arterial dilatation or perihilar pneumonia, is a frequent finding, paratracheal lymphadenopathy should alert one to the possibility of mycobacterial infection (Figure 9.7).

Recurrent infection in a specific lobe or segment might indicate localised bronchiectasis benefiting from resection. If this is suspected, consider chest CT and ventilation scanning to assess the extent of disease elsewhere.

Figure 9.7   Mycobacterial infection: marked hilar and paratracheal lymphadenopathy.

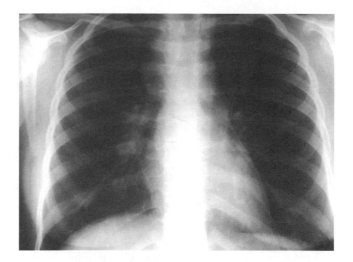

Figure 9.8   Coned view showing 'gloved finger' mucoid plugging.

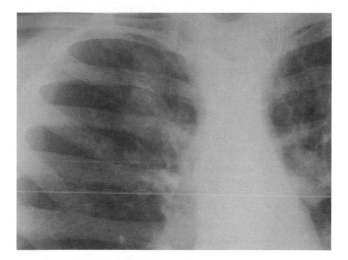

Allergic bronchopulmonary aspergillosis can be recognised by a central distribution of bronchiectasis and 'gloved-finger' mucoid plugging (Figure 9.8). Other features of ABPA leading to recognition in other patients include peribronchial thickening, mucoid impaction and perihilar infiltrates, which might already be present. Always consider ABPA in the presence of extensive consolidation.

Cor pulmonale can be recognised by noting right ventricular dilatation and evidence of pulmonary hypertension. The latter can be difficult to recognise as enlargement of the central pulmonary arteries is hard to differentiate from hilar lymphadenopathy and peripheral vascular pruning is difficult to detect in the presence of existing background radiographic changes. With hyperinflation the mediastinum is elongated and the heart appears relatively small. Even with the development of cor pulmonale, heart size can be within normal limits. It is important to look for changes in cardiac size on successive radiographs (CF 1993).

Obliterative bronchiolitis may present following lung transplantation.

Figure 9.9 (Expiratory) CT showing inhomogenous aeration in bronchiolitis obliterans (courtesy of Dr Richard Coulden).

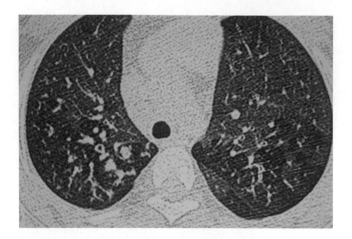

Chest CT Indications for chest CT include:

- Assessment of severity and location of bronchiectasis, for example if lobectomy is being considered.
- Assessment prior to heart/lung and double lung transplantation. This includes evaluation of chest shape, vascular anatomy, the presence of consolidation and mycetoma.
- Complications of lung transplantation. These include infection and bronchiolitis obliterans. The latter has many manifestations but bronchial dilatation in the lower lobes and airspace consolidation, with inhomogenous aeration and peribronchial thickening are indicative (Figure 9.9).
- Equivocal or confusing findings on plain chest X-ray.

Unless detailed mediastinal assessment is required, low dose techniques should be employed, as the intrinsic contrast of lung provides good quality images with lower milliamperage.

Recommended protocols are as follows (Lucaya 1996):

- For general assessment of severity of lung involvement and localisation of bronchiectasis:
  120 kVp
  high resolution filters
  50 mAS
  1 second scan time
  1 mm collimation
  20 mm intervals.
- For detailed assessment of focal disease, either as above but reducing scan interval to 10 mm or, if helical scanning is available:
  120 kVp
  high resolution filters
  130 mAS
  5–10 mm slice thickness
  pitch of 1.2–1.5.
- Multidetector CT is now widely available and has the advantage of rapid scanning during single breath-holds, and superior multiplanar

Figure 9.10 Severe cystic bronchiectatic change.

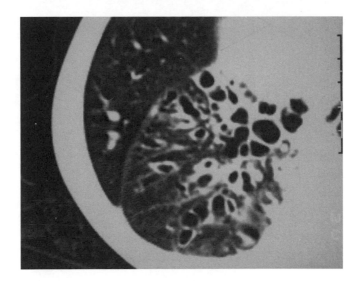

reconstruction. Guidelines for optimising imaging parameters whilst minimising dose have recently been published (Donnelly & Frush 2003).

If intravenous contrast enhancement is required the following injection timings are suggested for helical scanning:

- Injection volume 2 ml per kg body weight (300 mg of iodine per ml)
- Injection rate 1 ml per second
- Start scanning approximately 17 to 20 seconds after the onset of injection.

Appearances of chest CT in CF

- Typical abnormalities (Figure 9.10). High resolution CT shows several of the common pulmonary manifestations of CF to better advantage. Typical findings include cystic or varicose bronchiectasis, peribronchial thickening, mucoid impaction, peripheral areas of centrilobular opacities, and subpleural bulla formation.
- Allergic Bronchopulmonary Aspergillosis. Look for focal central bronchiectasis associated with mucous plugging.
- Fungal infection/pulmonary aspergilloma. These rarely present as areas of non-specific consolidation, however, occasionally cavitating nodules may be demonstrated (Figure 9.11).
- Obliterative bronchiolitis (Figure 9.9). See above.

SINUS DISEASE

The paranasal sinuses are not fully developed and pneumatised until the age of 10 years. Moreover, plain radiographs of the sinuses are notoriously unreliable in assessing the presence and severity of disease. Mucosal thickening varies from hour to hour as assessed by all forms of imaging modality and does not necessarily parallel pathology. Over 2 years of age, most individuals with CF have complete opacification of the paranasal sinuses, without evidence of clinical sinusitis. Nasal polyps can lead to facial deformity. In addition to conventional sinus views, a lateral view of the postnasal space is used to assess polyposis and mucosal hypertrophy.

Figure 9.11   Pulmonary aspergilloma. Note cavitation within an area of focal consolidation.

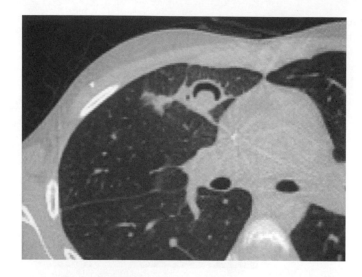

Figure 9.12   CT demonstrating expanded, mucous filled ethmoid sinuses.

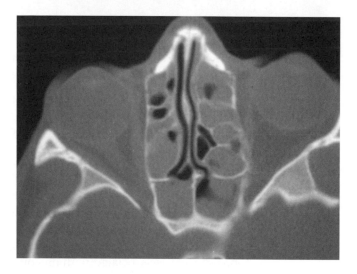

If surgery is contemplated, adequate assessment involves detailed demonstration of the paranasal sinuses, nose and osteomeatal complex, best achieved by high resolution coronal (+/− axial) CT (Figure 9.12).

GASTROINTESTINAL DISEASE

Meconium ileus

Plain abdominal X-ray   Approximately 10% present with meconium ileus at birth. Plain radiograph findings depend on whether secondary complications are present. Uncomplicated meconium ileus typically demonstrates:

- Dilated loops of small bowel without air fluid levels. It can be difficult to differentiate large and small bowel in neonates as the bowel is featureless (Figure 9.13).
- A bubbly appearance representing air trapped within the inspissated meconium (Figure 9.14).

Figure 9.13 One day old neonate. Abdominal; X-ray shows a single markedly dilated small bowel loop.

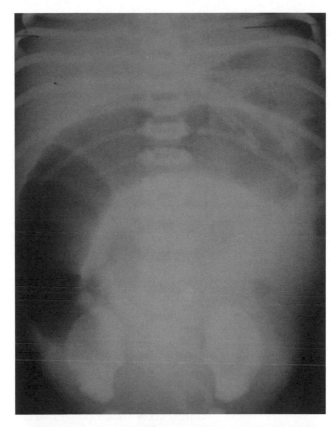

Figure 9.14 Note the bubbly appearance in the right side of the abdomen representing air trapped within meconium.

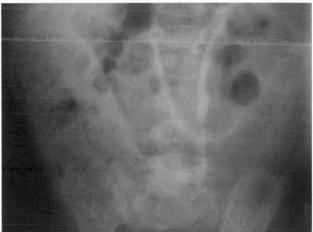

Potential complications can give the following appearances:

- Ileal or jejunal atresia – air fluid levels in small bowel above the level of the atresia.
- Meconium peritonitis – intraperitoneal calcification. This can be scrotal in the presence of a patent processus vaginalis at the time of perforation (Figure 9.15).

Figure 9.15 Calcified meconium within the abdomen.

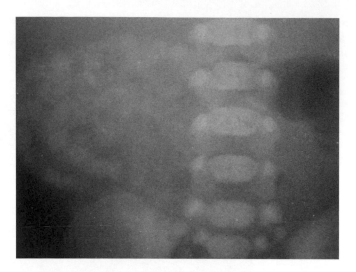

- Pseudocyst – abdominal distension with air-filled loops of bowel displaced by a soft tissue mass.

Ultrasound Abdominal ultrasound can distinguish meconium ileus from ileal atresia. In meconium ileus, sonography shows multiple loops of bowel containing very echogenic, thick meconium, whereas those with ileal atresia have dilated, fluid-filled loops of bowel with no echogenic contents.

Contrast enema – choice of medium If meconium ileus is suspected, the next investigation of choice is contrast enema. This can be both diagnostic and therapeutic. Barium should not be used as this might cause further inspissation. Full strength Gastrografin was previously advocated. It was thought that its hyperosmolality drew fluid into the bowel to dilute the meconium and make it less viscid. It has since been shown that iso-osmolar agents or dilute Gastrografin are equally effective in treating meconium ileus and that the surfactant agent added to the contrast medium (Tween 80) is probably the active component (Kao & Franken 1995).

Use of a hypertonic contrast agent can lead to the rapid shift of fluid from the vascular compartment into bowel lumen. This can cause an increased haematocrit, decreased pulse rate and decreased cardiac output. For this reason, dilute Gastrografin or iso-osmolar contrast media with additives are recommended.

Regardless of which contrast medium is used, preparation of the patient prior to therapeutic enema must include adequate hydration, intravenous infusion and continuous monitoring of heart rate and oxygen saturation.

Contrast enema – diagnostic features
- Microcolon
- Inspissated meconium seen as filling defects within undilated small bowel (Figure 9.16).

Therapeutic enema Contrast must be seen to fill the dilated small bowel proximal to the meconium obstruction for maximum effect.

Figure 9.16 Contrast enema. Inspissated meconium is visible within both large and small bowels. Note the microcolon.

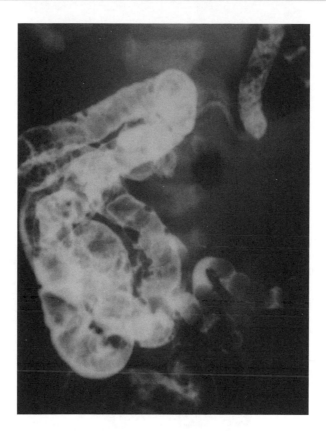

Success rates vary from 0–25% if only the colon is filled, to 51–100% when the dilated ileum is filled. It is worth several attempts, several hours apart, if obstruction is not initially relieved. Overall 50–60% of uncomplicated cases can be successfully treated with contrast enema. Perforation rates during the procedure are approximately 3% (Kao & Franken 1995).

Constipation

Plain abdominal X-ray results in a significant radiation dose and should be used with discretion. If confirmation of constipation will alter management this is probably justified. Look for faecal loading throughout the colon or in the rectum. This suggests constipation or distal colonic impaction.

Distal intestinal obstruction syndrome

Plain abdominal X-ray can suggest the diagnosis by a speckled faecal gas pattern in the right iliac fossa, or occasionally by demonstrating small bowel obstruction.

Ultrasound may show an impacted faecal mass in the right iliac fossa.

Contrast enema might rarely be necessary to confirm the diagnosis. Remember to use water soluble contrast if at all possible. This will show an inspissated right iliac fossa mass.

Appendicitis

Plain abdominal X-ray is frequently unhelpful, but may demonstrate:

- A soft tissue mass in the right iliac fossa
- A visible appendicolith (Figure 9.17).

Ultrasound should always be attempted. This might confirm the diagnosis or suggest alternatives. In appendicitis one can demonstrate:

- An inflamed, enlarged appendix (Figure 9.18)
- An appendix mass
- An appendicolith
- Free fluid in the pelvis.

Remember that although an abnormal appendix on ultrasound is a highly specific finding, the presence of a sonographically normal appendix does not exclude appendicitis (Sivit 1992).

Figure 9.17 Appendicitis. There is marked narrowing of the caecum and ascending colon and a calcified appendicolith is visible opposite the L4/5 interspace.

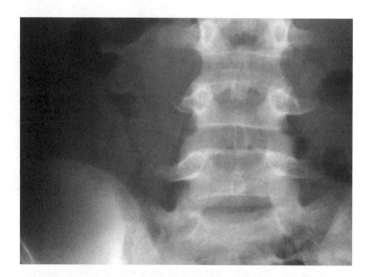

Figure 9.18 Ultrasound showing a sausage shaped inflamed appendix surrounded by bright fat.

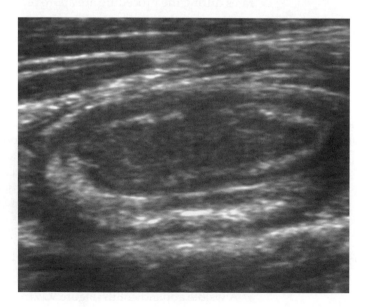

Intussusception

Plain abdominal X-ray may demonstrate:

- A soft tissue mass
- A paucity of gas in the large bowel
- Small bowel dilatation.

Plain abdominal radiograph can be non-specific in up to 50% of cases. Ultrasound is almost always diagnostic and demonstrates:

- The 'target' sign of echo-poor thickened bowel wall alternating with echogenic mucosa (Figure 9.19)
- Varying amounts of free intraperitoneal fluid.

Fibrosing colonopathy

Plain abdominal X-ray is unhelpful, except in showing faecal loading proximal to the site of narrowing.

Ultrasound may demonstrate bowel wall thickening (Figure 9.20).

Figure 9.19 Intussusception. Concentric hypo and hyper echoic rings on ultrasound.

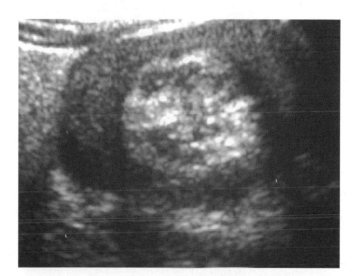

Figure 9.20 Ultrasound of ascending colon. The individual muscle layers can be identified.

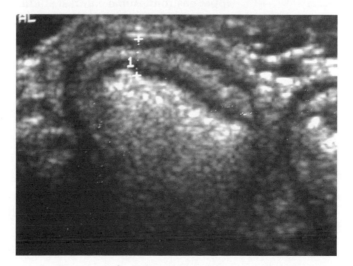

Figure 9.21   Barium enema showing extensive stricturing of the transverse colon and splenic flexure.

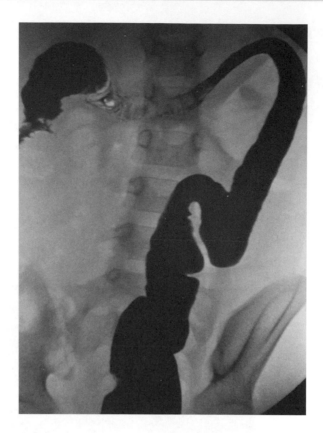

Contrast enema will identify the site and extent of large bowel strictures (Figure 9.21).

Gastro-oesophageal reflux

Barium meal is not the most sensitive investigation for reflux. If this is the only suspected diagnosis, alternative examinations such as pH monitoring will give a more definitive answer.

Upper gastrointestinal contrast studies can demonstrate:

- Hiatus hernia (not diagnosable with pH monitoring)
- Peptic ulcer disease
- Oesophagitis.

Non specific features include:

- Prominent duodenal folds
- Irregular small bowel dilatation, bowel wall thickening and prolonged transit time
- Evidence of malabsorption.

Pancreatitis

Pancreatitis is rare and usually confined to those retaining some exocrine pancreatic function. Features visible on ultrasound include:

- Progressive fatty replacement and fibrosis leading to diffusely increased echogenicity. This can be underestimated because of the concurrent

Figure 9.22 Coronal ultrasound showing a markedly enlarged, echogenic pancreas containing multiple hyperechoic cysts.

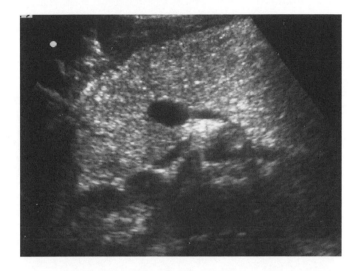

Figure 9.23 Axial CT at the level of the body of the pancreas showing speckled calcification.

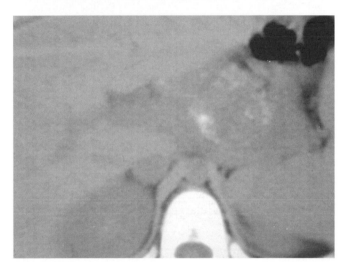

increase in hepatic echogenicity which also occurs (Paediatric Sonography 1995)

- Pancreatic atrophy
- Macrocysts or microcysts (Figure 9.22)
- Calcification
- Rarely, pancreatic duct dilatation.

There are often no sonographic changes to suggest pancreatitis although the pancreas can be enlarged and hypoechoic.

Extensive fatty replacement produces a striking appearance (Figure 9.23) on CT scan. Calcification can be demonstrated more accurately than by ultrasound, as can macrocystic changes.

LIVER DISEASE

Hepatobiliary complications are best imaged with ultrasound. CT is occasionally helpful.

Figure 9.24   Coronal ultrasound showing increased echogenicity around the portal tract.

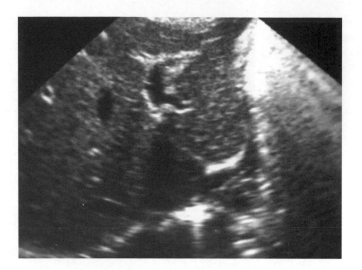

Cirrhosis

Abnormalities in echotexture can be detected in early childhood and include:

- Inhomogeneity of echogenicity
- Increased periportal echogenicity (Figure 9.24).

With the development of cirrhosis, look for:

- Atrophy of the right lobe and medial segment of the left lobe with compensatory hypertrophy of the lateral segment of the left lobe and caudate
- Irregular hepatic margins
- Further coarsening of hepatic echotexture
- Nodular regeneration causing compression of hepatic and portal veins.

Portal hypertension

When suspecting portal hypertension look for:

- Splenomegaly
- Reversal of flow in the portal or splenic vein on Doppler sonography
- Porto-systemic collaterals, for example dilated left gastric vein or gastro-oesophageal varices.

Gall bladder and biliary tree disease

Possible changes include:

- Gall bladder atrophy
- Gall stones (10%)
- Bile plug syndrome.

Bile plug syndrome presents as obstructive jaundice in the neonatal period caused by inspissated bile blocking the ducts. It manifests on ultrasound as dilated ducts containing sludge (Figure 9.25). Remember that the normal neonatal common bile duct is often invisible and never exceeds 2 mm in diameter.

Figure 9.25 Two week old infant. The common bile duct is dilated and contains echogenic sludge.

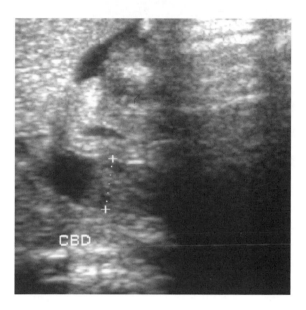

MAGNETIC RESONANCE IMAGING

Whilst attractive as an imaging modality both for its multi-planar capabilities and its lack of risk from ionising radiation, the applications of magnetic resonance imaging in CF remain limited. In order to overcome motion artefacts from respiration and cardiac pulsation, the signal must be gated so that it is only acquired during the same fraction of each respiratory and cardiac cycle. This results in prolonged scanning times that can exceed the endurance of those with respiratory compromise. Any coughing during an acquisition sequence, which can last in excess of 8 minutes, will render the images from that sequence uninterpretable. The development of rapid sequences and more widespread availability of higher field strength magnets will inevitably extend the role of MRI in CF in the future. Pancreatic changes have already been well documented (Kinsella 1991) although the information obtained does not currently improve on that gained with ultrasound. The greatest potential advantage of MRI would be the development of a reliable system for quantifying lung parenchymal disease. Lung imaging with MR is currently limited, but it is already possible to identify bronchial wall thickening and plugging (Kinsella 1991). Hilar adenopathy is much better demonstrated with MR than with plain chest X-ray or CT. Once it becomes possible to resolve parenchymal detail it might be feasible to develop a magnetic resonance scoring system to chart progression of disease without the need for repeated radiation exposure.

References

Bhalla M, Turcios N, Aponte V et al 1991 CF: scoring system with thin-section CT. Radiology 179:783–788

Brasfield B, Hicks G, Soong S et al 1979 The chest roentgenogram in CF: a new scoring system. Paediatrics 63:24–29

CF 1993 Clinical update for radiologists. In: Newman B The Radiologic Clinics of North America. WB Saunders p 623

Chrispin A R, Norman A 1974 The systematic evaluation of the chest radiograph in CF. Pediatric Radiology 2:101–106

Conway S, Pond M, Bowler I et al 1994 The chest radiograph in CF: a new scoring system compared with the Chrispin-Norman and Brasfield scores. Thorax 49:860–862

Donnelly L, Frush D 2003 Pediatric multidetector body CT. In: Boiselle P M (ed) The Radiologic Clinics of North America. W.B. Saunders 41(3):637–655

Kao S C, Franken E A 1995 Non-operative treatment of simple meconium ileus: a survey of the Society for Paediatric Radiology. Pediatric Radiology 25:97–99

Kinsella D, Hamilton A, Goddard P et al 1991 The role of magnetic resonance imaging in CF. Clinical Radiology 44:23–26

Lucaya J, Garcia-Pena P, Sotil J et al 1996 Low dose chest CT in children. Presented at IPR meeting. In: Siegel M J Pediatric Sonography. Raven Press, p 331

Sivit C, Newman K, Boenning D et al 1992 Appendicitis: usefulness of US in diagnosis in a paediatric population. Radiology 185:549–552

Weatherley M R, Palmer C G, Peters M E et al 1993 Wisconsin CF chest radiograph scoring system. Paediatrics 91:488–495

Chapter **10**

Psychological issues

Judi Maddison

INTRODUCTION

Living with a chronic disease can be stressful for the individual involved and their family. Physical and psychological health are interdependent and psychological concerns should not be overlooked. Some problems require the specialist attention of a psychologist or psychiatrist, whilst a trusted team member, such as a nurse, can address others. Establishing and maintaining good rapport with the family from the outset can be invaluable when attempting to help at particular times of need (Whyte 1994).

Remember

The confidential sharing of information amongst all team members is important. Families need to be made aware of this when confiding in individual team members.

There are several excellent books providing more comprehensive reviews about the psychological problems in CF (see Further reading). This chapter addresses the major issues that are commonly encountered.

COPING STRATEGIES

CF repeatedly challenges the affected individual and their family. Coping strategies will be used throughout life to address the psychological stresses these challenges bring. Families use different strategies at different times but often have an underlying strategy that they repeatedly return to. Identifying such behaviour, which might not be immediately obvious, can make it easier to work effectively with the individual and their family.

The coping strategies a family uses are a vital part of their ultimate coping mechanisms (McCubbin 1983). Respecting and working within them can help develop strong working relationships but it is important to recognize whenever these strategies become destructive and impede care.

Strategies can be categorized as adaptive or maladaptive.

Adaptive strategies

These place emphasis on normalising situations and take the emphasis away from the disease.

Establishing a routine

Incorporating treatment into normal daily life is a way of reducing its impact. It enables the family to achieve a sense of normality in an otherwise abnormal situation. It also has the practical advantage of ensuring treatment actually gets accommodated into the daily routine.

Filtering information

Families might sort and prioritise all information they receive, making adaptations if their situation changes. Some will avoid any information that is not directly relevant to them at the time. Other filtering strategies include:

- Reluctance to meet other affected families
- Preference for home care
- Unwillingness to participate in local groups or with the CF Trust.

Pushing the positive

Families might resent the differences that CF brings and long for a normal life. Understandably they draw attention to achievements such as sporting activities or academic prowess, whilst underplaying health problems. Whilst a positive approach is to be encouraged, a reluctance to acknowledge clear limitations can be destructive.

Maladaptive strategies

Denial and non-compliance

When individuals are well, denial can be a healthy adaptation. Similarly after the shock of diagnosis or a new complication, temporary denial can be part of a normal grief reaction. Persistent denial, manifest as non-compliance, needs addressing.

Over zealous adherence to treatment

Some families are so consumed by the health needs of their child that they become obsessed with treatment and highly anxious about minor complications (Wilson 1990). Families can develop inflexible routines. These ensure necessary care is given but destroy any chance of normal family life. Rarely, such obsessional behaviour, coupled with abnormal belief systems, can cause Munchhausen's syndrome in the child and Munchhausen's syndrome by proxy in the family (Rolles & Maddison 1995).

Alternative/ complementary therapies

Families desperate for a cure are vulnerable to the unsubstantiated claims of alternative and complementary therapists. Families will choose to believe these claims as they are often told what they want to hear. Such therapies might be of benefit, as part of the holistic approach to chronic illness, but must not be to the exclusion of conventional medicine. It can become a child protection issue if parents choose to go exclusively down the alternative therapy route.

ADHERENCE

Treatment recommendations are made on the assumption that they will be adhered to. However, a degree of non-adherence is very common and needs to be considered. Those who apply a sensible degree of flexibility to their treatment tend to be healthier and live fuller lives than their strictly adherent counterparts (Lask 1994). The main issues with non-adherence are the extent to which it occurs and the reasons why.

Non-adherence by parents

There are many reasons why parents do not adhere to their child's treatment and the motivation behind this is very individual. Issues that might usefully be explored include the following:

Failure to understand the treatment regime

An important starting point is to determine whether the family understands the importance of the treatment and how to carry it out. Lack of understanding may be due to poor explanation, language or intellectual barriers. Simple explanations with written and/or diagrammatical information may be helpful. The annual review offers an excellent opportunity to re-explore basic treatment regimes and reinforce understanding.

Inability to perform the treatment

For various physical or social reasons it can be difficult for a family to undertake certain aspects of treatment. For example, the competing needs of other children in the family might limit time available for treatment, or a back injury might make it difficult for a parent to carry out physiotherapy. Practical support might be all that is required. Other problems might require more ingenuity to resolve.

The child refusing treatment

If the child is getting upset or refusing treatment, parents might lack the emotional reserve to persevere. Most children learn how to manipulate their parents. Parents who do not understand the importance of the treatment will find it particularly difficult to persevere. Child psychology or psychiatric input can be helpful.

Denial   Some families experience difficulties accepting the diagnosis and subsequent treatment. Some never accept it. Ideally with a good team and support, especially at the time of diagnosis, this situation will be avoided. If denial is intractable and non-adherence is continuous, this can become a child protection issue.

Non-adherence by the individual with CF

Children sometimes refuse treatment from a very early age. This can continue throughout their lives and needs addressing as soon as it is recognised (Sharp, Strauss & Lorch 1992).

Understanding the need for treatment   It is often assumed that because individuals have always had treatment, they understand its basis. Continuing education should avoid this assumption. Compliance increases in those who feel they can talk to their doctors and know about their illness. It is important to realise that some parents will co-opt responsibility for informing their child about their disease to the CF Team. If this is not made clear a chronic lack of understanding will prevail.

Teenage rebellion and 'why me?'   Teenagers commonly reject rules and authority. Daily treatment is restrictive and they resent being different from their peers. Denial and treatment rejection is common at this age without thought about the implications. Teenagers need to have their views acknowledged and should be encouraged to participate in decisions about their treatment. Whilst compromising on all treatment is not possible, discussion and compromise in some areas can help towards better compliance in the future.

Fear of losing face   Many teenagers who are rebellious find it hard to back down over an issue. They might believe that complying with treatment gives their parents a moral victory and this can prevent them from asking for help. Parents and CF Teams should always try to ensure that there is a 'way back' for the teenager without them having to admit they were wrong or suffering 'I told you so' comments. Keeping lines of communication open and trying not to be judgemental is helpful.

Fear of the future and growing up   Children might fear the future and retain childlike dependency on their parents. Indeed, parents may encourage this dependency and over protection is not uncommon. With increasing survival well into adult life this is to be discouraged. Teenagers should be given clear and accurate information about their disease and its likely impact, thus ensuring their views are based on fact not myth.

Extreme adherence to treatment

Individuals who perform their treatment with religious zeal might not achieve the high standard of health they are hoping for. Minor non-adherence (for example, missing physiotherapy to attend a birthday party) surely benefits overall wellbeing.

It should be recognised that some of the problems with over-adherence can be caused by the CF Team's emphasis on performing treatment conscientiously. Over zealous parents can take these requests to extremes and out of the context in which they were given.

TIMES OF PARTICULAR STRESS

These are unique to each family but the following vulnerable periods can stretch the ability to cope:

- Diagnosis
- First major exacerbation or hospitalization
- Development of complications, for example the need for gastrostomy or increased intravenous antibiotics
- Growing up and adult issues, for example employment and pregnancy
- Terminal phase and bereavement.

DIAGNOSIS

When a child is born, the life of the family changes forever. During pregnancy parents' thoughts turn to the future, wondering what it will hold for their new arrival. The diagnosis of CF changes all this and holds only the promise of uncertainty and disruption to normal living. Life for the family becomes a juggling act as they try to coordinate daily treatments with the demands of everyday family life.

Following the introduction of national screening, most patients will be diagnosed prior to them having a health problem. The diagnosis of a life-threatening disease will be entirely unexpected. There will be a small number who will have a false negative result from screening. When their diagnosis is finally made their parents may find it even more difficult to come to terms with this information having been told that the disease had been ruled out (see Table 10.1).

Introduction to the team and available services

Centres vary, but it is our practice to admit newly diagnosed patients to hospital and ensure the following are adequately addressed:

- All team members are introduced and have time to get to know the family.
- All components of treatment are gradually phased in.
- The family has a breathing space to adjust to their new situation – although external pressures such as other children and employment need considering.
- The family becomes familiar with the in-patient environment for subsequent care.
- Direct observation, teaching and feedback can occur to ensure that the family is competent with recommended treatment regimens.
- A fuller assessment of the family's needs can be made and assistance with financial or social problems addressed.

Table 10.1   Relating the
diagnosis.

DO'S	DON'TS
• Introduce every person present and explain why he or she is there. • Come to the point of the consultation quickly, be positive and honest. • Give clear, concise information and be prepared to repeat it. • Use emotionally neutral language; it helps parents to have a more positive outlook. • Start the consultation with a brief review of past medical history and how they have reached the point they are at now. • Keep information to key issues that are important to the immediate future: include a simple explanation of the pathology, basic inheritance, initial treatments and future expectations. • Warn against reading conflicting and outdated information. Give information in a media that is accessible to the parents. • Ensure the parents have an opportunity to ask questions or request information is repeated. • Ensure the family understand what will happen next. • Be available to see the family again. • Give the parents an opportunity to be alone together after the consultation. • Refer to the child by the name used by the family.	• Start the consultation by 'I'm sorry to say' as parents find it hard to be positive after negative statements. • Waffle around the reason for the consultation – this can increase parental anxiety. • Forget that families might have prior knowledge or experiences of CF. Make sure you know what these are. • Make the parents feel rushed and unable to ask questions. • Forget to emphasise that new improved treatments are becoming available all the time. • Use medical jargon, abbreviations or long, complex explanations. What you may not consider to be jargon parents might. Use plain, simple language and explain terms used. • Use offensive words such as 'he is a cystic'. • Overload the family with too much information initially. • Forget the value of local and national support groups so that families can make contact if desired. • Forget to reassure parents that stories they hear in the media might not accurately reflect well-being of the majority. • Make predictions in years about long term survival.

Diagnosis is a time of extreme stress and evokes mixed emotions:

Shock and Disbelief   'Our child looks well' so how can this result be true? Such families often suffer considerable morbidity in anticipation of the complications that might follow.

Relief   'Finally we know what is wrong and have an explanation for our child's problems.' These families often cope better as a result of the health benefits that their child accrues following diagnosis.

Anger   … towards professionals who they perceive as not having listened or caused delay in reaching the diagnosis.

Guilt   … for not being more assertive at an earlier stage and for failing to get the best possible care.
    … for passing on the gene.

Grief   … for the loss of a 'normal' child and all the expectations that accompany this.

Denial   The diagnosis might be rejected or doubted and alternative opinions requested.

Difficulties experienced by families prior to diagnosis affect:

- The way they cope with the diagnosis
- The long-term adaptation to the condition
- The relationships they form with the multidisciplinary team.

The CF Team must acknowledge the family's experiences and feelings about the time prior to the diagnosis and allow them to be discussed. Feelings of anger and guilt are common and need to be expressed. In the long term these can be harmful and parents need help to resolve these issues as soon as possible. Encouraging parents to take positive action can prove useful but they should be encouraged to avoid 'knee jerk' reactions that might subsequently be regretted.

Breaking the news (Blum 1996)

The timing and way in which the diagnosis is related is crucial. It can colour the family's expectation for life. Forward planning is vital. Regional policies should be in place for ready access to specialist services.

Remember

Research has shown that families attach more importance to information given at diagnosis than at any other time.

In the community   Most infants diagnosed through screening will be at home and the family unaware of impending news. Regional laboratories processing blood spot tests should have an established policy for dealing with positive results. One important issue is to get families promptly to a specialist centre for diagnostic confirmation, and to meet the CF Team.

In many areas a health visitor and the CF nurse specialist will visit the family's home to inform them about positive results. Infants with raised IRT results will have been screened for common CFTR mutations on the same blood spot (see Chapter 3). Those who are heterozygotes will undergo repeat IRT testing and will be referred for sweat testing if there is sustained hypertrypisnogenaemia. Parents need to know that until a positive sweat test (or the discovery of two gene mutations) has confirmed the diagnosis, their child does not definitely have CF. Ideally, families should be able to have a sweat test and get the results within

48 hours of being notified about a positive blood spot test. Many centres will perform confirmatory sweat tests on all children with a positive blood spot test, even if they have two identifiable genes, and will relate the diagnosis only after the sweat test result is available.

Having the CF nurse undertake a joint visit with the health visitor ensures that any immediate questions can be answered accurately and that current information is given. This also enables the CF and community teams to make contact and establish a working partnership.

It is important to consider how the diagnosis is related to the family.

Setting the scene

The right person (Buckman 1992)   Ideally, this should be the consultant who is going to provide care for the child and another member of the CF Team – usually the nurse, who has already met the family.

If the child is already under the care of another consultant they should relate the diagnosis and introduce the CF Team. Onlookers including ward staff must be avoided unless there are specific reasons for their presence or they have developed a very close relationship with the family.

The right place   The room should be quiet and comfortable. It should be a place where the family can remain without a member of staff needing to be present. Consultant offices should be avoided.

The right time   The appointment should be convenient for the family and as soon as possible after initial contact. Appointments made for the day after the initial home visit allow parents the time to make any necessary arrangements but do not leave them in suspense for too long. Allow plenty of time for the appointment.

No distractions and interruptions   Ensure no interruption by bleep, telephone, or people wanting to access the room.

Consider children in the family   Consider alternative supervision for accompanying children. The presence of children can make it difficult for parents to talk openly and express their feelings. If of an appropriate age, the affected child and their siblings will need explanations and reassurances but it is not appropriate to do this when relating the diagnosis to the parents.

Avoid information overload   It is impossible for the family to absorb all the necessary information instantaneously. Aspects of treatment need to be introduced gradually. Prioritise the introduction of different aspects of treatment according to their relative need.

Select supportive information   Leaflets, pamphlets and booklets should be available. Audio-visual information can be helpful and given to families to take away. The previous contact with the health visitor can be helpful in determining the most appropriate type of information.

Identify special needs   Special needs such as deafness, language difficulties or learning difficulties must be identified and catered for. Use hospital translator services when necessary.

How to tell (Williams 2001)

Families construct belief systems based on information given at diagnosis, which can prove difficult to contradict in the future – even in the event of good news about an aspect of the disease. This can have a significant impact on long-term management.

Families also come to the diagnosis interview with preconceived ideas about medical staff and the health service in general. Whilst consultants might try hard to appear friendly and approachable their intelligence and verbal eloquence can seem threatening to some parents. Many parents will attach social stereotypes to members of the CF Team, based purely on their perceptions about how a doctor, a nurse or a social worker should be or what they do. This can make it difficult for some team members to access families, particularly social workers and those working in mental health.

Every parent has a different view about how they would like to be told their child has CF. By following a few simple rules and observing the parents' body language, the informing consultant should be able to give the news in an acceptable way that marks the beginning of a constructive working relationship.

FIRST MAJOR EXACERBATION OR HOSPITALISATION (Lingham 1996)

In most cases, following diagnosis and treatment, there is a stable period and families begin to regain control of their lives. The daily demands of treatment become part of family life. Parents often comment: 'we hardly notice it now, it is just a way of life to us.'

When the child's health is stable, parents often gain confidence in their ability to keep their child healthy. They sometimes drift away from support groups or parents' meetings, thus avoiding the possibility of exposure to the more negative aspects of the condition.

Parents find it easy to emphasise the 'normal' aspects of their child's life and may actually neglect to mention disturbing symptoms to professional staff for fear of the consequences.

Well meaning comments from the outside world, such as '...doesn't he/she look well' or 'you would never know that there was anything wrong' tend to reinforce this strategy.

Inevitably medical problems, needing increased treatment, will occur. Once again the spectre of CF intrudes on family life. Daily routines change and confidence can be lost. Carefully avoided reminders about the condition are brought back into focus and the family is forced to confront hidden concerns.

A first exacerbation is a source of major stress and anxiety. Parents usually need extra support at this time. They will have memories from the time of diagnosis and returning to hospital might evoke the emotions they experienced at that time. All staff should be aware that this is a first admission.

The stress of admission for a first respiratory exacerbation might be increased if the parents have not appreciated the change in health until a routine outpatient visit. It is important that an admission is not perceived as punishment by the child and that the whole family is supported throughout their stay.

> **Remember**
>
> Hospital admission is an opportunity for the family to learn new skills and enhance old ones. A positive experience enables families to return to their usual routines more quickly and with confidence.

Follow up

- Home visits following discharge allow progress to be monitored and new skills to be reviewed. These offer support to the family.
- The child should be encouraged to return to their previous level of activity if possible. Parents are at risk of overprotecting their children following exacerbations.
- Out-patient review shortly after discharge gives the opportunity to ensure symptoms have not returned. Parents can be reluctant to admit that a problem is still ongoing or recurring if the admission has been a stressful one.

ADAPTING TO THE PROGRESSION OF ILLNESS

There comes a time when the patient and their family are unable to reconcile the demands of treatment with 'normal' daily living and must adapt accordingly. How and when they recognise these changes varies, as does the acceptance of the need to change life styles.

Problems for the individual

The need for increasingly complex and invasive treatment can be frightening. Respiratory compromise impacts on many aspects of daily life and can result in low self-esteem. Major individual concerns are often not the same as those surmised by health care professionals or parents. All need the opportunity to discuss such issues.

Children of all ages often mask their true concerns for fear of upsetting their parents. Young children in particular can find it difficult to discuss issues they think their parents have tried to hide. It is not uncommon for young children to know a lot more about their disease and prognosis than their parents believe.

Problems for the family

Parents often feel frustrated and angry when, despite their best efforts, there has been an increase in morbidity.

Parents might feel guilty about lapses in treatment regimes. The level of noncompliance at which they feel guilty varies considerably. Some have serious concerns about every minor lapse. Others project their guilt onto the CF Team and blame them for not pushing harder to increase compliance.

Family dynamics can be complex. Often one parent bears the burden of treatment and has most dealings with the CF Team. Attempts should be made to involve both parents in care decisions whilst being clear about access rights and custody orders to ensure unwitting mistakes are not made.

Siblings are often under a lot of strain. There might be physical separation from a parent who has to spend a long time in hospital. It is not uncommon for siblings to have their own psychological problems and these can present as physical symptoms. Many of the services set up to support the affected child will now extend help to siblings (Bluebond-Langner 1996).

Managing this phase

Maintaining communication (Lessing & Tatman 1991)

Access   Any family performing specialised home treatment must have 24-hour access to advice and know there is the chance to 'bail out' through hospital admission.

Community support   Two-way communication with the family's doctor can improve understanding about family issues.

Extra support from the CF Team   Informal discussion with a trusted team member in the home can reveal family difficulties, fears and anxieties.

Intravenous antibiotics at home

Home care is often a popular choice and provides:

- Continuation of more normal home life
- Easier support for the family, by extended family and friends
- The family feel they are in control and have an essential role
- Schooling may be easier to maintain.

> **Remember**
>
> Home therapies can be stressful and a high level of continuous support is essential. It is not an option for all and careful assessment is required before commencing treatment (see Chapter 1, Figures 1.2–4).

Parents may have uncertainties about their own abilities because of disease progression and can find these difficult to voice – especially if they have previously undertaken similar therapies without difficulty. It must never be assumed that because the family normally undertakes home therapy that it will be appropriate on every occasion.

Using inpatient stays

Whilst most families will avoid an admission whenever possible, occasionally an inpatient stay can have beneficial psychological as well as physical effects.

When a patient needs more intensive treatment it is important to consider all of the following before making a decision:

- The nature of the treatment
- Where can it best be carried out
- What training is required
- What support is available
- What else is happening to the family
- The wishes of the individual and their family
- Where and when does the CF Team think treatment would be most appropriate and why.

ADOLESCENCE

The parent–child conflict (Pownceby 1997)

The teenage years are challenging. When the teenager has CF, normal problems can be accentuated by:

- Burden of treatment
- Fears about prognosis
- Rebellion against treatment
- Parental fear of letting go
- Physical immaturity.

Teenagers long for independence but CF imposes many restrictions. Ignoring therapy is a frequently used tactic resulting in family conflicts. Parents feel that all their previous hard work is being wasted. Giving increased responsibility to their child to care for themselves can be very difficult. Increasing symptoms may be taken as evidence of poor compliance. CF Teams sometimes have similar feelings of frustration. Nagging is rarely effective and can block lines of communication. Honest and open discussion can help prevent misunderstanding and enable fears about the future to be expressed.

It is particularly important for adolescents to have an opportunity to be involved in decisions about their health. They often cope better if they feel they have participated in this process.

Remember

Parents might still have outdated expectations of an early death that are resistant to change despite professional reassurance. This problem can be made worse by the popular press or outdated books.

Teenagers can believe that there is a conspiracy between their parents and professionals to present an over-optimistic prognosis.

TRANSITION TO ADULT CARE

A positive move

An important part of moving to an adult service is the acknowledgment that survival into adult life is anticipated. The transfer process is a turning point and a time for the CF individual to look to the future and realise that much of what it holds will be within their control (Miller 1996).

Problems related to transfer

The young adult:

- Will be leaving a team they have known all their life
- May have to accept a new hospital as well as new staff
- Will be expected to meet the professionals without their parents being present
- May find an adult ward a very different environment with more rigid rules (such as visiting times) and older patients.

The parents:

- May feel excluded by the adult team
- Lose friendship and support from the paediatric team they have known over many years
- May be anxious about how their child will manage without them.

The paediatric team:

- May also feel a sense of loss for the patient that they have cared for and nurtured for many years.

The adult team:

- May feel adversely judged after any difference in approach to treatment
- May be blamed by parents if there is a deterioration in health.

Careful planning and good liaison between the paediatric and adult teams can largely overcome these problems.

Timing of transition

- Transition should be a gradual process and never abrupt.
- It should occur when patients are in a stable phase.
- For each individual there is an appropriate time. Age is less important than maturity. The opinions of the young adult are paramount.

> **Remember**
>
> - Avoid times of other major life events such as moving to college or university.
> - Transfer of the terminally ill patient is inappropriate.

Adolescent clinics

A clinic where the paediatric and adult team work together allows gradual familiarisation with the new team whilst still maintaining contact with the old. Individuals can be ready to join this clinic at any time from 13 years. Attendance at this clinic will continue for several years. During this time the following can also take place:

- Visits to the adult ward
- Discussions with the adult team to learn about their service

- The young adult becomes more autonomous and starts to see the team without their parents
- Issues such as contraception can be discussed.

REPRODUCTIVE HEALTH
(See Chapter 16)

Issues concerning sex, fertility and pregnancy should have been discussed before they become practical issues. Parents should be prepared to give information to their child to supplement general sex education in schools. There is no right age at which such discussions are appropriate. Once individuals start showing signs of puberty discussions should certainly take place (Smith 1997).

> **Remember**
>
> It is the role of the Paediatric team to have discussed with the patient sexual issues relating to CF prior to transfer.

Males

It is important for boys to know the difference between infertility and impotence as this is frequently muddled. Virtually all CF men are infertile and this can be confirmed by semen analysis. The value of barrier contraceptive devices for safe sex, not just the prevention of pregnancy, should be made clear.

Females

Girls should be told that their fertility is usually unaffected and warned about the risks of an unplanned pregnancy. Discussions should include safe sex and not just pregnancy.

THE TERMINAL PHASE
(See Chapter 23)

Despite optimal care there comes a time when health deteriorates irrecoverably. For some there will be a significant event, which will be seen as a turning point, whilst for others it will be a gradual decline. However it happens, acknowledging the process and what it means can be incredibly difficult for all those involved.

Effect on the family

By this stage CF can no longer be incorporated into normal life. Its intrusion into daily routines becomes increasingly time consuming. Major changes in lifestyle are needed for all those involved. A family member may have to consider stopping work and become a primary carer. Those who have previously left home may have to return.

Emotional response

Families commonly feel a mixture of emotions as they face the terminal decline of a loved one.

Frustration   This is a disheartening time for the family. If they have been compliant they might feel cheated. If awaiting transplantation there might be frustration because this has not come to fruition, leading to poor acceptance of terminal care.

Guilt Where compliance has been poor some might feel guilty for having missed treatments and regret not doing more. Even compliant families often wonder if they could have done more.

Resentment Commonly families feel a sense of injustice with questions such as 'why me?'

Denial Persistent denial makes it very difficult to manage the family. Hopefully this will be a transient phase.

The CF team should offer help and support throughout this difficult time (see Chapter 23). For all it is a period of readjustment – to reorganise priorities and alter expectations. Transplant options should have been explored before entering this phase but they may need to be discussed again (see Chapter 19).

OTHER AREAS OF CONCERN
Needle phobias

Many experience needle phobias. Whilst this is frequently considered when dealing with children, many adults experience the same feelings of anxiety. The type of intervention needed will depend on the degree of anxiety. The following techniques can be tried:

- Allow the individual some feeling of control, for example participating in choice of access site used.
- If the patient would like to know what will happen, give a careful explanation. Some prefer a running commentary of what is happening.
- Entonox can be highly effective. It is important that individuals are assessed carefully as some of the medical complications associated with CF contraindicate its use (see Chapter 24). In suitable patients it offers a quick method of reducing anxiety and pain throughout the procedure.
- Topical anaesthetic creams work well at numbing the skin, but children will often spend the time needed for the cream to work worrying about what happens next.
- Ethyl chloride spray is a cold spray that numbs the skin instantly, although it can cause veins to disappear!
- Distraction techniques – used in combination with one of the above. Give the patients something else to think about whilst the procedure is carried out.
- Oral sedation can be useful, if plenty of time is available for it to take effect. It is most effective when used with topical anaesthetic creams.
- Intravenous sedation is usually only used to place larger lines and is generally given via a butterfly into the back of a hand.
- Play therapy or psychologists (depending on age) help individuals work through their fears and teach them how to remain calm.
- In extreme cases the use of totally implantable venous access devices should be considered if the patient is requiring repeated venepuncture. This will not completely obviate the need for needles and the need for monthly flushing must be considered.
- Parents should be advised against using needles as threats, this will increase the child's fear: 'if you don't take your medicine you will have to have an injection'.

Nocturnal enuresis

This is surprisingly common, easily overlooked by medical staff and can be debilitating. Regular nocturnal enuresis after the age of 5 years should be identified and treatment offered. The child might find it impossible to sleep away from home (due to the wetting) thus having to miss out on many social activities. Parents are likely to have disturbed nights and extra washing resulting in tiredness and irritability. There are a number of treatments available (Rogers 1996), ideally used in conjunction with advice and support from an enuresis clinic.

Initial assessment

Identifying the extent of the problem and possible trigger factors.

- Assess the parents' and child's attitude towards the problem.
- Assess 'functional pay offs' when wetting occurs, for example sleeping in the parental bed.
- Keep a diary of episodes for at least four weeks.
- Reassure and advise that this is common in CF and will improve.

Specific therapy:

- Stop functional 'pay offs'
- Scheduled arousal methods (lifting).

If there is no improvement after 4 weeks involve an enuresis clinic.

Enuresis Alarms

- Can be worn on the body or as a bed pad
- Use for 16 weeks with fortnightly review.

Desmospray

- Can be used for 12 weeks then stopped for a week
- If relapse occurs, longer term use should be considered
- Very useful for nights away from home, school trips, camping, etc.
- Should be used in conjunction with other training methods.

It is important to recognise the impact that this condition can have on the family and the psychological effect it has on the child. Parents might ignore the problem, assuming the child will grow out of it. Whilst this might be true, early intervention can save a lot of misery for the entire family.

ERIC (Enuresis Resource and Information Centre) is a national organisation providing literature and resources for families (see Chapter 25).

Stress incontinence

Many adult females experience stress incontinence, especially during respiratory exacerbations (White, Stiller & Roney 2000). Other occasions that might cause involuntary leakage include performing spirometry, coughing and some physiotherapy techniques. Many suffer in silence, too embarrassed to mention their problem.

Stress incontinence also occurs among children and some as young as seven years have reported symptoms. Some have also reported problems with stress faecal incontinence – usually an involuntary leakage of oily liquid. Few will voluntarily discuss their problems, although most have resorted to using some sort of sanitary protection.

Problems with urinary and/or faecal incontinence are not obviously related to the severity of lung disease, although the severity of incontinence symptoms can be linked to respiratory exacerbations. Some might under perform lung function tests and suppress their cough in attempts to avoid leakage.

It is important that CF Teams ask direct questions about incontinence. This is not exclusively a female problem and males often find it even harder to discuss. Pelvic floor exercise might be an effective intervention to address symptoms. Referral to urology services may be appropriate for some patients.

References

Bluebond-Langner M 1996 In the shadow of illness. Princeton, New Jersey.

Blum R W 1996 Compliance with therapeutic regimes among adolescents with chronic conditions. Presentation, International CF Conference, Jerusalem.

Buckman R 1992 How to break bad news. Papermac, London

Lask B 1994 Non-adherence in CF: methods, meanings and management. Journal of the Royal Society of Medicine 21:25–27

Lessing D, Tatman M 1991 Paediatric home care in 1990s. Archives of Diseases in Childhood 66:994–996

Lingham S, Newton R 1996 Right from the start. BPA Standing Committee on Paediatric Practice Guidelines. Ref No PPG/96/02, London

McCubbin H, McCubbin M, Patterson J et al 1983 Coping Health Inventory for Parents: an assessment of parental coping patterns in the care of the chronically ill child. Journal of Marriage and the Family 45:359–370

Millor S 1996 Transition of care in adolescence. Paediatric Nursing 8:9 NOV

Pownceby J 1997 Coming of age project. CF Trust, Kent

Quittner A 1996 Identifying sources of parent – teen conflict and targets for intervention. Presentation at International CF Conference, Jerusalem

Rogers J 1996 Cognitive bladder training in the community. Paediatric Nursing 8(8) OCT

Rolles C J, Maddison J 1995 Is this Münchhausen Syndrome by Proxy. Poster presentation, European CF Conference, Brussels

Sharp M C, Strauss R P, Lorch S C 1992 Communicating medical bad news: parents' experiences and preferences. Journal of Pediatrics 121:539–546

Smith R 1997 Promoting the sexual health of young people. Paediatric Nursing 9(2) MARCH

White D, Stiller K, Roney F 2000 The prevalence and severity of symptoms of urinary incontinence in adult CF patients. Physiotherapy Theory & Practice 16:35–42

Whyte D A 1994 Family nursing: The case of CF. Avebury, Aldershot

Williams D P 2001 The well siblings' perspective. In: Bluebond-Langer, Lask, Angst (eds) Pyschosocial aspects of cyctic fibrosis. Arnold, London

Wilson J, Fosson A, Kanga J et al 1990 Longitudinal relationships between family environment and clinically significant deterioration of pulmonary function. Pediatric Pulmonology 5:285

Recommended reading

'Psychosocial Aspects of CF'. Ed Bluebond-Langner M, Lask B & Angst DB, 2001 Arnold – London. ISBN 0-340-75891-0

'Living in the Shadow of Illness' Bluebond-Langner M, 1996, Princeton – New Jersey

Chapter **11**

Diabetes and glucose intolerance

Fiona Regan, Peter Betts

INTRODUCTION

Cystic Fibrosis Related Diabetes (CFRD) is the most common co-morbidity affecting individuals with CF. The onset is insidious. Diagnosis is typically preceded by a long prodromal phase of glucose intolerance during which the early insulin response to a glucose load is delayed. Individuals can become diabetic during infective episodes but revert to normal glucose tolerance. By the time of CFRD diagnosis, insulin deficiency is the primary problem. Evidence is accruing that early treatment with insulin improves quality of life and life expectancy. Diagnosis is often delayed.

EPIDEMIOLOGY

- The CF centre in Copenhagen has reported prevalence figures of 1.5%, 13% and 50% in individuals aged 10, 20 and 30 years (Lanng 1994).
- There is an age-dependent incidence rate of around 5% per year starting in the teenage years (Lanng 1991a).
- CFRD has been reported in children as young as 2 years (Rodman, Doershuk & Roland 1986).

Large variations in the prevalence of CFRD between CF centres are probably a result of different screening methods.

PATHOLOGY

- On histology there is significant pancreatic fibrosis, inter and intra islet cell fibrosis, and a greater reduction in insulin-producing beta cells compared to glucagon-producing alpha cells.
- Islet amyloid polypeptide is present. This is also found in the islets of non-CF patients with type 2 but not type 1 diabetes.
- Islet cell antibodies (Stutchfield, O'Halloran & Smith 1988) and glutamic acid decarboxylase antibodies (Nousia-Arvanitakis 2000) are variably reported but autoimmunity is not thought to be aetiologically significant.
- There is poor association between HLA genetic markers and CFRD.
- CFRD is much more common in the more severe class I–III mutations associated with pancreatic insufficiency.
- There is a slight female preponderance.

AETIOLOGICAL FACTORS

Factors that influence the onset and course of diabetes in the patient with cystic fibrosis include:

- High energy expenditure
- Respiratory infection: further increasing energy requirements and causing insulin resistance
- Liver dysfunction: affecting gluconeogenesis and liver insulin sensitivity
- Malnutrition: impairing insulin synthesis
- Malabsorption
- Abnormal intestinal transit time: affecting food absorption
- Increased insulin clearance by 30–40%
- Glucagon deficiency
- Dose-dependent oral corticosteroid treatment.

CLINICAL FEATURES

Impaired glucose tolerance is usually asymptomatic. During the prodromal phase of diabetes, a reduced dietary intake can mask symptoms although such individuals usually fail to gain weight. Episodes of reactive hypoglycaemia can also occur prior to treatment. Glucose intolerance or diabetes can become clinically overt when:

- The individual becomes unwell, for example with a severe chest infection
- Supplemental enteral feeding is started
- Oral corticosteroids are given
- A woman becomes pregnant.

Remember

- Always perform a GTT when there is unexplained weight loss or deterioration in respiratory or nutritional status.
- Monitor blood glucose levels when supplemental feeding or systemic steroid treatment is commenced.
- Monitor blood glucose levels routinely during the first 24 hours of hospital admission for respiratory exacerbations (see Chapter 1).

Whilst symptomatic diabetes is readily recognised by the triad of polyuria, polydipsia and weight loss, these typical symptoms of hyperglycaemia can be absent for many years prior to diagnosis. Ketoacidosis is rare.

CFRD often has a significant impact on pulmonary function. There can be deterioration in overall clinical status for up to 5 years before CFRD develops. CFRD can increase mortality by up to six fold (Cystic Fibrosis Foundation 1998, Lanng 1992, Lanng 1991b).

COMPLICATIONS

As a result of increased life expectancy, the long-term microvascular complications of diabetes are increasingly recognized (Sullivan & Denning 1989). Macrovascular complications are rare but might increase in the future.

Screening for complications should be part of a CFRD modified annual review and include:

- Enquiry into episodes of hypoglycaemia, eyes, feet, skin and genitourinary problems
- Fundal photography for retinopathy in children aged >12 years
- Measurement of blood pressure and urinary albumin excretion for nephropathy
- Testing of tendon reflexes, vibration sense and symptom enquiries for neuropathy
- Examination of foot pulses
- Fasting lipid profile.

DIAGNOSIS

When overt symptomatic diabetes is present the diagnosis is rarely in doubt and is simply confirmed by blood glucose determination. Treatment with insulin is mandatory.

Ideally, glucose intolerance should be diagnosed before deterioration in health and growth through screening.

There is no satisfactory single test to reliably identify those without overt symptoms. The following investigations can be useful for screening and monitoring:

Blood glucose monitoring

Several analyses of glucose intolerance detected by standard oral glucose tolerance testing have shown fasting blood glucose measurements to be poorly sensitive (Lanng 1994, Solomon 2003, Moran 1998, Yung 1999). However, pre- and 2 hour post-prandial blood glucose monitoring might usefully identify hyperglycaemia during initial treatment of acute respiratory exacerbations (see Chapter 1). Individuals receiving oral corticosteroids and enteral feeds should be monitored shortly after commencing treatment. Initial pre- and post-feed monitoring should also be routine for enterally fed patients whenever they are admitted to hospital. Preliminary studies have validated the use of continuous glucose monitoring systems which might prove useful in the early detection of clinically significant insulin deficiency (Dobson 2002).

HbA1c

The level of glycosolated haemoglobin as measured by HbA1c is routinely used to assess diabetic control. Normal levels pre-diagnosis do not exclude the possibility of impaired glucose tolerance or CFRD.

The test has poor sensitivity and should not be used for screening without additional glucose tolerance testing.

Oral glucose tolerance test (OGTT)

This remains the gold standard for the diagnosis of glucose intolerance and frank diabetes. The 1999 WHO criteria (WHO 1999) are:

Impaired fasting glucose	fasting venous plasma glucose 6.1–6.9 mmol/L
Impaired Glucose tolerance	2 hour venous plasma glucose 7.8–11.0 mmol/L (after oral glucose load)

> **Note**
>
> Up to 58% of individuals with impaired glucose tolerance revert to normal on subsequent testing but are at increased risk of developing CFRD.

Diabetes	fasting venous plasma glucose >7.0 mmol/L 2 hour venous plasma glucose >11.1 mmol/L (after oral glucose load)

The GTT consists of:

- Unrestricted diet for three days prior to test
- Fasted 10–16 hours. Plain water only to drink for the duration of the test.
- Take basal venous plasma sample for glucose concentration.
- Give orally 1.75 g/kg of anhydrous glucose (to a maximum of 75 g glucose) or 9.1 ml/kg of chilled Lucozade (not Lucozade Sport) to a maximum of 390 ml. The chilling is useful in reducing nausea.
- Diagnosis confirmed on venous plasma glucose taken at base line and after 2 hours.

RECOMMENDATIONS FOR SCREENING FOR CYSTIC FIBROSIS RELATED DIABETES

Perform an oral glucose tolerance test in:

- All individuals over the age of 10 years as a routine investigation at annual review
- Any individual with symptoms suggesting frank diabetes
- Any individual with unexplained failure to gain weight, weight loss or deterioration in respiratory function
- Before a planned pregnancy
- At the time of confirmation of pregnancy
- Middle of the second and third trimester.

MANAGEMENT

Impaired glucose tolerance

- These individuals are at increased risk of progression to CFRD. They should be provided with equipment to monitor their blood glucose when unwell.
- If truly asymptomatic no other specific interventions are indicated. OGTT should be repeated annually or sooner if there is any decline in well-being.

- Consider insulin treatment for those with weight loss or worsening lung problems. A small series of individuals with normal OGTT but high random glucoses have shown marked clinical improvement in weight and lung function when treated with insulin (Dobson 2002).

As yet there is little evidence to recommend oral therapy. A small study showed that a subgroup of individuals could be managed adequately on the oral sulphonylurea glibenclamide without worsening clinical deterioration compared to a group treated with insulin (Rosenecker 2001). New oral agents such as repaglinide, which stimulates first phase insulin secretion in a glucose dependent fashion, have yet to be fully evaluated in CF. A recent study demonstrated that it was less effective in normalising hyperglycaemia and hypoinsulinaemia than insulin Lispro. The dose might not have been large enough to demonstrate full potential (Moran 2001). Metformin is contraindicated in cystic fibrosis.

Cystic Fibrosis Related Diabetes

Individuals with CFRD should be reviewed by a multidisciplinary team, ideally with diabetic and cystic fibrosis teams in a joint clinic.

Insulin is the mainstay of treatment. Some oral hypoglycaemic agents promote first phase insulin release and might have a role in asymptomatic CFRD. Further studies are needed.

When insulin is initiated to meet the demands of an increased energy supply such as an enteral feed and the feed is subsequently discontinued or reduced, the need for insulin may disappear. These individuals need careful ongoing surveillance and probably will require long-term insulin at some point in the future.

Insulin treatment promotes protein catabolism and can reverse declining weight and lung function. Insulin frequently improves appetite and the dose might need to be increased as food intake improves.

Starting insulin

- A regime that best fits the individual's lifestyle should be used.
- Doses will need adjusting according to blood glucose values. These should be measured before and 2 hours after meals until stable. The aim is to keep pre- and post-prandial blood glucose values above 4 mmol/L and below 8 mmol/L.
- The basal insulin requirement is relatively low when not acutely unwell.
- Ideally insulin regimes should focus on meal coverage with rapid acting insulin given before food and a long acting insulin given at bedtime. 0.5–1 U of rapid acting insulin is usually adequate to cover 15 g carbohydrate.
- For those unwilling to have four injections a day, a twice daily subcutaneous injection of medium acting Isophane or mixed insulin such as Mixtard 30 can be used. 0.2 units/kg/day is a suitable starting dose. Two-thirds of the total daily dose should be given in the morning and one-third in the evening.
- The use of a single injection of one of the new long acting insulin analogues, might be sufficient for some patients.

- Those receiving overnight enteral nutrition will probably need a larger proportion of insulin at night. If a regime of quick acting insulin before meals is being used during the day, a mixture of medium and quick acting insulin given at the start of the feed should result in adequate insulin cover for the whole feed.
- An increase in insulin requirements up to 1–2 units/kg/day can occur, particularly during puberty.
- Insulin doses might need increasing at times of acute infection or when oral steroids are given.

Remember

Treatment with insulin should be considered in any individual failing to thrive or exhibiting unexplained clinical deterioration.

Monitoring

Individuals receiving insulin should monitor their blood glucose daily. They should include pre and post-prandial readings after different meals throughout the day.

Those with impaired glucose tolerance should check their blood glucose when unwell.

Those prone to developing intermittent CFRD when unwell should check their blood glucose 3–4 times daily during periods of deterioration.

Pregnant women who develop gestational diabetes should check their sugars 4–6 times a day.

NUTRITION

It is important to ensure an adequate calorie intake to sustain normal growth. Insulin requirements need to be tailored around dietary intake. This is particularly relevant to overnight enteral feeding. Conflicts between dietary advice for CF and diabetes should usually be resolved in favour of the CF diet.

Remember

CFRD is best treated with insulin. Nutritional management should be tailored to the cystic fibrosis dietetic needs and the administration of insulin matched accordingly.

Dietary guidelines

- Ensure complex carbohydrate is eaten at each meal, especially at bedtime.
- Ensure regular meals and snacks are eaten.
- Puddings containing normal sugar should be allowed.
- Do not restrict the fat content of the diet.
- Encourage chocolate biscuits or cakes for snacks (i.e. foods containing fat and sugar).
- Encourage sugar-free drinks between meals (except during acute illness).
- Encourage 'eat to appetite'.

- Drink no more than 2–3 units of alcohol at any time and never on an empty stomach.
- 'Diabetic' products such as diabetic chocolate should be discouraged because of the laxative effect of their sorbitol content.

PSYCHOLOGY

The diagnosis of CFRD can evoke anxiety and fear at a difficult time (see Chapter 10). Some families might believe that the diagnosis of a second chronic disease indicates inevitable decline and that death is imminent. The teams involved need to actively seek out and address such misconceptions. If the potential complication of diabetes has been fully discussed before it occurs, this might help improve acceptance of the diagnosis.

CFRD imposes an additional burden of care at a time when some young adults are rejecting standard therapy. Injections of insulin, regular blood glucose testing and regular meals can be hard to reconcile with a busy lifestyle. Fortunately ketoacidosis as a result of missed insulin injections rarely occurs in CFRD.

Difficulties with compliance might occur because of a relative lack of symptoms prior to diagnosis.

Psychology input from professionals with prior knowledge of both conditions can help address these issues.

As more data becomes available about the consequences of CFRD it is likely that even tighter diabetic control will be recommended in the future.

> **Remember**
>
> It is very important to stress the long-term health benefits that are expected from treatment.

References

Cystic Fibrosis Foundation Patient Registry 1988 Annual Data Report. Cystic Fibrosis Foundation, Bethseda, MD

Dobson L, Hattersley A, Tiley S et al 2002 Clinical improvement in cystic fibrosis with early insulin treatment. Archives of Diseases in Childhood 87:430–431

Lanng S, Thorsteinsson B, Erichsen G et al 1991a Glucose tolerance in cystic fibrosis. Archives of Diseases in Childhood 66:612–616

Lanng S, Thorsteinsson B, Nerup J et al 1991b Diabetes mellitus and lung function in cystic fibrosis. Diabetes 40(suppl 1):525A (abstract)

Lanng S, Thorsteinsson B, Nerup J et al 1992 Influence of the development of diabetes on clinical status in patients with cystic fibrosis. European Journal of Pediatrics 151:684–687

Lanng S, Thorsteinsson B, Lund-Andersen C et al 1994 Diabetes mellitus in Danish cystic fibrosis patients: prevalence and late diabetic complications. Acta Paediatrica Scandinavia 83:72–77

Moran A, Doherty L, Wang X et al 1998 Abnormal glucose tolerance in cystic fibrosis. Journal of Pediatrics 133:10–17

Moran A, Phillips J, Milla C 2001 Insulin and glucose excursion following pre-meal insulin lispro or repaglinide in cystic fibrosis-related diabetes. Diabetes Care 24:1706–1710

Nousia-Arvanitakis S, Galli-Tsinopoulou A, Dracoulacos D et al 2000 Islet autoantibodies and insulin dependent diabetes mellitus in cystic fibrosis. Journal of Pediatric Endocrinology and Metabolism 13:319–324

Rodman H M, Doershuk C F, Roland J M 1986 The interaction of the two diseases: diabetes mellitus and cystic fibrosis. Medicine 65:389–397

Rosenecker J, Eichler I, Barmeier H et al 2001 Diabetes mellitus and cystic fibrosis: Comparison of clinical parameters in patients treated with insulin versus oral glucose-lowering agents. Pediatric Pulmonology 32:351–355.

Solomon M, Wilson D, Corey M et al 2003 Glucose intolerance in children with cystic fibrosis. Journal of Pediatrics 142:128–132

Stutchfield P R, O'Halloran S M, Smith C S 1988 HLA type, islet cell antibodies and glucose intolerance in cystic fibrosis. Archives of Diseases in Childhood 63:1234–1239

Sullivan M M, Denning C R 1989 Diabetic microangiopathy in patients with cystic fibrosis. Pediatrics 84:642–646

WHO 1999 Diagnosis and classification of diabetes mellitus Geneva

Moran A, Hardin D, Rodman D et al 1999 Diagnosis, screening and management of CFRD: a consensus conference report. Journal of Diabetes Research and Clinical Practice 45:55–71

Yung B, Kemp M, Hooper J 1999 Diagnosis of cystic fibrosis related diabetes: a selective approach in performing the oral glucose tolerance test based on a combination of clinical and biochemical criteria. Thorax 54:40–43

Recommended reading

The National Service Framework for Diabetes
http://www.doh.gov.uk/nsf/diabetes/index.htm

Diabetes UK
www.diabetes.org.uk

Cystic Fibrosis Trust Guidelines for the Management of Cystic Fibrosis Related Diabetes 2004.

Chapter 12

Liver disease

June Abay, Mark Beattie

INTRODUCTION

Liver and biliary tract disease are well recognised in CF. Careful counselling and appropriate information for both the child and family are essential. The most serious complications are related to portal hypertension rather than synthesis failure. The main aspects of treatment are:

- Prevention of hepatic and biliary complications
- Treatment of variceal bleeding
- Nutritional support
- Liver transplantation.

PATHOLOGY

The CF transmembrane regulator (CFTR) is located in the apical membrane of epithelial cells lining the intra-hepatic bile ducts. CF is the only inherited metabolic disease of the liver with primary pathology in the intra-hepatic bile ducts rather than the hepatocyte. This makes the diagnosis of CF-related liver disease difficult because there is currently no biliary cell function test. Pathogenesis is thought to be related to inspissation of ductular secretions and changes in components of the bile acid pool. This leads to bile duct obstruction, destruction and focal biliary cirrhosis.

Figure 12.1
Hepatosplenomegaly.

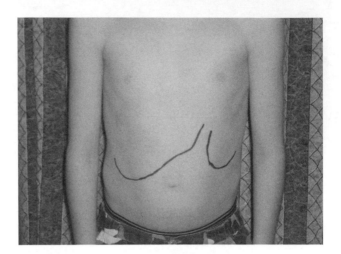

EPIDEMIOLOGY

Most individuals with CF will have at least minor abnormalities of their intra-hepatic biliary system. Prospective studies using ultrasound and biochemical testing for detection report prevalence figures between 18–37%. Liver disease develops in the first 2–10 years of life and presents less commonly thereafter. Approximately 5% will develop cirrhosis with portal hypertension and up to a half of this group will have variceal bleeding. Two to three per cent might ultimately proceed to liver transplantation (Colombo 2002).

> **Remember**
>
> Liver disease usually occurs within the first decade. Screening for liver complications should focus on early childhood.

Risk factors for CF related liver disease are:

- Pancreatic insufficiency (rare in sufficiency)
- Male sex (3:1 preponderance)
- Meconium ileus (5 fold increase).

There is poor concordance of liver disease within CF sib-ships. Other genetic factors include:

- Alpha-1-antitrypsin phenotype
- HLA type
- Variants of mannose binding lectin and transforming growth factor beta expression.

TYPES OF CF LIVER DISEASE

Neonatal cholestasis

- Occurs in less than 5%.
- Associated with meconium ileus.
- Presents with conjugated jaundice with or without hypoalbuminaemia.
- Median duration of jaundice is around 7 months.
- Consider investigations to exclude biliary atresia.
- Good medium term prognosis, if no co-existent problems, after treatment with ursodeoxycholic acid (Shapira 1999).

Hepatic steatosis (fatty liver)

- Is a cause of hepatomegaly in CF identified by ultrasound scanning.
- Can be associated with poor nutrition.
- Does not progress to biliary cirrhosis and requires no specific therapy.
- Is associated with alcohol ingestion and diabetes in non-CF patients.

Biliary tract disease

- Symptomatic biliary disease is rare.
- A non-functioning micro-gallbladder occurs in up to 30% of patients and is usually asymptomatic.
- Gallstones occur in 5–15% of patients; the incidence increases with age. Stones contain calcium bilirubinate and proteins, not a preponderance of cholesterol. Ursodeoxycholic acid is ineffective for dissolving gallstones in CF patients.
- Cholecystitis is rare.
- Pain is severe, colicky and located in the right upper quadrant or epigastrium. Occasionally the pain will be referred to the right subscapular region. Symptoms are thought to occur when a stone impacts in the cystic or common bile duct producing obstruction and proximal distension of the biliary tree or gallbladder. Serum bilirubin, alkaline phosphatase and transaminases may be elevated during or just after pain.
- Laparoscopic cholecystectomy is recommended because of the risks of recurrence and the potential for ascending cholangitis.

Cirrhosis

- Macronodular, multilobular cirrhosis with portal hypertension develops in up to 5% of patients.
- It can be the initial presenting feature of CF.
- Meconium ileus is a risk factor.
- Most patients have pancreatic insufficiency.
- Regular clinical evaluation is the key to early detection. Cirrhosis is frequently asymptomatic and develops insidiously.

SCREENING FOR LIVER PROBLEMS

Liver disease progresses slowly in CF. The following routine screening is recommended:

Abdominal examination at 2-monthly clinic visits

- A palpable liver is most likely due to hepatomegaly rather than displacement by hyperinflated lungs.
- Selective left lobe enlargement is characteristic. This is easily missed if the epigastrium is not palpated.
- The right lobe might feel normal or might even shrink.
- Cutaneous signs of liver disease are rare.
- Jaundice is generally limited to neonatal cholestasis, symptomatic gallstones or end stage liver disease.
- Splenomegaly indicates portal hypertension rather than infection.
- Digital clubbing and oxygen desaturation can occur with cirrhosis without significant pulmonary disease. Cirrhosis can initiate precapillary pulmonary shunting by an unknown mechanism (hepatopulmonary syndrome).

Annual serum liver function tests and prothrombin time

These can be misleading because:

- Transaminases and alkaline phosphatase can be normal in some cases of cirrhosis.
- Transient elevations can occur with respiratory infections, hypoxia and antibiotic exposure.
- Sustained abnormalities of liver function on repeat testing require further investigation and treatment with ursodeoxycholic acid. Follow-up tests should be performed to ensure abnormalities are normalised (see below).
- Prolonged prothrombin time and hypoalbuminaemia are late findings indicative of hepatic decompensation.
- Bilirubin levels are only elevated in advanced liver disease.

Routine liver ultrasound

This should be performed every 2 years during childhood up to the age of 10, and more frequently if there are abnormal findings, or abnormal liver function tests.

- Characterizes the reasons for abnormal abdominal findings.
- Can detect minor abnormalities. Serial scans can be the most sensitive way of detecting disease progression.
- Can detect gallstones, ascites and dilatation of bile ducts or hepatic veins.
- Doppler ultrasound can detect raised hepatic venous and portal venous pressures, but is poorly predictive of the risk of variceal bleeding.

HIDA scanning

Hepatobiliary Scintigraphy (HIDA scanning) uses iminodiacetic acid derivatives to visually assess biliary excretion and provide anatomical definition. Scintigraphy has been used to evaluate the efficacy of choleretic treatment but its place in routine practice is not yet clear. Scanning could be considered in children who have reached 10 years of age with no evidence of liver disease to exclude insidious problems and thus limit the need for further routine ultrasound scanning.

FURTHER INVESTIGATIONS

Barium swallow

This is an insensitive investigation for oesophageal varices and not routinely indicated.

Direct oesophagoscopy

This is mandatory following haematemesis to assess the presence of oesophageal varices, plan treatment and to identify oesophagitis or gastritis which may be a further risk factor for re-bleeding.

Endoscopic retrograde cholangio pancreatography (ERCP)

This should be done in a specialist centre for clear indications (i.e. stones in the common bile duct or suspicion of common bile duct stenosis).

Table 12.1 Investigations to exclude other causes of liver disease.

Investigation	Disorder
Alpha-1-antitrypsin phenotype	Alpha-1-antitrypsin deficiency
Hepatitis serology	Viral hepatitis
Autoimmune profile	Autoimmune hepatitis
Serum copper and caeruloplasmin	Wilson's disease
Serum ferritin, iron and TIBC	Haemochromatosis

Remember

Endoscopy should only be carried out in specialist centres where there is continuing experience in upper GI endoscopy and the ability to treat varices if present.

Liver biopsy

This is not often performed. Liver disease is focal and percutaneous needle biopsy can miss the patchy early lesions thus correlating poorly with overt disease.

MANAGEMENT OF LIVER DISEASE

This should be in conjunction with a Paediatric Hepatology unit. The aims of management are to:

- Prevent progression
- Prevent malnutrition
- Prevent complications
- Intervene early to treat variceal bleeding, fat soluble vitamin deficiency and prevent hepatic decompensation.

Newly diagnosed liver disease

Diagnosis may follow clinical findings/indicative ultrasound features and/or a sustained alteration of liver function tests.

Ursodeoxycholic acid

Initiate treatment with ursodeoxycholic acid 15–25 mg/kg/day divided into 2–3 doses with meals with dose adjustments to achieve normal liver transaminases. Some centres will also give Taurine 30 mg/kg/day in divided doses.

The Cochrane meta-analysis of the benefits of ursodeoxycholic acid to treat CF related liver disease did not find evidence favouring clinically important outcomes. Its use will 'normalise' elevated serum liver enzymes (Columbo 1996). It has also been shown to improve liver morphology on biopsy after two years treatment (Lindblad, Glavmann & Strandvik 1998).

Vitamin K

This should be given routinely to all children once liver disease is identified in addition to other fat-soluble vitamins. Assessment and

Figure 12.2 A Medic Alert bracelet. Medic–Alert Foundation. 1 Bridgewarf, 156 Caledonian Road, NU1 9UU.

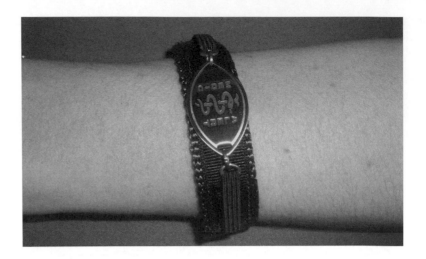

treatment of coagulopathy is essential in patients undergoing surgical procedures.

Monitoring

Liver disease needs careful monitoring to detect the development of portal hypertension. Regular abdominal ultrasounds should be performed. Liver function tests and fat-soluble vitamin status should be checked 6-monthly.

Nutrition

Absolute weight is an insensitive measure of nutritional status because of the increased weight that can occur from hepatosplenomegaly, mesenteric oedema and ascites. More detailed evaluation of lean body mass using anthropometry is recommended. Aggressive use of supplemental feeds can improve nutritional status. Improved nutrition improves survival, quality of life and the outcome of liver transplantation. There is a risk of gastric varicocoeles around gastrostomy tubes in children with advanced liver disease.

Splenomegaly

Splenomegaly is occasionally massive and can cause functional hypersplenism with anaemia and thrombocytopenia. The latter might aggravate a bleeding tendency. Although usually asymptomatic, pain from splenic infarction or perisplenitis can occur. There is a small risk of splenic rupture and affected patients should be discouraged from participating in rigorous contact sports.

Management of acute haematemesis

Bleeding oesophageal varices are a life threatening complication. For those at risk ensure that:

- They and their family are aware of the signs and symptoms of gastrointestinal haemorrhage
- Their blood group is documented

- The individual carries some form of instruction in the event of a bleed such as a Medic-Alert bracelet (see Figure 12.2)
- They have open access to the nearest hospital
- Aspirin and non-steroidal anti-inflammatories are avoided.

Everyone with bleeding should be admitted to a regional specialist centre, even if the bleed is small, because they might have a slow initial bleed followed by a massive bleed.

- Assess the site and extent of the bleed. Melaena might not appear for up to 24 hours.
- Ensure good venous access and monitoring.
- Resuscitate with albumin, fresh frozen plasma and red cell transfusions.
- Correct any coagulopathy with IM Vitamin K 2–5 mg and FFP.
- Administer H2 antagonists and/or proton pump inhibitors.
- Use intravenous octreotide and/or glypressin or vasopressin to reduce portal pressures. Octreotide does not produce systemic vasoconstriction unlike vasopressin.
- Bleeding can be a feature of bacterial peritonitis. Administer broad-spectrum antibiotics.
- As soon as haemodynamically stable, consider diagnostic endoscopy and therapeutic sclerotherapy or band ligation.
- If bleeding continues, balloon tamponade with the modified Sengstaken-Blakemore tube may be necessary although this might be poorly tolerated.
- H2 antagonists or sucralfate may reduce bleeding from gastritis.

Treatment of varices

This is the same as treatment of oesophageal varices from any other cause of liver disease and should be in a specialist centre. The risks of a re-bleed are 60–80% in the next two years. Recurrent variceal haemorrhage is an indication for liver transplantation although temporizing procedures might be necessary in the short term.

- Band ligation has largely replaced injection sclerotherapy.
- Repeat haemorrhage might also be controlled by insertion of transjugular intrahepatic portosystemic stent shunt (TIPSS). This procedure can help stabilize prior to liver transplantation.

Ascites

Ascites often occurs with GI bleeding and the family should be pre-warned of this. Treatment is required if abdominal distension becomes troublesome. Spironolactone (2–3 mg/kg/day) is useful for initial therapy but takes a few days to become effective. Thiazides and frusemide work more quickly but often produce hypokalaemia, hypochloraemia and mild hyponatraemia.

Bacterial peritonitis

Fever, abdominal pain, worsening ascites, diarrhoea and vomiting would suggest spontaneous bacterial peritonitis.

Paracentesis demonstrates a neutrophil count > 250 neutrophils/mm^3. At least 10–30 mls of ascitic fluid should be sent for culture as the density of organisms may be quite low.

Gram-negative bacteria, mainly *E. coli*, are most commonly implicated although individuals with CF are at risk from pseudomonas infection.

Peritonitis requires prompt treatment with broad-spectrum intravenous antibiotics.

Bacterial peritonitis often recurs. Prophylactic therapy with oral norfloxacin has been effective in adults.

LIVER FAILURE

Hepatic decompensation is a late feature of CF liver disease. Liver transplantation should not be delayed until signs of hepatic decomposition.

Principles of treatment are:

- Prevent the accumulation of ammonia
- Remove or correct identifiable precipitating factors
- Improve liver function by reducing protein intake
- Use neomycin and lactulose.

LIVER TRANSPLANTATION

Indications

- Recurrent variceal bleeding
- Progressive hepatic dysfunction e.g. falling albumin <30 g/dl, increasing coagulopathy not corrected by Vitamin K
- Development of ascites and jaundice
- Worsening malnutrition unresponsive to energy supplements
- Deteriorating quality of life related to liver disease
- Encephalopathy
- Hepatorenal failure
- FEV1 above 60% predicted.

Liver transplantation replaces the diseased liver and decompresses the portal venous system. Assessment should establish whether a combined heart/lung/liver transplant is more appropriate than liver transplantation alone. Preoperative assessment of pancreatic endocrine function is important because immunosuppressives including steroids and tacrolimus have a diabetogenic effect. Survival post-liver transplantation is similar to other groups of children (90% short term). Higher doses of immunosuppressives might be required to obtain therapeutic levels due to abnormal CF pharmacokinetics. Post-operative improvements in nutritional status and pulmonary function are common.

References

Colombo C, Battezatti P M, Podda M et al 1996. UDCA for liver disease associated with CF: a double blind multicentre trial Hepatology 23:1484–1490

Colombo C, Battezzati P M, Crosignani A et al 2002 Liver disease in CF: a prospective study on incidence risk factors and outcome. Hepatology 36: 1374–1382

Lindblad A, Glaumann H, Strandvik B 1998 A two year prospective study of the effect of ursodeoxycholic acid on urinary bile excretion and liver morphology. Hepatology 27:166–174

Shapira R, Hadzic N, Francavilla R et al 1999. Retrospective review of CF presenting as infantile liver disease Archives of Diseases in Childhood 31:125–128

Chapter **13**

Ear, nose and throat

Christopher Randall

INTRODUCTION

The upper respiratory tract, with its mucous-producing respiratory lining, has the same potential to be affected by abnormalities of secretion that occur in the rest of the respiratory tract (Berman & Coleman 1997).

The resulting problems are not potentially life threatening, but deserve attention because of their significant morbidity, and relationship to lung pathology.

PATHOLOGY
Primary pathology

The nose and nasal sinuses rely on mucociliary transport and this is particularly important for the drainage of small ostia. Although the ciliary mechanism is unaffected, the mucous may be too viscid resulting in obstruction.

Secondary pathology

- Stasis and bacterial infection of mucous (Pseudomonas species, *Staphylococcus aureus, Haemophilus influenzae*)
- Nasal polyps
- Mucoceles (mucous filled cysts)
- Facial deformity: mucoceles can impart pressure within the thin walled ethmoidal sinuses resulting in:
  - Widening of the nasal bridge
  - Reduced nasal lumen
- Poor development of frontal sinuses due to poor sinus aeration.

> **Remember**
>
> Children with CF are just as likely as unaffected children to have
> - allergic rhinitis
> - tonsillitis
> - nasal foreign bodies
> - acute rhinitis
> - secretory otitis media.

Relationship to the lower respiratory tract

Stasis of mucous in the nose and sinuses almost invariably causes low-grade infection. It remains to be proven whether upper respiratory tract disease can significantly affect lung pathology by acting as a septic reservoir. Studies have failed to show that surgery of the sinuses improves lung function (Madonna 1997). However, there is a consensus that the lower respiratory tract suffers if upper respiratory tract disease is poorly controlled (Umetsu 1990).

Transplanted lungs are commonly infected by CF pathogens that have colonised the nasal cavity.

NASAL PROBLEMS

In a survey by Brigade and Clement (Brigade and Clement 1995) the following symptoms were recorded:

● Nasal blockage	73%
● Recurrent rhinitis	72%
● Rhinorrhoea	61%
● Headache	57%
● Anosmia	23%
● Recurrent sinusitis with fever & malaise	27%

The following signs were found:

● Purulent secretions	57%
● Broadening of the nasal bridge	34%
● Middle meatal polyps	36%
● Medial bulging of the lateral nasal wall	13%

History and examination

History

- Family history of atopy
- Nasal discharge or epistaxis
- Snoring, noisy breathing
- Loss of taste.

Examination

- Inspection of facial shape for evidence of chronic obstruction
- Simple inspection in the nose with otoscope (Figure 13.1)
- Consider sinus X-ray, CT scan (see Chapter 9, Figure 9.12), endoscopic examination.

Treatment

There is continuing debate about what degree of nasal disease in cystic fibrosis should be actively treated.

Figure 13.1   Nasal polyps.

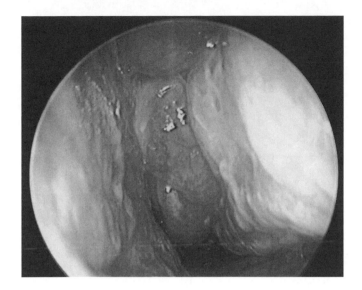

> **Remember**
>
> Children with long standing symptoms might not recognise their problem as abnormal.

- Symptomatic disease, particularly with evidence of obstruction, should always be treated.
- Saline douches made with one teaspoonful of salt and one teaspoonful of sodium bicarbonate in a pint of water and then syringed or sniffed up the nose can be helpful. Douches can physically remove some of the pus and secretions but are only suitable for older children.
- Purulent nasal secretions and post-nasal discharge might require antibiotics. Often symptoms are alleviated at the same time as lower respiratory tract infections are treated. If the nasal passages are patent, inhaled antibiotics such as Colomycin can be topically applied to the nasal passages by encouraging nose breathing of nebulised solutions through a mask rather than a mouthpiece.
- Nasal polyps can be treated with topical corticosteroids but if there is complete obstruction by polyps these are often ineffective. Beta-methasone drops can be tried to improve local deposition. Some nasal steroid sprays are thixotrophic and this may improve adhesion to the nasal mucosa.
- If medical management does not improve polyps, intranasal surgical removal will immediately improve airways with consequent relief of symptoms.
- Sinus washouts can usefully resolve persistent symptomatic infections but the clearing of secretions is generally short lived.

Figure 13.2 An algorithm for the management of nasal obstruction.

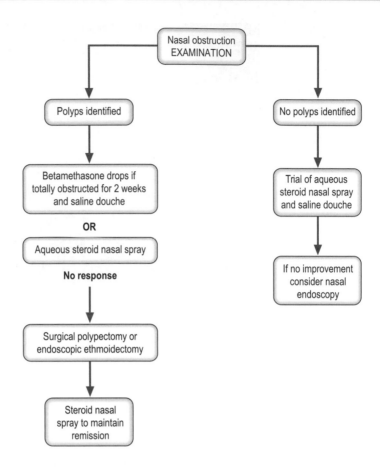

Remember

The benefits of repeated surgical interventions must be balanced against the hazards and complications of repeated anaesthesia.

Endoscopic surgery

The advent of endoscopic surgical techniques has opened up the possibility of more proactive treatment of nasal disease.

- It requires a high degree of surgical skill.
- CT scanning of sinuses when surgery is contemplated can be of use for pre-operative planning but there is significant radiation exposure with each scan (see Chapter 9).
- Nasal polyposis, causing widening of the ethmoidal complex medially or widening of the nasal bridge, requires an opinion from an ENT surgeon with expertise in treating these conditions.
- Endoscopic surgery can significantly improve symptoms but there is a fairly high recurrence rate requiring re-operation within 2–4 years (Yung 2002). Benefits are greater when used to treat symptoms as a result of infection than predominantly nasal blockage (Rowe-Jones & MacKay 1996).

- Although there have been concerns about whether surgery on the lateral nasal wall might significantly alter subsequent facial growth, there is now evidence that the risks are small and that growth is usually normal (Bothwell 2002).

> **Remember**
>
> Many of the problems in the upper airways recur even following good surgical management.

SUMMARY

- Nasal and sinus problems are not in themselves life threatening but can add considerably to misery and interference with well being.
- All patients should have regular assessment of the upper respiratory tract including inspection of nasal passages.
- Endoscopic inspection in experienced hands can be useful diagnostically and therapeutically.
- Nasal steroids and/or polypectomy should treat uncomplicated nasal polyposis.
- Endoscopic sinus surgery might improve symptoms for longer than simple polypectomy.
- Severe polyposis, medialisation of the lateral nasal wall, or widening of the nasal bridge, requires CT scanning with a view to endoscopic sinus surgery.
- Ethmoidal sinus surgery does not seem to cause significant facial growth problems.

References

Berman J, Coleman B H 1997 Nasal aspects of cystic fibrosis in children. Journal of Laryngology and Otolaryngology 91:133

Bothwell M R, Piccirillo J F, Lusk R P et al 2002 Long term outcome of facial growth after functional endoscopic sinus surgery. Head and Neck Surgery 126(6):628–634

Brigade P, Clement P A R 1995 Endoscopy and CT in Cystic Fibrosis. Abstract 20th European Cystic Fibrosis Conference, Brussels

Madonna D, Isaacson G, Rosenfeld R M et al 1997 Effect of sinus surgery on pulmonary function in patients with cystic fibrosis. Laryngoscope 107(3):328–331

Rowe-Jones J M, Mackay I S 1996 Endoscopic sinus surgery in the treatment of cystic fibrosis with nasal polyposis. Laryngoscope (12.1):1540–1544

Umetsu D, Moss R, King V et al 1990 Sinus disease in patients with severe cystic fibrosis: relation to pulmonary exacerbation. Lancet 335:107

Yung M W, Gould J, Upton G J 2002 Nasal polyposis in children with cystic fibrosis: a long term follow up study. Annals of Otolaryngology Rhinology and Laryngology 111 (12.1):1081–1086

Chapter 14

Osteoporosis and joint disease

Lee Wisby, Gary Connett

INTRODUCTION

Up to 14% of CF children will have significant musculo-skeletal problems (Massie 1998). Such complications occur more frequently in adult life.

OSTEOPOROSIS

Decreased bone mineral density is a well recognised complication of cystic fibrosis. Significant osteoporosis does not usually occur until adulthood and results in part from failure to achieve expected peak bone mass during puberty.

The magnitude of the peak bone mass determines how much bone an individual can lose in a lifetime before the development of negative clinical consequences. Prevalence of osteopenia in adults has been reported as 31–51% with osteoporosis in 20–31% (Moran 2002). Fracture rates among adults are up to twice that of the general population. Rib fractures are a particular problem complicating the treatment of pulmonary complications. Vertebral osteopenia may be an important contributing factor to thoracic kyphosis. Bone pain can occur as a result of spinal compression fractures and result in reduced height.

Causal factors include:

- Severity of lung disease
- Malnutrition
- Vitamin and mineral deficiency
- Decreased physical activity
- Delayed puberty

- Diabetes
- Treatment with glucocorticoids.

Aetiology is multifactorial resulting in increased bone degradation and diminished new bone formation (Baroncelli 1997).

Monitoring

- Annual measurement of calcium, phosphorus, 25-OH vitamin D
- Annual parathormone levels in those at increased risk
- Regular assessment of pubertal status
- Some centres now carry out dual energy X-ray absorptiometry (DEXA) scans 1–2 yearly in all adolescent and adult individuals. Control data is essential and results corrected for short stature to ensure accurate interpretation. Z or T scores of < -2 are concerning.

Management

Prevention is the primary aim. Maximising nutrition and pulmonary function will help achieve expected peak bone mass during pubertal growth. As far as possible minimise treatment with oral glucocorticoids.

> **Note**
>
> Peak bone mass occurs at around 15 years compared with 30 years in non-CF individuals.

- Calcium intake should achieve at least age related requirements.
- Give routine Vitamin D supplements (Chapter 7, Table 7.4). Titrate serum levels of 25-OH Vitamin D to the high end of the normal range. Levels are typically higher in summer months. Regular exposure to sunlight should be encouraged.
- If there is reduced bone mineral density, calcichew D3 forte 1–2 daily should be given.
- Delayed puberty should be treated as appropriate (see Chapter 15).
- Weight bearing exercises should be encouraged.
- Vitamin K is an important co-factor in bone turnover. There is accumulating evidence that deficiency is common in CF suggesting the need for routine supplements of 10 mg daily.
- Pharmacological agents for treating osteoporosis have not been evaluated in children.
- Biphosphonates have been used in adults with CF. Pamidronate given by three monthly intravenous infusions can increase the mineral density of spinal bone. Troublesome bone pain can be minimised by concomitant oral steroid therapy around the time of treatment.
- Oral biphosphonates have also been used but absorption can be erratic and there are concerns about worsening gastro-oesophageal reflux and oesophageal lesions. There are concerns about teratogenicity.

JOINT DISEASE

Three main types of arthropathy occur in cystic fibrosis:

- Cystic fibrosis arthritis (CFA) (also called episodic arthritis)
- Hypertrophic pulmonary osteoarthropathy (HPOA)
- Coincidental arthropathies unrelated to CF.

Cystic fibrosis arthritis

Incidence

- The most common joint disease in CF affecting 5–10% of children.
- Can occur any time after infancy but typically during the second decade of life.

Clinical features

- Episodes are usually of sudden onset over 12–24 hours.
- Joint involvement can be mono, pauci or polyarticular.
- Most commonly affects knees, ankles and wrists. PIP joints, shoulders, elbows and hips can also be affected.
- Episodes are not usually associated with pulmonary exacerbations or deteriorating lung function.
- Fever, and a maculopaular, vasculitic or erythema nodosum rash can also occur.
- Episodes generally last 5–7 days and recur after weeks or months with symptom-free intervals.
- Prognosis is variable but spontaneous long-term remission can occur.

Pathology

An increase in circulating immune complexes, associations with pseudo-monas colonization and higher levels of serum IgG have been observed in some but not all studies. Autoantibodies might also be relevant.

Radiological features

Joint effusions might be demonstrable but erosive arthritis with bone destruction is rare.

Hypertrophic pulmonary osteoarthropathy

HPOA is a syndrome characterized by:

- Digital clubbing
- Chronic, usually symmetrical, distal long bone and joint pain/swelling
- Periostitis in the distal portion of long bones.

Incidence

- Rare in paediatrics
- Age-related increased incidence and association with progressive suppurative lung disease
- 2:1 male predominance.

Clinical features

Joints

- Gradual onset of joint pain, stiffness and swelling with effusion
- Joints are warm to the touch but not usually erythematous
- Knees and ankles are most commonly affected
- Less commonly involves wrists, proximal interphalangeal joints and elbows.

Long bones

- Gradual onset of dull bone pain and tenderness
- Tibia, fibula, ulna and radius are most commonly affected.

Symptoms typically increase in cold weather and after activity. Pains are worse during pulmonary exacerbations but swelling persists between episodes. Autonomic dysfunction with flushing, blanching, sweating and burning pain in the hands and fingertips can occur.

Bone and joint disease tend to progress with the increased occurrence of pulmonary exacerbations.

Pathology

Pathogenesis is unclear but there may be a causative role for platelet-derived growth factors from megakaryocytes reaching the distal micro-circulation as a result of intrapulmonary shunting of blood. Symptoms have been improved after lung transplantation and lobectomy for focal bronchiectasis.

Radiological findings

- Characteristic layers of new bone are seen adjacent to the line of the cortex. These extend into the cortex with disease progression.
- Changes might not occur until some months after the onset of symptoms.
- Earlier findings are apparent on radioisotope bone scanning with accumulation of tracer along the cortical margins of the diaphyses and metaphyses of distal long bones.

Management of CFA and HPOA

- Exclude other causes (see below).
- Use regular non-steroidal anti-inflammatories and bed rest. (These do not alter the course of the disease.)
- HPOA often responds to aggressive management of underlying respiratory disease.
- Steroid therapy may be of benefit for resistant cases and erosive disease.
- Liaison with an experienced paediatric rheumatologist is invaluable in difficult-to-manage cases.

> **Note**
>
> Osteoporosis and hypertrophic pulmonary osteoarthropathy are related to disease severity and can be minimised through good nutrition and aggressive management of underlying chest disease.

Coincidental arthropathies unrelated to CF

A number of important clinical entities may coincidentally occur in cystic fibrosis. Differential diagnoses which should not be missed include:

- Septic (bacterial) arthritis (usually mono-articular)
- Haematological malignancy
- Non-accidental injury.

Clinical assessment and discriminating use of further investigations should readily differentiate the above diagnoses. Full blood count and film, and acute phase marker (ESR/CRP) and X-ray are important first line investigations. Synovial fluid aspiration and blood culture are mandatory if infection is suspected.

Juvenile chronic arthritis (JCA)

Any of the following sub-types of JCA can coexist with cystic fibrosis:

- Polyarticular JCA: Usually rheumatoid factor-negative and erosive.
- Pauciarticular JCA: Affects up to four joints, often asymmetrical. Important association with chronic uveitis in ANA-positive cases.

- Systemic JCA: Acute onset polyarticular arthritis with characteristic fever pattern, rash, splenomegaly, lymphadenopathy and leucocytosis.

Reactive arthritis

- May follow clinical history of previous infection, e.g. Group A beta haemolytic streptococcus pharyngitis.
- HLA B27 individuals are at increased risk following gastrointestinal or genitourinary infection.
- Investigation includes appropriate bacterial cultures, ASO and viral titres.

Autoimmune connective tissue diseases, rheumatoid arthritis, sarcoid arthropathy and psoriatic arthropathy have all been described in cystic fibrosis. Diagnosis depends on suggestive clinical findings and appropriate investigation.

VASCULITIS

Rarely older CF individuals have developed vasculitic lesions in the form of a purpuric rash, usually on the lower limbs. Lesions can be associated with arthritis and a severe deterioration in pulmonary status. The possibility of a drug reaction should be considered. There is an association with increased serum IgG concentrations and there are similarities with the lesions seen in hypergammaglobulinaemic purpura.

Investigation

This should include a full blood count, ESR, acute phase reactants, and an autoimmune profile. Further investigations to exclude other organ involvement should include urinalysis, renal and liver function.

Treatment

This should include aggressive treatment of lung disease and immuno-suppression with corticosteroids and/or more potent agents.

OTHER MUSCULOSKELETAL CONDITIONS

Chest wall deformity

Sternal deformities such as pectus excavatum and carinatum are not uncommonly seen in cystic fibrosis but are generally not clinically significant beyond the cosmetic implications. Kyphosis is possibly an under-recognised manifestation of musculoskeletal disease with up to 77% of females and 36% of males over the age of 15 years having a degree of kyphosis greater than the upper limit of the normal range (Henderson and Specter, 1994). Whilst this rarely affects lung function testing, it can contribute to significant discomfort and posture problems (see Chapter 5).

References

Baroncelli G, De Luca F, Magazzu G 1997 Bone demineralization in cystic fibrosis: evidence of imbalance between bone formation and degradation. Pediatric Research. 41:397–403

Henderson R, Specter B 1994 Kyphosis and fractures in children and young adults with cystic fibrosis. Journal of Pediatrics 125(2):208–212

Massie R, Towns S, Bernard E et al 1998 The musculoskeletal complications of cystic fibrosis. Journal of Paediatrics and Child Health 34:467–470

Moran A 2002 Endocrine complications of cystic fibrosis. Adolescent Med 13:145–159

Recommended reading

Cassidy J, Petty R, Ed. Textbook of Pediatric Rheumatology, 4th Ed. WB Sanders co, Philadelphia, Pennsylvania. ISBN 0-7216-8171-9.

Phillips BM, David TJ. 1986 Pathogenesis and management of arthropathy in cystic fibrosis. Journal of the Royal Society of Medicine (Suppl 12) 79:44–49.

Turner MA, Baildam E. 1997 Joint disorders in cystic fibrosis. Journal of the Royal Society of Medicine (Suppl 3) 90:13–20.

Chapter **15**

Growth and puberty

Fiona Regan, Peter Betts

CHAPTER CONTENTS

GROWTH

Some children with CF have poor growth despite optimal CF care.

The Oxford CF population had a mean height SDS of −0.54 and BMI SDS −0.24 (Taylor 1999). American data shows that 29.3% had a height <10th centile and 18.1% a height <5th centile. Weight is also reduced, with 25.9% <10th centile and 17.7% <5th centile (CF Foundation 2000). Reduced height velocity is particularly marked during puberty.

The reasons for reduced growth are multifactorial and include:

- Antenatal effects; the average birth weight of children with CF is reduced and there are increased numbers of constitutionally small individuals forming a fishtail distribution at the lower centiles for weight and height.
- Nutritional status; this has improved in recent years and has resulted in increased BMI but mean height SDS has remained static (CF Foundation 2000, Laursen 1999).
- Pulmonary infection.
- Diabetes.
- Gastro-oesophageal reflux.
- Liver disease.
- Treatment with corticosteroids.

There has been recent interest in the relationship between growth hormone, insulin-like growth factor 1 (IGF-1) and insulin-like growth factor

Figure 15.1 Calculation of target height range.

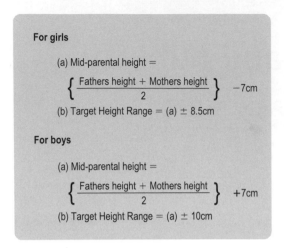

For girls

(a) Mid-parental height =

$$\left\{ \frac{\text{Fathers height} + \text{Mothers height}}{2} \right\} -7\text{cm}$$

(b) Target Height Range = (a) $\pm$ 8.5cm

For boys

(a) Mid-parental height =

$$\left\{ \frac{\text{Fathers height} + \text{Mothers height}}{2} \right\} +7\text{cm}$$

(b) Target Height Range = (a) $\pm$ 10cm

binding proteins (IGFBP3) and their relationship to poor growth (Ripa 2002). However there are complex interactions between nutrition, liver function and insulin secretion affecting IGF-1 and IGFBP3 production and function. Studies are conflicting, with IGF-1 and IGFBP3 reported as either normal or decreased.

Monitoring

Anthropometric measures should be used with attention to the following:

- Linear length/standing height measured and plotted on appropriate centile charts (Child Growth Foundation 1996) at least 3–6 monthly to identify growth problems.
- Weight should be measured and plotted at every clinic visit to monitor nutritional status.
- BMI can be calculated from the equation $BMI = Wt/Ht^2$ and plotted on an appropriate chart.
- Measurements should preferably be made by the same observer to minimise measurement error.
- Determine and plot target height range on the centile chart calculated from mid-parental centile (Figure 15.1).

When to be concerned (Hall 1996)

Pre-school child (<5 years of age)

Falling across one height centile band over a period of 12–18 months may herald the onset of problems. Falling across two centile bands should prompt reassessment.

School age (>5 but <10 years of age)

Falling across half a height centile band over a period of 12–18 months may herald problems. Falling across one centile band should prompt reassessment (see below).

At any age

Less than target height range (small for family size).

- Prior to puberty, growth velocity slows until the rapid growth spurt begins as puberty progresses. Thus children with delayed puberty may fall across one or more centile bands as they drift away from their peers.
- There is a degree of individual variation in longitudinal growth. In school age children a deviation up to one centile band may be normal.

Investigation of growth failure

- Exclude uncontrolled malabsorption or insufficient calorie intake and consider enteral feeding.
- Review respiratory status.
- Exclude diabetes mellitus with a Glucose Tolerance Test (see Chapter 11).
- Consider effects of medication (for example, effects of inhaled corticosteroids on individuals unusually sensitive to their effects on growth).
- Be aware that other pathologies not related to CF may co-exist and cause growth failure.
- Tests should include FBC, U&E, LFTs, CRP, ESR, thyroid function tests and a coeliac screen.
- Parameters to assess the growth hormone axis include IGF-1, IGFBP3 and overnight urinary growth hormone measurements. These investigations should be ordered in conjunction with a paediatric endocrinologist.

Treatment of poor growth

- Optimise treatment of CF and any complications.
- Treat impaired glucose tolerance or diabetes if present (see Chapter 11).

PUBERTY

Children with CF can have delayed puberty by up to 1–4 years compared to their peers (Sinnema 1993, Reiter 1981).

Menarchal age in females is delayed to a mean of 14.9 years. In one study patients homozygous for ΔF508 had later menarche than those who were not (15.2 years compared to 14.7 years) (Johannesson 1997).

There may be a delayed rise in spontaneous luteinizing hormone (LH) and follicle stimulating hormone (FSH) secretion but normal hormonal responses to stimulation tests.

Aetiological factors in delayed puberty include:

- Poor nutrition; decreased essential fatty acids, important for the synthesis of bioactive metabolites for sexual maturation.
- Deficiency of insulin which interacts with LH and FSH receptors and possibly their activity.
- Decreased IGF-1 and IGFBP3.
- Delayed maturation of the hypothalamic-pituitary-gonadal axis.
- Direct effects of abnormal CFTR, which may have a regulatory function for neuroendocrine secretion in the brain (Arrigo 2003).

Pubertal status

Monitoring (see Figures 15.2–15.4)

Figure 15.2 Genital development stages. Stage 1: Pre-adolescent. Testes, scrotum and penis are of about the same size and proportion as in early childhood; Stage 2: Enlargement of scrotum and of testes. The skin of the scrotum reddens and changes in texture. Little or no enlargement of penis at this stage; Stage 3: Enlargement of the penis, which occurs at firstly mainly in length. Further growth of testes and scrotum; Stage 4: Increased size of penis with growth in breadth and development of glans. Further enlargement of testes and scrotum; increased darkening of scrotal skin; Stage 5: Genitalia adult in size and shape. Reproduced and adapted by permission of Blackwell Science Limited.

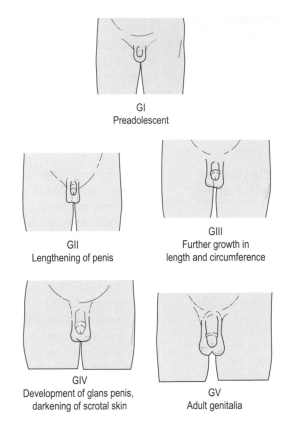

GI
Preadolescent

GII
Lengthening of penis

GIII
Further growth in length and circumference

GIV
Development of glans penis, darkening of scrotal skin

GV
Adult genitalia

Male

- Tanner staging for genital development (Figure 15.2)
- Testicular volume using Prader Orchidometer
- Height measurements.

Approximately 90% of normal boys achieve testicular volume of 4 ml (indicating pulsatile gonadotrophin secretion and onset of puberty) by the age of 14 years and achieve genital stage 2 by 14.5 years.

Peak height velocity usually coincides with genital stage 3–4 and a testicular volume of approximately 10 mls.

Females

- Tanner staging using breast and pubic hair development (Figures 15.3 & 15.4)
- Height measurements.

Approximately 90% of females achieve breast stage 2 (usually the earliest sign of pubertal development in girls) by the age of 13.8 years.

Peak height velocity usually coincides with breast stage 2–3, menarche usually at breast/genitalia stage 4.

Lack of pubertal development

In either sex by 14 years warrants assessment.

Figure 15.3 Pubic hair stages. Stage 1: Pre-adolescent. The vellus over the pubes is not further developed than that over the abdominal wall, i.e. no pubic hair; Stage 2: Sparse growth of long, slightly pigmented downy hair, straight or only slightly curled, appearing chiefly at the base of the penis or along labia; Stage 3: Considerably darker, coarser and more curled. The hair spreads sparsely over the junction of the pubes; Stage 4: Hair now resembles adult type, but the area covered by it is still considerably smaller than in the adult. No spread to the medial surface of the thighs; Stage 5: Adult in quantity and type with distribution of the horizontal (or classically 'feminine') pattern (Dupertuis, Atkinson & Eftman 1945). Spread to medial surface of thighs, but not up linea alba or elsewhere above the base of the inverse triangle. Reproduced and adapted by permission of Blackwell Science Ltd.

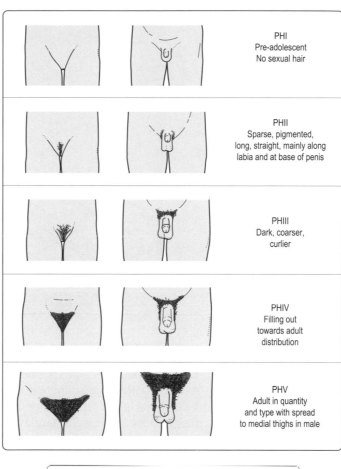

Figure 15.4 Breast development stages. Stage 1: Pre-adolescent: elevation of papilla only. Stage 2: Breast bud stage: elevation of breast and papilla as small mound. Enlargement of areolar diameter. Stage 3: Further enlargement and elevation of breast and areola, with no separation of their contours. Stage 4: Projection of areola and papilla to form a secondary mound above the level of the breast. Stage 5: Mature stage: projection of papilla only, due to recession of the areola to the general contour of the breast. Reproduced and adapted by permission of Blackwell Science Ltd.

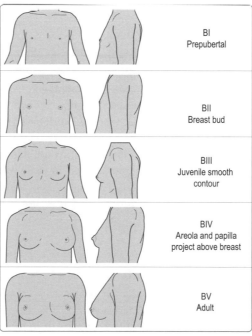

Figure 15.5 A UK growth chart showing the slowing of growth during delayed puberty in boys. (1) A boy normally growing on the 50th percentile. (2) A boy normally growing on the 2nd percentile.

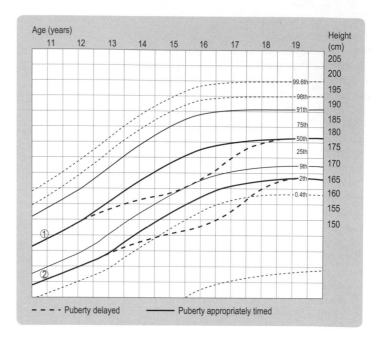

Discordant pubertal development

Genital stage, testicular volume and height velocity in boys should follow a logical pattern as should breast, pubic and axillary hair stages and height velocity in girls. Breast development without concomitant increase in height velocity implies organic pathology and requires expert assessment, as does pubic and axillary hair development without breast development.

> **Remember**
>
> - The gap in height between an adolescent with delayed puberty and their peer group is more noticeable in small subjects (for example those growing along the 2nd–9th centile). The slowing of growth due to pubertal delay might then result in a height drift to <0.4th centile.
> - Conversely individuals growing normally above the 50th centile might not notice their height is not increasing as expected around this time (Figure 15.5). While this group may suffer less psychologically, pubertal delay beyond 14 years warrants assessment.
> - Pubertal delay might add to the psychological problems coping with a chronic disease at this vulnerable age.

Puberty and lung growth (Rosenthal et al 1993)

Lung volumes increase proportionately more around puberty and especially in males (dis-synaptic growth). Inducing puberty in boys with added testosterone or its derivatives, when natural development is delayed, can result in improved lung function.

Figure 15.6   Delayed puberty algorithm.

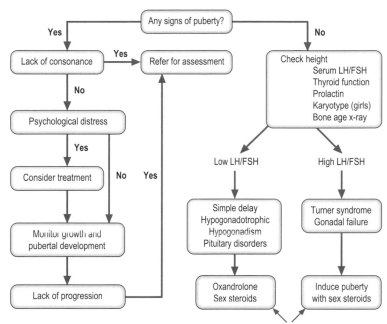

Investigation of abnormal pubertal development

- Ensure optimal treatment of CF and exclude associated pathology such as diabetes.
- A suggested algorithm is outlined overleaf (Figure 15.6 – Delayed Puberty Algorithm: Adapted from Brook CDG, Clinical Paediatric Endocrinology (Brook 1995)).
- The majority will have simple 'constitutional' delay. There might be a family history of delayed puberty. Ask the age of maternal menarche and whether the father thinks he started shaving and had his teenage growth spurt at the same age as his peers.

Treatment options

There are differences in practice about when to intervene and what medications to use. Consideration must be given to the young person's perception of the problem and their expectations of treatment.

Males

If growth is the primary concern consider oral Oxandrolone. Oxandrolone:

- Is a synthetic anabolic steroid, with weak androgenic effects
- Promotes skeletal growth without significantly advancing bone age
- May stimulate natural puberty to occur earlier
- Does not significantly affect genital development other than an increase in penile length but not pubic hair
- Side effects are rare in low dosage
- Usual duration of treatment is 6–12 months
- Treatment should be discontinued when evidence of natural puberty (for example pubic hair) occurs.

If lack of genital development is the primary concern then sex steroids can be used to induce puberty (this will also stimulate height gain).

- Testosterone esters are usually given by IM injection, for example, Sustanon.
- Start at 50 mg monthly, increasing in stages.

Females   The most practical current option is to use oral oestrogens starting at a dose of 1–2 mcg per day, increasing dose at appropriate intervals. Oestrogens do not promote a growth spurt.

> **Remember**
>
> - The induction of puberty in males and females requires close monitoring and should be supervised by a paediatric endocrinologist.
> - In both sexes the aim is to mimic the tempo of natural puberty. Inducing too rapid a progress may limit final adult height by advancing skeletal maturation out of step with linear growth; there may be reduced pubertal development, especially in girls, who run the risk of inadequate breast and uterine size.

References

Arrigo et al 2003 Pubertal development in CF: an overview. Journal of Pediatric Endocrinology and Metabol 16:267–270

Brook C G D (ed) 1995 Clinical Paediatric Endocrinology, 3rd edn. Blackwell Frome, England.

Child Growth Foundation 1996/1 (Charity Reg. No 274325) Harlow Printing Limited, South Shields

CF Foundation 2000 CF 2000 Annual Report. Bethesda, MD

Hall D M B (ed) 1996 Health for all children. Report of the third Joint Working Party on child health surveillance, 3rd edn. Oxford University Press, Oxford

Johannesson et al 1997 Delayed puberty in CF despite good clinical status. Pediatrics 99:29–34

Laursen et al 1999 Secular changes in anthropometric data in CF patients. Acta Paediatrica 88:169–174

Reiter et al 1981 The reproductive endocrine system in CF1. Basal gonadotrophin and sex steroid levels. American Journal of Diseases in Children 134:422–426

Ripa et al 2002 The relationship between insulin secretion, the insulin-like growth factor axis and growth in children with CF. Clinical Endocrinology 56:383–389

Rosenthal M et al 1993 Lung function in white children aged 4 to 19 years – Spirometry. Thorax 48:794–802

Sinnema et al 1983 Adolescents with CF in the Netherlands. Acta Paediatrica Scandinavia 72:427–432

Taylor et al 1999 The relationship between insulin, IGF-1 and weight gain in CF. Clinical Endocrinology 51:659–665

Chapter 16

Fertility

Sucheta Iyengar, Matthew Coleman

INTRODUCTION

As individuals with CF live longer, issues concerning fertility and pregnancy are becoming increasingly relevant. It is important for CF adolescents to have information about fertility, sexuality, self-esteem, expected body image and safe-sex practices.

SEXUAL HEALTH

Discussions about fertility and contraception should begin during adolescence. Individuals are often reluctant to raise these issues and health professionals should be prepared to actively initiate discussions.

Men

Subfertility is generally accepted as inevitable and is usually due to congenital bilateral absence or atrophy of the vas deferens (CBAVD) resulting in azoospermia. However, spermatogenesis can be normal. As a result of advances in assisted reproductive technologies, it is possible for men to father children. Genetic counselling is essential before proceeding with either microscopic epididymal sperm aspiration (MESA) or Testis Sperm Extraction (TESE).

These techniques involve aspirating sperm from the testes or epididymis and intracytoplasmic sperm injection (ICSI) using microscopic techniques. Both have been successful.

Women

Apart from the mechanical barrier of thickened cervical mucus, impairing the passage of sperm beyond the cervix, there is little evidence for reduced fertility. Women need to be counselled about contraception should they wish to avoid pregnancy. The combined oral contraceptive pill or injectable progesterones are the preferred contraceptive choices. When antibiotics are given, barrier contraceptive protection may be needed for the duration of treatment and for a further seven days.

Both men and women need to be aware of the additional benefits of using barrier methods of contraception to prevent sexually transmitted diseases.

PREGNANCY

Women need to understand how pregnancy might adversely affect their health and how their CF might affect the unborn child.

Effects of pregnancy on CF

- Increased mortality with moderate to severe lung disease. Maternal survival is positively correlated to pre-pregnancy FEV1.
- Women need to consider their morbidity and possible mortality while their child is still young and discuss these issues with their partner and the CF team.
- The main reasons for maternal morbidity are poor maternal weight gain and deterioration in lung function. A 10–15% decline in FEV1 and pulmonary infective exacerbations should be anticipated.

Effects of CF on pregnancy

- There is no increased risk of miscarriage or congenital anomalies.
- Pre-pregnancy FEV1 is the most useful predictor of outcome. Pregnancy is not advisable in women with pulmonary hypertension, cor pulmonale, or an FEV1 of less than 50% of predicted. Poor nutritional status will adversely impact on pregnancy outcomes.
- Individuals who have had transplants should be advised against pregnancy because of the risks of precipitating acute rejection.
- Risks to the baby include prematurity and chronic hypoxia causing intrauterine growth retardation.
- Consideration should be given to the CF status of the unborn child.

Pre-pregnancy

Potential risks to the mother and baby need to be discussed clearly and honestly. Discussions should include the risks of maternal deterioration after pregnancy because of the extra physical demands of child-care. It is important that the partner and possibly the extended family are included and fully understand the implications.

Genetic counselling is important. All children will either be carriers or are at risk of having CF.

Women should be advised about the importance of additional folic acid (400 μg/day) and the need to maintain good nutritional status during pregnancy. They should be reminded about the importance of adhering to prescribed treatment regimes and reassured about safety issues in relation to drugs and effects on the foetus.

Immunisation against rubella should be confirmed before pregnancy and early glucose tolerance testing performed.

Pregnancy

Specialist multidisciplinary care is essential. The team should include obstetricians, physicians and midwives experienced in looking after high-risk pregnant women and who have a good understanding of CF.
Specific recommendations include:

- Close adherence to chest physiotherapy regimes and adequate intake of antibiotics (except tetracyclines).
- Early recognition and aggressive treatment of acute infections.
- Close nutritional monitoring and maintenance of a high calorie diet.
- Vitamins A and E and trace element levels should be measured, in addition to routine antenatal blood tests.
- Repeat monitoring of glucose tolerance.
- Pulmonary and cardiovascular status should be regularly monitored.
- Regular scans to monitor foetal growth are essential. Intrauterine growth retardation is common.

Nutritional advice

Weight gain of at least 10 kg (0.5 kg/week from 20 weeks gestation) during CF pregnancy has been associated with a good outcome (Cohen & Di Sant'Agnese 1980, Geddes 1992). Regular dietetic monitoring 4–6 weekly at clinic visits and early aggressive management of sub-optimal weight gain is essential. Deterioration in lung function during pregnancy can compromise weight gain (UK CF Working Group 2002). Oral or enteral nutritional supplements might be required (Hilman, Aitken & Constantinescu 1996).

Supplements

- Folic acid supplements (400 mcg/day) should be commenced pre-conceptually and continued for up to 12 weeks of pregnancy (Department of Health 1992).
- Iron supplements might be required, especially in late pregnancy
- Retinol is potentially teratogenic. It is prudent to discontinue Vitamin A supplementation throughout pregnancy and restart once the baby is born.
- All other supplements, including Vitamin D, should be continued.
- All foods at risk of bacterial contamination e.g. soft cheeses should be avoided (as for all pregnant women).

Delivery

If there is resting hypoxia towards the end of pregnancy, bed rest and oxygen are necessary.

There are no contraindications to vaginal delivery. Epidural analgesia might be preferable to opiates, thus avoiding respiratory depression. Entonox should not be given to those with a history of pneumothorax or large bullae.

The second stage of labour can be shortened by assisted vaginal delivery. Spontaneous pneumothorax can occur as a result of prolonged pushing. If Caesarean is necessary, regional anaesthesia is preferable.

Post partum

Breast feeding should be encouraged, although the mother might need nutritional supplements to meet additional demands.

Contraception should be discussed so that future pregnancies are planned and spaced appropriately.

Unwanted pregnancies High-risk or unwanted first trimester pregnancies may be terminated using the oral prostaglandin mifepristone. This might avoid the need for a general anaesthetic.

SUMMARY Pregnancy can be well tolerated by women with cystic fibrosis although a lot of issues need to be addressed. These should be discussed preconceptually.

References

Cohen L A, Di Sant'Agnese P A 1980 Cystic fibrosis and pregnancy. A national survey. Lancet 2:842–844

Department of Health 1992 Folic acid and prevention of neural tube defects. Report from an expert advisory group. Health Publications Unit, HMSO, London

Geddes D M 1992 Cystic fibrosis and pregnancy. Journal of the Royal Society of Medicine 85(Suppl 9):36–37

Hilman B C, Aitken M L, Constantinescu M 1996 Pregnancy in patients with cystic fibrosis. Clinical Obstetrics and Gynaecology 39:70–86

UK Cystic Fibrosis Trust 2002. Nutritional management of cystic fibrosis. CF Trust, Bromley

Recommended reading

Nelson-Piercy C 1997 Handbook of Obstetric medicine 60–64. ISIS Medical Media, Oxford

Chapter 17

Surgical issues

Mervyn Griffiths

INTRODUCTION

Individuals with CF can require routine or emergency surgery unrelated to their condition.

Remember

The CF team should be involved with all surgical admissions, including non-CF conditions.
Surgery requires specialist anaesthetic input (see Chapter 18).

GASTROSTOMIES

A gastrostomy is an iatrogenic fistula between the skin and the stomach. It has long term advantages over naso-gastric feeding.

Indications

A combination of the need for supplemental enteral feeds (see Chapter 7), and failure of naso-gastric (NG) tube feeding because of either tube problems or cosmetic problems.

Tube problems:

- Insertion problems. For example trauma or recurrent naso-bronchial intubation.
- Displacement problems. Some cough up their tubes. Unco-operative children may pull them out.
- Nasal irritation or sensitivity to adhesive.

Cosmetic problems:

- NG tubes are often socially unacceptable. They are a marker of disease in an otherwise normal-looking child.

Contraindications

Gastro-oesophageal reflux

Fixation of the stomach to the anterior abdominal wall tends to make the gastro-oesophageal junction more incompetent thus increasing pre-existing reflux. A simultaneous fundoplication should be considered.

Portal hypertension

Opinions differ about the risk of gastric varices at the gastrostomy site. If the nutritional need is sufficient, the benefits outweigh the risk.

Types of gastrostomy

Gastrostomy tube

Insertion Percutaneous tube (percutaneous endoscopic gastrostomy; PEG) is the most common tube. Sedation or general anaesthesia can be used. There are numerous tubes differing significantly in ease of replacement, right angled connectors at skin level, omnifunctional adapters and resistance to splitting.

Open laparotomy takes at least 45 minutes and carries significant risks of post-operative respiratory complications. The upper abdominal wound is painful and restricts coughing. The insertion is performed under direct vision and the stomach is sutured to the anterior abdominal wall.

Radiological insertion is possible, and ultrasound and screening combined have a high success rate for simple short-term catheters. This technique is rarely used in CF. Advantages include percutaneous insertion requiring only local anaesthetic.

> ### Note
>
> - Tubes with flanges are difficult to displace but require general anaesthesia to change.
> - Tubes with balloons can fall out, but are easy to replace.
> - Cutting the tube as short as possible reduces the chances of accidental pulling and improves cosmetic appearance.
> - If the tube fractures easily this will require more frequent changes.

Gastrostomy button

Although tubes are suitable for those who are immobile, buttons are better for long-term use in active individuals.

Insertion Insertion may be single stage or two stage. Single stage insertion includes open insertion at laparotomy. The development of buttons with inflatable Foley-type balloons (Figure 17.1) has allowed their insertion by a Single stage, Percutaneous, Rapid INsertion of a Gastrostomy button (SPRING) procedure (Figure 17.2).

Historically, all button insertions were two stage procedures. An initial gastrostomy track was created using a suitable PEG tube, which was left in situ for eight to twelve weeks. This allowed the stomach to weld to the anterior abdominal wall. Under a second general anaesthetic the tube was removed and replaced with a button.

Figure 17.1 Gastrostomy button with inflatable balloon.

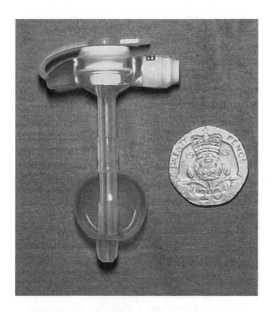

Figure 17.2 Button in situ. Note sutures used to ensure stomach closely opposed to anterior abdominal wall.

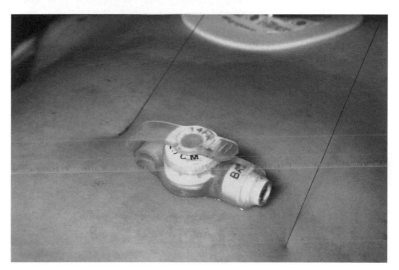

Table 17.1 Relative benefits of tubes and buttons.

		Tube	Button
1.	Single stage insertion	✓	✓
2.	Easy replacement	x	✓
3.	Anti-reflux valve	x	✓
4.	No dangly bits	x	✓
5.	Tube with two flanges	✓	✓

Balloon buttons fulfil four of the ideal criteria for a gastrostomy and when inserted by a SPRING only one general anaesthetic is required (see Table 17.1).Balloon devices can be expensive but the cost is offset by the reduced need for surgery.

General complications of gastrostomies

Technical

Wound dehiscence after open insertion   This requires general anaesthesia and re-suture.

Separation of the stomach from the anterior abdominal wall   This requires general anaesthesia, a laparotomy and suture of the stomach to the anterior abdominal wall with peritoneal lavage.

Bleeding   If intraperitoneal, this might be from a gastro-epiploic artery and cause rapid circulatory collapse requiring laparotomy. If from the superior epigastric artery it might stop with compression between the flange and the skin but can require formal exploration.

Infection (Figure 17.3)   Cellulitis needs systemic and local antibiotics (i.e. intravenous antibiotics and Fucidin cream). MRSA will probably not be eradicable without gastrostomy removal.

Injury to other organs   Pancreatic and liver trauma have occurred with no lasting harm. The colon is likely to be transfixed percutaneously following both underinflation of the stomach (causing the colon to remain in the way) and over-inflation (rotating the colon up and allowing insertion into the posterior gastric wall). Easy visualisation of the gastroscope light suggests that there is nothing in the way. If diagnosed, do not do a laparotomy but treat conservatively with intravenous antibiotics and remove the gastrostomy tube or button. Allow to settle and reinsert the gastrostomy percutaneously.

Omentum appears through the anterior abdominal wall   A general anaesthetic and mini-laparotomy will enable its replacement and placing of a stay suture in the anterior gastric wall.

Button extrudes (Figure 17.4)   If the button is too short, it may extrude. Re-measure and replace with the correct length button.

Care–related

The tube falls out   As a gastrostomy is a fistula, it will close remarkably quickly, making reinsertion difficult or impossible. A general anaesthetic and formal reinsertion will be required for a tube. Dilation under local anaesthesia might be possible for a button.

Less than eight weeks after insertion

- The tube needs to be replaced in hospital, as there is a risk that the stomach will be pushed off the anterior abdominal wall.

More than eight weeks after insertion

- Balloon type catheter: parents should be instructed to immediately reinsert a spare Foley-type catheter previously provided, blow up the balloon and tape it in position.
- PEG type tube: this will always require formal reinsertion under GA.

Skin excoriation   This is either due to leakage of gastric juice around the tube or problems with sweatiness or allergy to adhesive tapes.

- The tube must be kept at 90 degrees to the skin as angulation guarantees leakage.
- Additional treatment with H_2 blockers or a proton pump inhibitor reduces gastric acid secretion which should help.

Figure 17.3 Cellulitis around gastrostomy button site.

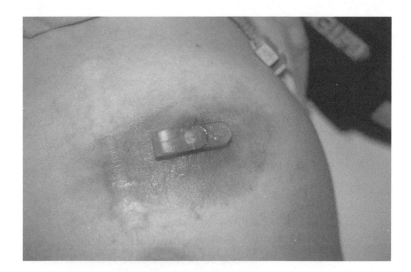

Figure 17.4 Protrusion of a button.

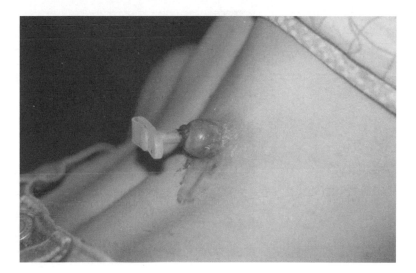

Persistent leakage can be treated by removing the tube and reinserting a temporary, smaller Foley-type tube overnight. The next day, following dilatation under general anaesthetic, the larger permanent gastrostomy tube or button is reinserted. This allows the track to contract down and fit more snugly.

Tube blockage   This can be prevented by flushing, before and after feeds, to remove debris. Tubes can be cleared using flat cola, meat tenderiser or gastrostomy brushes (see Chapter 7).

Tube-related   **Granulation tissue (Figures 17.5, 17.6)**   Most gastrostomies produce granulation tissue around the skin hole. This might be reduced if the skin incision is large initially. Lesions can be resistant to treatment. Silver nitrate pencils ($AgNO_3$), Sofradex ointment (Roussel) and Lyofoam dressing (Seton) have their advocates.

Figure 17.5 Granulation tissue around gastrostomy tube site.

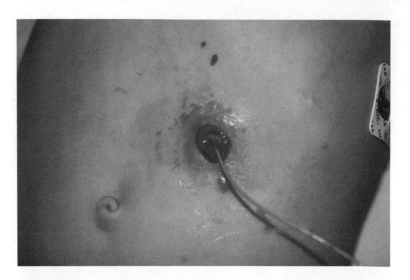

Figure 17.6 After treatment with silver nitrate.

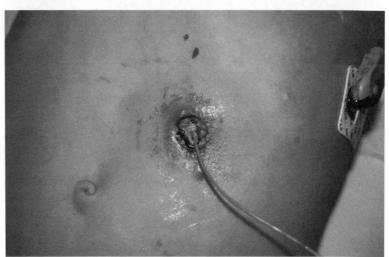

Leakage   Tubes, and not buttons, have no anti-reflux valve. If connectors are faulty, gastric juice or feed will leak out into the clothes or bedding.

Duodenal obstruction   Foley catheter-type gastrostomy tubes are prone to peristaltic passage through the duodenum if they are not securely fixed on the anterior abdominal wall. This can cause impaction in the third part of the duodenum and the bizarre symptom complex of pure green bile vomit with perfectly normal feeds through the gastrostomy (Rosie's Sign).

Balloon deflation causes fall out   See above.

Psychological   The visible presence of a tube, which is difficult to hide, can cause problems with body image although this is usually much less of a problem than a naso-gastric tube.

Long term   **Gastro–oesophageal reflux**   In some series, up to 50% of adults with gastrostomies start to vomit following insertion, even though there was no initial problem with vomiting. This reflux is presumably due to the fixation of the stomach to the anterior abdominal wall and should respond to medical management (antacids, prokinetic agents). Fundoplication can be required if the gastrostomy is sufficiently important and the reflux uncontrollable.

Complications specific to buttons and their treatment

After a SPRING

Initially the balloon is all that holds the stomach in position against the anterior abdominal wall. If it deflates very early, the stomach will almost certainly fall away and a laparotomy is required.

Should the button fall out in the first eight weeks the individual should be brought to hospital urgently for replacement as the stomach will not be stuck firmly.

After a couple of weeks, if the stomach is empty it might remain stuck long enough to allow careful replacement under general anaesthetic by the original method.

After eight to twelve weeks the individual or their parent can simply replace the button without risk, or tape the old one in place to hold the track open.

Traumatic reinsertion

With a mushroom ended Corpac button, reinserting this into a well established tract without sedation or general anaesthetic is tempting. This is cruel and may cause nightmares or hospital-phobia.

TOTALLY IMPLANTABLE VENOUS ACCESS DEVICES (TIVAD) (PORTACATH/ VASCUPORT)

Subcutaneous ports with lines inserted into the right atrium via the superior vena cava have become standard treatment for venous access problems in CF. They are much more acceptable then a percutaneous Hickman or Broviac line because of the patients' normal lifestyle requirements and the ports' repeated short term use for intravenous (IV) antibiotics.

Indications

- Established respiratory infection requiring IV antibiotic courses at least three or four times a year
- Peripheral intravenous lines lasting less than two days (for example, three or four peripheral lines needed per week)
- Absence of usable veins
- Severe needle-phobia (although TIVADs do not obviate the need for needles).

Contraindications

- Superior vena cava obstruction or severe pulmonary hypertension. Both of these can be complications of previous central lines.
- Social reasons – inability to look after the device.

Pre-operative care

The optimal position of the TIVAD Port is level with the nipple in the anterior axillary line of the non-dominant axilla (Figure 17.7). This position has many advantages. It allows the individual to get at the dressing easily and to help with self-care. Cosmetically, it is not in the breast and is out of sight. It does not restrict arm movement.

Figure 17.7   Optimal position of TIVAD.

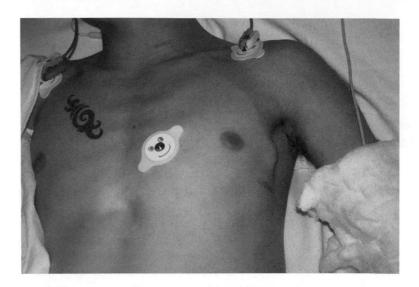

There is no point in positioning the scar to attempt denervation. Local anaesthetic creams such as Emla (Astra) or Amitop (Rousell) are efficient and effective.

Per-operative points

Insert the line by low cut down into the internal jugular vein. High insertions have a greater kink and retraction rate. The subclavian, percutaneous route is contraindicated because of pulmonary hyperinflation.

Make the incision for the pocket well below its actual site so that the scar is nowhere near the needle puncture site. Avoid the temptation to make the pocket just big enough for the port as a snug fit – the pocket needs to be comfortably larger than the port as this makes insertion easier. Mobilise the caudal skin flap to remove any tension.

Fix the port to the muscle fascia.

Screen the catheter tip per-operatively for position and make a hard copy. This obviates the need for a further check radiograph on the ward.

Position the tip just at the SVC-right atrial junction. Estimate the life of the port to be at least two years. There might be significant retraction of the tip with the growth of the child. It is unfortunate if a port has to be replaced just because it is too short.

Flush with Teicoplanin (Merrell 10 mg/kg) (not heparin) at the end of the procedure and leave this in situ to help prevent *Staph. epidermidis* infection (remember not to shake it, as it froths uncontrollably).

After skin closure:

- Insert the correct length of Huber needle and fix with opsite. This fixes the port and allows the pocket to shrink around it.
- Inject local anaesthetic around the port and cutdown site.

Remember

Insertion of the needle post-operatively is very painful. Insert it per-operatively.

Figure 17.8   Huber needle inserted into port.

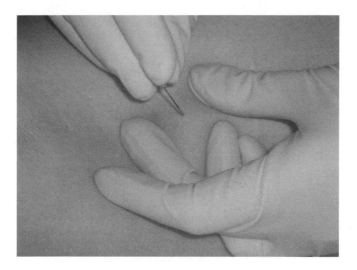

Post-operative points

TIVADs need careful maintenance to ensure longevity. Monthly flushes are required in the intervals when intravenous antibiotics are not given. The following are guidelines and not instructions.

Monthly flushing

- Use strict aseptic technique.
- Anaesthetise the skin over the port with local anaesthetic cream.
- Position the individual comfortably – preferably leaning or lying against something.
- Prime the Huber needle with heparinised saline.
- Clean the port with antiseptic solution using circular motions from the inside outwards and allow to dry.
- Stabilise the port with one hand and with the other insert the Huber needle firmly into the middle of the port at a right angle to the skin (Figure 17.8).
- Inject 5 ml of heparinised saline (100 u/ml) observing for signs of swelling. Leave 0.5 mls of solution in the syringe. Clamp the line if using an extension set.
- Whilst supporting the port remove the needle (maintaining pressure on the syringe plunger if the line has not been clamped).
- Clean the skin and apply a plaster if required.

Remember

TIVADs should only be accessed by individuals who have received training. Huber needles must be used when accessing the port because failure to do so can result in a 'coring' of the port's silicone block, necessitating premature removal.

Meeting resistance in the line when attempting to flush

Check for obvious obstructions (for example, line kinked, gate clamp or needle dislodged). Get the individual to:

- Move head and/or arm and look away from the port
- Take some slow deep breaths
- Perform a valsalva manoeuvre.

Remove the needle and insert a new one. If these do not help try unblocking the line (see complications and their treatment, below).

Inserting indwelling Huber needles

The technique is identical but the needle must be secured using padding and occlusive dressing (Figures 17.9 and 17.10).

Remember

Needles can be left in for a maximum of 14 days, but sites should be inspected regularly for signs of inflammation or swelling.

Blood sampling

The method is the same as for monthly flushing but the line should be primed with saline not heparinised saline.

- With a clean syringe draw back a minimum of 3 mls of blood and discard.
- With a second clean syringe draw back the amount of blood required.
- Flush with 5 mls of heparinised saline.

Figure 17.9 Huber needle in situ with wings.

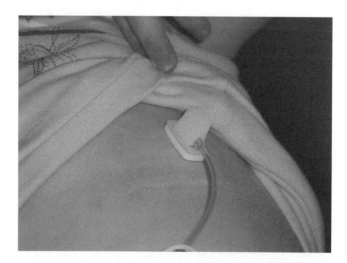

Figure 17.10 Gauze padding between Huber needle (wings removed) and skin, secured with occlusive dressing.

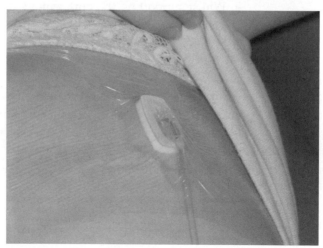

> **Remember**
>
> Aminoglycosides coat the inside of TIVADs and sampling directly from the line can give falsely high levels. Peripheral venous sampling is recommended.

Drug administration

- Morphine and heparin solutions cause precipitations in the line. If morphine is used, normal saline flushing before and after injection is recommended.
- TPN should not be given because of the high risks of sepsis.
- Penicillins and aminoglycosides cause precipitation if mixed. Ensure adequate flushing with normal saline between these drugs.

Treatment of complications

Infection   This is rare if families and nursing staff take scrupulous care. TIVAD devices should only be used by trained staff.

Bacterial infection is treatable with high dose antibiotics in 80% of cases and the line can be maintained. The remainder will require line removal. Fungal infections are incurable, and ports must be removed.

Mechanical   Blockage can occur if the child has grown rapidly and the line has migrated out of the SVC.

Blood clots rarely cause problems. They can occur if blood is aspirated with insufficient flushing – backflow with clots is less common with TIVADs than non-implanted Hickman and Broviac lines. Echocardiography can be useful if clots are suspected.

Treating a blocked TIVAD

This can be difficult. Unclogging with a guide wire is impossible and the use of a high pressure flush is usually unsuccessful. Urokinase can be injected:

- Mix 500 units in 2 ml of normal saline.
- Expel all air and connect to the port needle.
- Before injecting the Urokinase, aspirate to attempt to draw some blood into the line and then inject even a small amount.
- If the Urokinase has gone in, leave in the line for up to 24 hours.
- Withdrawal of 5 mls of blood/Urokinase prior to reusing will minimise the drug's systemic effects.

If flushing is easy, but aspiration is impossible:

- Try gentle aspiration with a 50 ml syringe.
- Check the position of the tip of the line.
- There might be a ball-valve clot at the tip – consider a Urokinase infusion.

Urokinase infusion

Under 5 years   2500 units in 4 ml of normal saline
Over 5 years   5000 units in 4 ml of normal saline

Infuse slowly over 4 hours using a syringe pump. If partially effective, repeat after two to three days. If these measures are unsuccessful replacement of the device may be the only option.

Large loops in the neck predispose to retraction of the line with neck movement. The tip might simply retract out of the vein or flick into the subclavian (where it can still work), or the azygos vein (where it will not). A kink can develop in the neck and cause blockage. Re-operation is usually necessary.

Separation of the tubing from the port is usually a technical error requiring re-operation. The tubing can fracture and migrate into the right atrium or pulmonary artery. This requires percutaneous removal by a cardiologist.

Extravasation occurs when the infusing fluid does not enter the chamber of the port. It is more common than leakage and due to incorrect needle insertion, or displacement. Often no treatment is required other than line removal and analgesics before the port is reused.

Pain over the tubing usually occurs in the neck, but only at the time of infusion. Pain can occur in a line that has migrated because of growth. Conservative measures are useless and replacement is inevitable. The replacement catheter must reach the right atrium/superior vena caval junction, where there is more tip movement. As a result the fibrin sheath, which grows around the line, is thinner and less likely to occlude the tip.

ACUTE ABDOMINAL PAIN

Abdominal pain and a palpable mass

If the pain is periumbilical and colicky or in the right iliac fossa there is usually a palpable mass. The differential diagnosis includes the following:

Distal intestinal obstruction syndrome (DIOS)

10–50% of individuals have occasional symptoms of mild recurrent intestinal obstruction. With good medical management these seldom require surgery (see Chapter 6).

The appendix

Non-inflamed   There is a CF syndrome of pain in a palpable appendix which is distended with inspissated mucus, but not actually inflamed. This is cured by appendicectomy.

True appendicitis   This often presents a diagnostic dilemma. DIOS can mimic appendicitis and there might be diagnostic delay. Up to 90% of CF children may perforate or have an abscess (non-CF perforation rate is 10–15%). The following help to differentiate:

- Always remember appendicitis with right iliac fossa pain, even though the individual has CF.
- Marked tenderness with a raised white cell count is unusual in DIOS.
- Ultrasound scan may well be 'normal' in DIOS.
- A contrast enema might demonstrate extrinsic compression of the caecum by an appendix abscess, and non-filling of the appendix.

Intussusception	The mass can be mistaken for faeces, due to DIOS rather than intussusception, if it is in the upper abdomen. The following should be noted:

- Intussusception in CF usually occurs in older children (peak age 8–10 years) rather than in infants.
- The classical symptom of redcurrant jelly stool is less common and thus intestinal obstruction is usually interpreted as DIOS.
- Ultrasound should distinguish between DIOS and intussusception if the differential diagnosis is considered.
- Plain abdominal X-ray may be unhelpful.
- As with non-CF intussusception, chronic intermittent colicky pain might occur with symptom-free intervals.
- Long standing intussusception is more likely to result in perforation of the bowel wall.

Other rarer causes of pain with a mass

- Crohns disease. Best diagnosed by barium meal – can be associated with peri-anal fistulae
- Ovarian cysts
- Volvulus and strictures secondary to previous surgery
- Constipation, although faeces are usually impalpable (see Chapter 6).

Acute abdominal pain with no mass

Epigastric pain

Gastro–oesophageal reflux and oesophagitis   (see Chapter 6).

Gastritis   Basal gastric acid output can be higher than normal. Ulcers can be precipitated by extreme physiological stress or the concurrent use of oral steroids. Investigation including gastroscopy and biopsy is required prior to treatment.

Central pain radiating to the back

Pancreatitis   This occurs in the pancreatic-sufficient. There might be recurrent mild acute attacks, which are self-limiting or respond to bowel rest or naso-jejunal feeds. It can be associated with biliary complications such as sclerosing cholangitis, common bile duct stenosis and cirrhosis. Chronic or burnt out pancreatitis can cause severe pain requiring pancreatectomy.

Large pancreatic cysts   These can be tense, causing chronic severe pain and associated with pancreatic stones. Treatment options include percutaneous aspiration, lithotripsy and pancreatectomy.

Intestinal obstruction without a mass or following adequate treatment for DIOS

Adhesion obstruction   Previous surgery, for example meconium ileus, makes adhesion obstruction a possibility but is usually diagnosed late as DIOS is more common.

Colonic stricture   (see Chapter 6).

Other causes   These include renal stones, urinary tract infection, gall stones, giardiasis and very rarely carcinoma.

Recurrent abdominal pain with no positive clinical findings

Psychosomatic abdominal pain is common (see Chapter 6).

Figure 17.11   Gastrograffin enema: the dilated ileum and microcolon are obvious.

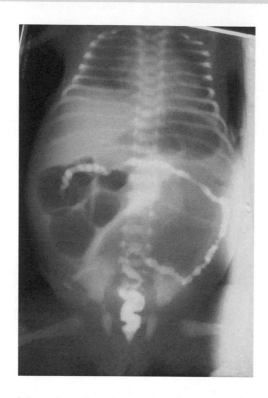

MECONIUM ILEUS AND MECONIUM PERITONITIS

Meconium ileus is a neonatal surgical emergency characterised by delayed passage of meconium, abdominal distension and green, bile-stained vomiting. The baby should be managed by the local regional neonatal surgical unit.

Conservative treatment

Gastrograffin enema (Figure 17.11)   The 'Tween 80' component in gastrograffin can emulsify the inspissated meconium (see Chapter 9).

Surgical treatment

Most surgeons prefer to clear out the bowel via an enterotomy (or enterotomies) in a reasonably normal piece of proximal ileum. The meconium is emulsified with acetylcysteine or gastrograffin. The microcolon is flushed through. The bowel can take some time to recover from the effects of surgical handling and chemicals.

Historically, a 'Bishop-Koop' ileostomy was constructed which required delayed closure.

Up to 30% of babies with meconium ileus require a bowel resection and anastomosis.

Diagnosis of CF

The regional surgical unit should work closely with the paediatric CF team (see Chapter 10). Not all affected children will have CF.

Remember

If the terminal ileum has been removed, Vitamin B12 absorption must be checked and supplements given by injection if necessary.

OTHER PROBLEMS RELEVANT TO SURGICAL CARE

Strictures/Adhesions

60% of neonates with meconium ileus undergo laparotomy. These children are at risk of strictures at the anastomosis and adhesion obstruction.

Because DIOS is common, the symptoms of intestinal obstruction are often treated medically. If there is no mass, adhesion obstruction or stenosis is more likely.

Strictures can cause diarrhoea unlike typical malabsorptive stools. If diarrhoea persists, radiological investigation is required to exclude a stricture.

Sodium loss

With obstruction, there is fluid loss into the peritoneum and bowel lumen. This fluid has a higher than usual sodium content. If pyrexial, sweating will increase sodium losses. Hyponatraemia can be severe and require large amounts of sodium.

Liver disease

Although cirrhosis can be asymptomatic there may be clotting abnormalities which require correction prior to surgery. Pre-operatively check the prothrombin time and correct with Vitamin K and fresh frozen plasma if needed.

Post-operative ileus

If there has been extensive adhesiolysis (especially after previous meconium peritonitis) there might be prolonged ileus. Prokinetic agents (e.g. rectal domperidone Motilium, Sanofi-Winthrop), can be helpful.

Post-operative dehydration

Pre-operative starvation and surgery are often followed by a variable period of post-operative starvation and possibly nausea and vomiting. This can make intestinal mucous more viscid and predisposes to post-operative DIOS. Per-operative intravenous rehydration, prophylactic anti-emetics and the early re-introduction of fluids should minimise this risk.

Rectal prolapse

Rectal prolapse occurs because of a combination of voluminous, frequent bowel actions, poor nutrition and increased intra-abdominal pressure from coughing.

It can occur in up to 18% of CF children, with a peak onset at 1–2 years of age. Most children with rectal prolapse do not have CF.

Treatment

If present at diagnosis most cases will resolve when enzyme treatment is introduced. The rest will usually improve more slowly.

If prolapse occurs in an adequately treated child then surgical treatment with 5% phenol in almond oil injections into the submucosa can be considered.

References

Gastrostomies

Gauderer M W L 1991 Percutaneous endoscopic gastrostomy: a 10 year experience with 220 children. Journal of Pediatric Surgery 26:288–294

Griffiths D M 1996 Single stage percutaneous gastrostomy button insertion: a leap forward. Journal of Paediatric Enteral Nutrition 20:237–239

Ruangtrakool R, Ong T H 2000 Primary gastrostomy button: a means of long-term enteral feeding in children. Journal of Medical Association of Thailand 83(2):151–159

TIVAD

Cassey J, Ford W D A, O'Brien L et al 1988 Totally implantable system for venous access in children with CF. Clinical Pediatrics 27:91–95

Deerojanawong J, Sawyer S M, Fink A M et al 1998 Totally implantable venous access devices in children with CF: incidence and type of complications. Thorax 53(4):285–289

Morris J B, Occhionero M E, Gauderer M W L et al 1990 Totally implantable vascular access devices in CF: a 4 year experience with 58 patients. Journal of Pediatrics 117:82–85

Abdominal pain

Atlas A B, Orenstein S R, Orenstein D M 1992 Pancreatitis in young children with CF. Journal of Pediatrics 756–759

Coughlin J P, Gauderer M W L, Stern R C et al 1990 The spectrum of appendiceal disease in CF. Journal of Pediatric Surgery 25:835–839

Dalzell A M, Heaf D P, Cart H 1990 Pathology mimicking distal intestinal obstruction syndrome in CF. Archives of Diseases in Childhood 65:540–541

Holmes M, Murphy V, Taylor M et al 1991 Intussusception in CF. Archives of Diseases in Childhood 66:726–727

Littlewood J M 1992 Gastrointestinal complications in CF. Journal of Royal Society of Medicine 85(Suppl 18):13–19

Stern R C, Izant R J, Boat T F et al 1982 Treatment and prognosis of rectal prolapse in CF. Gastroenterology 82:707–710

Recommended reading

Freeman N V, Neill V et al 1994 Surgery of the neonate. Edinborough, New York: Churchill Livingstone

Chapter **18**

Anaesthesia

Catherine Wood

INTRODUCTION

Most individuals require general anaesthesia (GA) at some stage and many will require multiple procedures. With improved long-term survival the numbers requiring anaesthesia will increase.

Typical procedures include:

- Insertion of totally implantable vascular access devices
- Insertion of gastrostomies
- ENT procedures
- Endoscopy and injection of oesophageal varices
- Laparotomy for intestinal obstruction
- Pulmonary surgery
- Incidental surgical procedures e.g. appendicectomy.

Neonatal intestinal obstruction and transplant procedures should be carried out in specialist centres and are beyond the remit of this chapter.

COMPLICATIONS OF GENERAL ANAESTHESIA

Reviews of anaesthesia in CF report a significant risk of complications (Doershuk 1972). These include:

- Ineffective mask ventilation necessitating intubation
- Endotracheal tube obstruction from excessive secretions
- Bronchospasm

- Slow induction and emergence
- Cardiac arrhythmias
- Postoperative atelectasis
- Pneumothorax
- Postoperative respiratory failure.

This list emphasises that, although CF is a multi-system disorder, pulmonary complications are of primary concern. The accumulation of bronchial secretions during anaesthesia can cause increased airways resistance, airway obstruction and gas trapping. Areas of increased V/Q mismatch result in hypoxia. Many will also manifest increased bronchial hypereactivity.

There is often a short-term deterioration in pulmonary function for up to 48 hours following GA. The most significant changes are in FEV1, resting lung volume and forced expiratory flow (Richardson 1984). GA should not cause long-term deterioration in the patient's condition (Lamberty & Rubin 1985, Olsen et al 1987, Robinson & Branthwaite 1984).

PRE–OPERATIVE EVALUATION

General considerations

Respiratory

GA should be avoided during acute respiratory tract infections. Individuals are generally good judges of their respiratory status and how much, if any, scope there is for improvement.

Pre-operative physiotherapy and bronchodilator inhalations up to the time of anaesthesia should reduce problems associated with excessive secretions and bronchospasm.

Cardiovascular

Long-standing hypoxia may have led to pulmonary hypertension and cor pulmonale.

Gastrointestinal

Gastro-oesophageal reflux is common (Scott, O'Loughlin & Gall 1985). If symptomatic, this needs to be considered when deciding on anaesthetic management.

Most individuals should not be malnourished but some will be undergoing surgical procedures such as gastrostomy tube insertion to address this problem.

Endocrine

Glucose intolerance or frank diabetes might necessitate the use of dextrose and potassium regimes combined with an insulin sliding scale during the immediate peri-operative period.

Liver function

CF-related liver disease might prolong the effect of opioid analgesics and muscle relaxants.

Liver disease might impair clotting; ensure Vitamin K has been given and fresh frozen plasma is available for those undergoing major surgery.

Fluid balance

Most will be able to drink clear fluids until 2 hours before anaesthesia.

There is an increased risk of sodium depletion and dehydration from hyperthermia. This can cause cardiovascular collapse.

Drug treatment   In general all medications should be continued until immediately prior to anaesthesia.

Some will be receiving high doses of inhaled corticosteroids and/or repeated courses of oral steroids. Steroid replacement therapy in the peri-operative period might be required.

History and examination

The pre-operative visit and discussion should cover all the standard aspects of anaesthesia as well as those concerned with CF. Concerns about respiratory status should not distract from checking for simple things such as wobbly teeth.

Respiratory and cardiovascular examinations are mandatory. Even in the absence of an acute infection there may be chest signs with added wheezes or crepitations and it is important to document a baseline assessment.

Investigations

- Recent pulmonary function tests: FEV1 usefully indicates the severity of lung disease (Kerem 1992). An FEV1 of <30% predicted may preclude elective surgery.
- Resting oxygen saturation in air.
- Recent sputum culture and sensitivity.
- Recent chest radiograph: looking particularly for bullae which might increase the risk of pneumothorax and choice of inhalational agent.
- Serum electrolytes: abnormalities might occur as a result of salt loss or diuretics. Renal disease is uncommon.
- In more severe cases consider blood gases and an ECG.

Pre-operative discussion and pre-medication

Many will be familiar with hospital routines, intravenous and inhaled drug administration and, in many cases, anaesthetics. Wherever practical, individual views about how procedures are carried out should be respected.

A pre-operative visit by the anaesthetist will generally remove the need for sedative pre-medication. If required, an oral benzodiazepine such as temazepam 0.5 mg/kg or midazolam 0.5 mg/kg can be considered. Opiates should be avoided.

There are theoretical contraindications to the pre-operative use of atropine, which can cause thickening of respiratory secretions.

H2 antagonists should be considered in those with reflux.

A local anaesthetic cream (EMLA or Amethocaine) should be applied when intravenous cannulation is anticipated (see Chapter 1).

INDUCTION

Although asymptomatic reflux is common, there are no reports of aspiration associated with anaesthesia. In the absence of other factors, a rapid sequence induction is not required.

Intravenous induction

If an implanted intravenous access device is present or if peripheral intravenous access can be readily established, intravenous induction is generally easier, and more controlled than inhalational induction.

If an implanted intravenous access device is used, strict asepsis should be observed.

Thiopentone or propofol are suitable induction agents. Propofol has possible advantages because of decreased airway reflexes and shorter recovery times. Lignocaine should be added to Propofol to decrease discomfort on injection.

Ketamine is contraindicated because it can lead to excessive production of secretions.

Inhalational induction

Many will be accustomed to using masks. Induction might take longer than anticipated because of V/Q mismatch and there is a high incidence of coughing and laryngospasm.

Sevoflurane is the agent of choice, offering a relatively smooth induction.

MAINTENANCE

For all but the shortest surgical procedures it is preferable to paralyse, intubate and ventilate. The advantages are:

- Reduced incidence of laryngospasm
- The ability to perform endotracheal lavage and suction during and at the end of the procedure
- More rapid awakening and return of airway reflexes.

Muscle relaxants

Suxamethonium should only be used if there is a specific indication because suxamethonium pains can hinder post-operative physiotherapy and coughing.

Any of the currently available non-depolarising agents are suitable.

Inhalational agents

Nitrous oxide is contraindicated if there are pulmonary bullae. Otherwise a nitrous oxide, oxygen and vapour technique is acceptable.

Intubation and ventilation

Nasal intubation should be avoided because of the risk of haemorrhage from polyps.

All inspired gases should be humidified to facilitate the clearance of secretions. Repeated suctioning of the endotracheal tube might be required.

Airway pressures must be monitored and adjusted to minimise the risk of barotrauma and pneumothorax.

The end tidal carbon dioxide should be maintained at values approximating the child's pre operative levels where known.

Monitoring

- Pulse oximetry
- Electrocardiogram
- Blood pressure
- Inspired/expired gas and vapour analysis
- Ventilator disconnect alarm
- Core temperature
- Peripheral nerve stimulator.

Reversal

Endotracheal suction with or without saline instillation should be performed before reversal and extubation. The place of formal physiotherapy under anaesthetic is being assessed. Extubation should occur only when fully awake and breathing spontaneously.

INTRA-OPERATIVE AND POST-OPERATIVE ANALGESIA

Many will return for further procedures. Adequate analgesia and good control of postoperative nausea and vomiting will help to reduce anxiety about future anaesthetics. Good analgesia, preferably without accompanying sedation, is important to enable effective chest physiotherapy and early mobility. Major surgical procedures often require opiates. Their use should be combined with other, less sedative, analgesia.

Local blocks

The first paediatric report of the benefits of epidural analgesia was in children with respiratory disease (Meignier, Souron & Le Neel 1983). Wherever possible the anaesthetic should incorporate either a formal local block or infiltration with local anaesthetic.

Simple analgesics

- Paracetamol
- Codeine phosphate.

Non-steroidals

- Diclofenac: Oral, rectal or intramuscular preparations
- Ibuprofen: Available as tablets or as syrup
- Piroxicam: Available as Feldene Melts which are useful if nil by mouth and may be preferable to suppositories.

Opiates

- Morphine infusion.
- Patient-controlled analgesia (PCA): After appropriate preparation, children as young as 7–8 years old are often able to master the use of a PCA regime. This gives them a measure of control over their management and enables background analgesia to be supplemented prior to potentially painful interventions such as physiotherapy. Children receiving a small background infusion have fewer episodes of oxygen desaturation than when receiving only boluses. A suitable regime is:
  - Morphine 0.5 mg/kg in 50 ml normal saline (1 ml = 10 mcg/kg morphine)
  - Background infusion   0.4 ml/hr
  - Bolus   2 ml
  - Lockout   5 min
  - Max in 4 hrs   40 ml
- In younger children, nurse-controlled analgesia is more appropriate with nursing staff assessing the need for bolus doses in addition to a background infusion. The pump is programmed with a longer lockout interval to prevent overdosing:
  - Morphine 0.5 mg/kg in 50 ml normal saline (1 ml = 10 mcg/kg morphine)

– Background infusion   1–2 ml/hr
– Bolus   1–2 ml
– Lockout   30 min

OTHER POST-OPERATIVE CONSIDERATIONS

Oxygen

Humidified oxygen should be given according to continuous pulse oximetry measurements to achieve normal saturations.

Chest physiotherapy

This should be reinstated as soon as possible.

References

Doershuk C F, Reyes A L, Regan A G et al 1972 Anesthesia and surgery in CF. Anesthesia and Analgesia 51(3):413–421

Kerem E, Reisman J, Corey M et al 1992 Prediction of mortality in patients with CF. New England Journal of Medicine 326(18):1187–1191

Lamberty J M, Rubin B K 1985 The management of anaesthesia for patients with CF. Anaesthesia 40:448–459

Meignier M, Souron R, Le Neel J C 1983 Postoperative dorsal epidural analgesia in the child with respiratory disabilities. Anesthesiology 59:473–475

Olsen M M, Gauderer M W L, Girz M K et al 1987 Surgery in patients with CF. Journal of Paediatric Surgery 22(7):613–618

Richardson V F, Robertson C F, Mowat A P et al 1984 Deterioration in lung function after general anaesthesia in patients with CF. Acta Paediatrica Scandinavica 73:75–79

Robinson D A, Branthwaite M A 1984 Pleural surgery in patients with CF. Anaesthesia 39:655–659

Scott R B, O'Loughlin E V, Gall D G 1985 Gastro-oesophageal reflux in patients with CF. Journal of Pediatrics 106:223–227

Chapter **19**

Lung transplantation

Julian Legg, John Warner

CHAPTER CONTENTS

INTRODUCTION

The first attempt at human lung transplantation was in 1963. The patient died 18 days post-operatively of sepsis and breakdown of the bronchial anastomosis. Improvements in survival only occurred after advances in immunosuppressive therapy. Transplant can now be considered an option in all cases.

In 1984 the first successful heart–lung transplants were performed in two CF adults in the UK. Following these initial successes an increasing number of individuals have undergone heart–lung transplantation and, more recently, bilateral sequential lung transplantation. Between April 1 1998 and March 31 2002 over 800 CF individuals underwent lung transplantation worldwide (United Network for Organ Sharing 2003). Within Europe, the survival rate was 80% at 1 year and 64% at 3 years (see Figure 19.1).

Most deaths following transplantation occur in the first months after surgery and relate directly to surgical complications, infection, multi-system organ failure with respiratory distress syndrome or post-transplant lymphoproliferative disease. The major long-term concern is bronchiolitis obliterans syndrome (BOS).

TRANSPLANTATION PROCEDURES

Single lung transplantation is unsuitable in CF, as the remaining native lung would be a source of infection. Bilateral sequential lung transplantation has

Figure 19.1 International actual survival after transplant (Source: Based on UNOS/ISHLT data as of December 2003 for transplants performed January 1990 to June 2001).

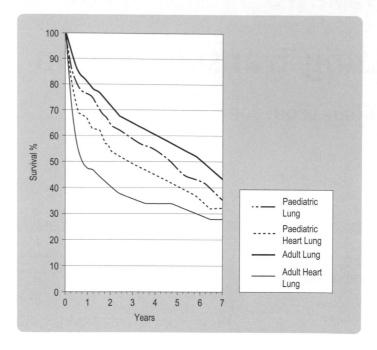

Legend:
- Paediatric Lung
- Paediatric Heart Lung
- Adult Lung
- Adult Heart Lung

now become the predominant operative approach as a result of improved techniques to establish the bronchial anastomoses. This procedure has comparable outcomes to heart–lung transplantation whilst enabling the donor heart to be used in a separate transplantation procedure and avoiding long-term complications related to coronary artery disease.

PATIENT SELECTION

The process of selection for lung transplantation should start locally. The physician should consider this as an option for those with poor quality of life and whose life expectancy is predicted to be less than 2 years. Early planning is advised as all transplant programmes have an inherent waiting time. The median waiting time for lung transplantation in the USA is currently 817 days.

In 1998 an international consensus committee developed guidelines for the selection of lung transplant candidates with CF (Starnes 1999, Maurer 1998). Objective criteria suggesting referral would appropriately include:

- FEV1 less than 30% of predicted despite optimal medical therapy
- Rapidly progressive respiratory deterioration
- Increasing numbers of hospitalizations
- Massive haemoptysis
- Recurrent pneumothorax
- PaO_2 <7.35 kPa (55 mmHg)
- $PaCO_2$ >6.7 kPa (50 mmHg)
- Increasing cachexia
- Young females with severe disease.

Absolute and potential contraindications

These vary between transplant centres and should be discussed directly with the relevant centre. Individuals who have been refused by one centre might be accepted by another.

Strong contraindications

- Invasive pulmonary aspergillosis
- Non-compliance with treatment
- Active *Mycobacterium tuberculosis* infection
- Major psychiatric illness
- Malignancy within 5 years
- HIV infection
- Hepatitis B antigen positive.

Potential contraindications

- Airway colonisation with a pan-resistant *Pseudomonas aeruginosa* or with *Burkholderia cepacia*
- Diabetes mellitus
- Hepatic impairment
- Previous pleural or thoracic surgery
- Ventilator dependence (excluding non-invasive ventilation).

Factors requiring pre-transplant intervention

- High dose systemic steroids (>1 mg/kg/day Prednisolone or equivalent) need reduction
- Poor nutrition – should be reversible using supplemental feeding regimens
- Atypical mycobacteria infection
- Methicillin-resistant *S. aureus* colonisation.

PRACTICAL ISSUES

At the referring centre

Teams should be objective in trying to recognise those at risk of dying in the next few years. In all cases, the option of lung transplantation should be discussed by the full team before formal discussion with the family. In some cases team members and families are unaware of disease severity and the poor long-term outlook. Families might find this news very difficult to accept. However, most families should be given the opportunity to consider this treatment option.

Transplantation might best be discussed at a planned visit outside of routine clinic times. Frank discussion about possible outcomes should include up-to-date information about the likelihood of a successful outcome and the rigorous demands that are inherent in assessment and acceptance onto a programme.

Individuals need to know that they will continue to need treatment for pancreatic insufficiency and other complications of the disease. Furthermore, because of the immuno-suppression necessary to maintain the transplanted organs, susceptibility to infection remains and is not just restricted to the lungs.

At the transplant centre

The selection procedure is protracted and for some may end in rejection from the programme. For the rest there is an agonising wait and an inexorable decline in lung function. The attrition on waiting lists is as high as 50% (Aurora 1999), with ever-increasing waiting times for suitable organs to become available.

The standard assessment programme involves a 3–4 day admission, which will include:

- Detailed lung function testing including exercise testing.
- Imaging of the upper and lower respiratory tract, often with CT scanning to detect any sources of infection particularly in the sinuses and teeth and also to establish whether there is any scarring, particularly in the pleura, which might complicate surgery.
- Blood sampling for bone marrow, liver and renal function as these will be compromised by the drugs administered after surgery to suppress immune rejection of the transplant.
- Blood and sputum specimens for serology and cultures taken to detect other underlying infections which might compromise surgery.
- Detailed nutritional assessment.
- Detailed psycho-social assessment looking for any factors which might influence medical compliance and success of the post-operative surveillance programme.
- In those having double-lung transplant, detailed cardiovascular assessment including echocardiography will also be necessary.

The decision about whether an individual is placed on the active list for transplant is dictated by many factors including lung function, quality of life, rate of decline of clinical status, aggressiveness of current treatment regimen and consideration of potential contraindications. The majority are placed on a provisional waiting list and reviewed by the transplant centre at least every 6 months before progressing to the active list.

WAITING FOR TRANSPLANT

Medical issues

Individuals on transplant waiting lists need continued aggressive management of nutrition and respiratory complications. Certain factors might require particular attention before transplantation. Nasal intermittent positive pressure ventilation (NIPPV) used judiciously for improving oxygen delivery (rather than treating hypercapnia) can increase survival by 6–9 months providing an extended window in which a donor organ may be found (Madden 2002).

There is inevitably a great temptation to delay the introduction of effective terminal care whilst continuing to wait in hope of the opportunity for a transplant. This has resulted in sub-optimal management when entering the terminal phase. The prospects of transplantation should not be allowed to affect decisions about palliative care. Relief of pain and distress must be a primary consideration at all times, even if this might reduce the time remaining to have the chance of a transplant (Warner 1991).

Social issues

Whilst waiting for a transplant a bleeper is issued so that contact can be made at all times. It is usual for the transplant centre to test the system periodically to ensure that families are maintaining contact. There will be occasions when the family will be contacted because of the potential availability of donor organs, only for this expectation to be thwarted hours later by unexpected events.

Support must be intensified. It may, for instance, be necessary to admit individuals for respite care because of the tensions generated whilst waiting.

Finding a donor

Donors and recipients are matched by:

- ABO blood group compatibility
- Size
- Cytomegalovirus (CMV) serological status.

Donor lungs should be slightly smaller than the recipient chest cavity to prevent atelectasis and uneven ventilation. Those who are CMV-negative should receive CMV-negative donor organs and blood products to prevent CMV infection – a major cause of morbidity and mortality in the post-transplant period.

POST-OPERATIVE MANAGEMENT

Immunosuppression

Survival after thoracic organ transplantation improved significantly following the introduction of Cyclosporin A. Maintenance immunosuppression following transplantation typically consists of three separate drugs:

- Cyclosporin A or Tacrolimus (FK-506)
- Azathioprine or mycophenolate mofetil
- Prednisolone.

Cyclosporin A and Tacrolimus are the mainstay for suppression of allograft rejection. Both drugs bind to proteins within cells to form complexes, which in turn inhibit the phosphatase activity of calcineurin, an important step in the activation of T lymphocytes. Both have a narrow therapeutic index and acceptable tolerance within a narrow range of blood concentrations. Dose ranges vary considerably because of a high degree of pharmacokinetic and pharmacodynamic variability. Blood level monitoring is essential. Nephrotoxicity is the main side-effect of excessive levels. Other complications include:

- Hypertension
- Hypercalcaemia
- Hepatotoxicity
- Gingival hyperplasia
- Hirsutism
- Convulsions.

Additional immunosuppression is achieved with a purine synthesis inhibitor (azathioprine or mycophenalate mofetil) and corticosteroids (intravenous methylprednisolone followed by oral prednisolone) perioperatively. Prednisolone doses are gradually weaned to minimise the complications of long-term steroid use. Other immunosuppressive agents are used depending on the clinical situation including anti-thymocyte globulin and monoclonal antibodies to a range of receptors on T lymphocytes.

Complications

Acute rejection

Acute pulmonary rejection is a common phenomenon occurring in 50% of cases. Clinical signs and symptoms include low-grade pyrexia, breathlessness, cough, bibasilar inspiratory crackles, bilateral interstitial infiltrates on chest X-ray and occasionally a pleural effusion. As these signs are non-specific, regular monitoring is essential. Monitoring is primarily based on daily spirometry. Significant changes are investigated by bronchoscopy, broncho-alveolar lavage and transbronchial biopsy in order to distinguish rejection from infection. Acute rejection is characterised by peri-vascular cuffing with mononuclear cells on biopsy.

Treatment includes high-dose intravenous Methylprednisolone, anti-thymocyte globulin and T-cell receptor antibodies. A change of maintenance immunosuppression (e.g. Cyclosporin to Tacrolimus) is considered after repeated episodes.

Infections

Post-operative infection can occur with similar organisms to those that occur in other immunosuppressed individuals, e.g. CMV and Aspergillus. Clinical and radiological findings are often identical to those of acute rejection and require investigation as detailed above. Bacterial organisms are usually isolated from broncho-alveolar lavage fluid whereas viral, fungal and protozoal infections are best diagnosed from transbronchial lung biopsy. Appropriate treatments include broad-spectrum anti-bacterial, protozoal, fungal and antiviral drugs. All patients receive life-long prophylactic Co-trimoxazole against *Pneumocystis carinii*.

Bronchiolitis obliterans syndrome (BOS)

This is the most feared long-term complication and can occur years after transplant (Estenne & Hertz 2002). Bronchiolitis obliterans is the pathological lesion. BOS is characterized by a late decline in FEV1 not attributable to acute rejection, infection or mechanical obstruction from bronchial anastomoses complications. BOS is the most common cause of death from lung transplantation after the first six months. Aetiology is unknown, but might be a chronic rejection process. Known pre-disposing factors include:

- Chronic local infection
- Airway stenosis
- CMV infection.

Symptoms include cough, shortness of breath and wheezing. On examination there are diffuse fine end inspiratory crackles. The chest radiograph is usually normal or demonstrates a modest degree of hyperinflation. Flow-volume loops demonstrate airflow obstruction poorly responsive to bronchodilators. Treatment includes increasing maintenance immunosuppressive drugs or the addition of other immune-modulating treatments. Unfortunately only 50% are responsive. The only option for severe unresponsive BOS is re-transplantation but survival rates are universally poor compared with first-time lung transplant recipients. Re-transplantation is controversial because of the limited availability of donor lungs (Hosenpud 1996).

Lymphoproliferative
disease

Post-transplant lymphocytproliferative disease (PTLD) is a heterogenous clinical entity manifested by an abnormal expansion of lymphoid cells. PTLD occurs in up to 20% of organ transplant recipients, most commonly within the graft lymphoid tissue (Cohen 2000). Clinical features include pyrexia, malaise, weight loss, anorexia or a detectable mass. Imaging demonstrates a well-defined mass and diagnosis is confirmed by open biopsy. Clonal proliferation of B-lymphocytes due to T-cell immunosuppressive therapy is felt to be the cause and Epstein-Barr viral infection may have a role. Treatment involves reduction of immunosuppression and radiotherapy or surgery.

THE FUTURE

The ultimate treatment aim is to prevent decline in lung function, thus avoiding the need for transplantation. In the foreseeable future, the demand for transplants will outweigh the provision of donor organs. This has led to consideration of two alternative strategies.

Surgeons in California have pioneered the technique of living lobar transplantation. The procedure involves harvesting a left lower lobe from one healthy donor and a right lower lobe from a second donor. Children have received a lobe from each parent with reported outcomes comparable to results obtained using cadaveric whole lung allografts (Starnes 1999). This raises enormous ethical issues particularly concerning whether a healthy donor should be subjected to the risks and morbidity of lobectomy.

An alternative strategy is to use non-human donors (i.e. xeno-transplantation). Uncontrollable humoral rejection usually accompanies cross-species transplantation and the very few attempts at transplants from baboon to man have failed. However, the development of transgenic pigs expressing human cell surface molecules that prevent activation of the immune system is now possible. This gives the opportunity to consider breeding transgenic animals to produce organs for transplantation. Unfortunately, the lungs are extremely susceptible to xenograft rejection and the prospect of pulmonary xeno-transplantation is some time away.

References

Aurora P, Whitehead B, Wade A et al 1999 Lung transplantation and life extension in children with cystic fibrosis. Lancet 354:1591–1593

Cohen A H, Sweet S C, Mendeloff E et al 2000 High incidence of post-transplant lymphoproliferative disease in pediatric patients with cystic fibrosis. American Journal of Respiratory and Critical Care Medicine 161:1252–1255

Estenne M, Hertz M I 2002 Bronchiolitis obliterans after human lung transplantation. American Journal of Respiratory and Critical Care Medicine 166:440–444

Hosenpud J D, Novick R J, Bennett L E et al 1996 The Registry of the International Society for Heart and Lung Transplantation: thirteenth official report 1996. Journal of Heart and Lung Transplantation 15:655–674

Madden B P, Kariyawasam H, Siddiqi A J et al 2002 Noninvasive ventilation in cystic fibrosis patients with acute or chronic respiratory failure. European Respiratory Journal 19:310–313

Maurer J R, Frost A E, Estenne M et al 1998 International guidelines for the selection of lung transplant candidates. The International Society for Heart and Lung Transplantation, the American Thoracic Society, the American Society of Transplant Physicians, the European Respiratory Society. Transplantation 66:951–956

Starnes V A, Woo M S, MacLaughlin E F et al 1999 Comparison of outcomes between living donor and cadaveric lung transplantation in children. Annals of Thoracic Surgery 68:2279–2283

United Network for Organ Sharing 2003 UNOS data. Online. Available: http://www.unos.org. Accessed December 2003

Warner J O 1991 Heart–lung transplantation: all the facts. Archives of Diseases in Childhood 66:1013–1016

Chapter **20**

Primary care

Simon Pennell

INTRODUCTION

General Practitioners (GPs) and their teams are well placed to make important contributions to the care of individuals with CF and their families. Holistic care and support at local level can enhance the delivery of care recommended by the regional centre. Involving GPs leads to their better understanding about the need for costly therapeutic options and action required for acute respiratory exacerbations.

The CF Trust have identified areas of care for which GPs are well placed to contribute.
These include:

- An important role in home care and terminal care
- An important role in communication and ongoing support
- Prescribing of routine medications*
- Ensuring CF individuals are routinely immunised and arranging annual influenza vaccinations each autumn
- Making appropriate referrals to address fertility issues
- Arranging referrals for direct family members and other relatives for genetic counselling
- Care and bereavement counselling.

---

*Repeat prescriptions of long-term therapies such as pancreatic enzymes and vitamin supplements should provide at least 1–2 months supply of medication.

> **Note**
>
> Individuals who are long distances from the CF centre might use their GP practice to send microbiological specimens for culture and obtain appropriate first line antibiotics. Clear delineation of responsibilities and training about obtaining adequate specimens are essential.

Negative attitudes about GPs who have a small number of CF patients under their care and a lack of clarity about areas of responsibility can undermine the primary care role. Improved primary care services might be achieved by enabling a GP within each locality to develop a specialist interest in CF care.

GPs should explore options for contributing to care along lines that have been successfully used for other chronic conditions. Specialist providers should facilitate the involvement of GPs. The GP provides stability throughout childhood into adult life. By contributing to all aspects of care for the whole family they are in a unique position to advise about appropriate options.

OPPORTUNITIES FOR THE GENERAL PRACTITIONER

Specialist hospital teams should make direct contact with an individual's GP soon after diagnosis. This might best be achieved by the CF nurse and/or paediatrician visiting the practice.

Opportunities for primary care input in CF management might include:

Support at specific times

- At diagnosis – The support of a known and trusted health care professional can be of benefit whilst adapting to new treatment demands and the attentions of an unfamiliar group of health care professionals.
- Terminal care – GPs can provide meaningful care at this time because of their involvement and understanding of family dynamics.

A role in continuous assessment

Routine consultations with the GP between visits to the specialist centre could be offered in addition to emergency appointments for acute symptoms. Direct discussion between the specialist and primary care teams should take place to establish clear responsibilities. Effective two-way lines of communication are essential if this is to happen. Such arrangements might be appropriate for families living in remote areas. Individuals are often poor at assessing their health status. A GP is well placed to say 'You are not as well as you think you are', and liase with the specialist centre over the best course of action.

Other benefits include:

- Input to improve concordance.
- A better understanding of the use of prescribed therapies.

An interpretive role

CF individuals might value the opportunity for the GP to interpret and reflect with them on the treatments advised by the specialist unit.

Supportive role

Supportive services for parents and siblings are an important part of holistic care. GPs are well placed to assess and access support in an appropriate local environment. Engagement in the continuity of CF care will increase recognition of when support is needed and reinforce confidence in the value of primary care input.

Prescribing

The GP has an important role in prescribing. Good facilities for prompt repeat prescriptions in appropriate quantities are essential. GPs should be familiar with the agreed prescribing protocols developed by specialists, understand the need for, and thus support the use of expensive drugs.

Immunisation

- It is recommended that children receive a standard immunisation schedule. Underlying medical conditions, however, need to be taken into consideration and may affect the timing of such injections.
- CF individuals on oral steroids should not receive live vaccinations (for example, MMR). However, it is important to ensure that they are given these at a later date.
- Influenza vaccination is recommended every autumn.
- Most children respond to childhood diseases in the same way as non-affected peers. They do run a slightly higher risk of chickenpox pneumonitis and some centres advocate the use of oral Acyclovir when infection is diagnosed.

Contribution to annual assessments

Some GPs might value the opportunity to formally provide information and feedback about CF individuals within their practice to the regional centre. This could be achieved by inviting GPs to provide a written contribution as part of the annual review process.

Anticipatory role

Anticipating CF individual and family needs is an everyday skill in general practice. This is often opportunistic. Such awareness develops through an appreciation of the individuality of each patient and family in their community setting. Some areas where it is possible to anticipate needs include:

- Obtaining airway microbiological cultures
- The use of contraception by female patients and the use of condoms by sexually active males as part of healthy sexual practice
- General health education about smoke avoidance and the use of alcohol
- Travel needs
- Family genetic issues
- Immunisation.

Responsibility to the family

GPs are well paced to share the burden of illness with a family. This might usefully reduce their vulnerability to the effects of stressful occurrences.

CONCLUSION   There are limitations in the extent to which specialist services can provide for all the health care needs of a CF individual. The involvement of general practice can enable a more comprehensive service for families. Individual arrangements will differ, but the primary care role should be clearly defined between GPs and secondary care services. CF individuals should be encouraged to make the best use of these resources.

Chapter 21

Social issues

Judi Maddison

INTRODUCTION

CF variably affects everyday life and activities. Regardless of the health of the individual the mere fact of having CF will influence and can sometimes prejudice opportunities. It is the carer's responsibility to provide families with ongoing information and support.

TODDLER AND PRE-SCHOOL YEARS

Social interaction with their peer group is an important part of a child's development, but can result in an increased number of infections. It is common for non-affected children aged under 2 years to get recurrent coughs and colds. Whilst this can be a nuisance, these viral illnesses do not usually have a significant impact on the child's health and do not require antibiotics. This is not the case for a CF child, who might require repeated courses of antibiotics, frequent clinic visits and suffer general disruption to everyday life. Concerns about the risk of infection can cause some parents to withdraw their child from activities involving others and might also impact on decisions about returning to work. It is important that the infection risk is sensibly weighed against the loss of social contact and the isolation this will cause (Nicholson, Hammersley & Kent 1996). Enforced social isolation can be a reminder about the child's illness and parents can lose their perspective on normal behaviour and illnesses. Engendering a sickness model in an otherwise healthy child can cause problems in later years and distortion of their actual prognosis (Simmons & Goldberg 2001).

For many parents there is no choice about returning to work and so childcare options need to be discussed. If childcare is needed in the first year of life, ideally it should be in a setting where there is a small number of peers. Parents might find it helpful if a member of the CF Team makes a joint visit with them to their child's possible placement, to allay any staff fears and discuss any specific needs. Some local authorities accept CF children into their special needs nurseries and pre-school groups and some offer subsidised or free places.

Since April 2003 parents of children under 6 years or, if the child is disabled, under 18 years have a legal right to ask their employer for a change to their working arrangements. Rules apply to either parent provided they have worked for their current employer for at least 26 weeks. Employers have a legal obligation to consider the request but they do not have to agree to it. However, they do have to notify the employee in writing about their decision. If they refuse an alteration to working times or haven't followed the correct procedure, an employee is entitled to take their claim to an industrial tribunal, or to make a claim under the Sex Discrimination Act.

There is also legislation relating to children aged under six years allowing parents to take unpaid leave for up to several months. This legislation is subject to a number of criteria and parents should be advised to contact the Social Services or the appropriate government department to discuss their individual case.

SCHOOL YEARS

Most schools now have the infrastructure in place for children with special needs. However, staff are often unfamiliar with CF and will need appropriate information and support. Parents should initiate good lines of communication at the earliest opportunity. Each school now has a Special Needs Coordinator (Special Educational Needs and Disability Act 2001) with responsibility to ensure that all pupils' specific needs are met. Parents should be encouraged to meet this person and maintain regular contact throughout the time their child attends the school.

A school visit by a CF Team member is often useful, particularly if the child has complex needs. It is important to encourage the school to regard the child as a normal pupil, with specific needs to be taken into account and not a sick child who needs to be restricted. Schools that have previously had a CF pupil should be reminded that every CF child is different.

The following common misconceptions often need to be addressed:

- *The child has a fatal condition and might suddenly collapse and die.* It needs to be stated explicitly that this will not happen.
- *The cough is infectious or is exaggerated by the child.* Staff must be reassured that although CF children may cough a lot, there is no risk of infection to their healthy peer group. Most will suppress rather than exaggerate their coughs.
- *The pancreatic enzymes are dangerous if taken by others.* It must be emphasised that the enzymes are not drugs and are a replacement therapy. Even if accidentally consumed by others they are of no risk.

- *Missed or inappropriate enzyme dosages will cause health problems.* Staff are often fearful about administering unfamiliar medication and need to be reassured that minor mismatch between enzyme intake and content of the meal is of little importance.
- *The CF diet is unhealthy.* Staff must understand that a healthy diet for CF children includes high calorie foods such as sweets and chocolate with meals and as snacks. School policies might need to be reviewed.

Should the child's peer group know?

Some parents and their children may wish to maintain secrecy about their condition. Whilst such wishes should be respected, the following should be considered:

- Maintaining secrecy is extremely difficult, particularly when the child is requiring regular medication.
- A child who has to keep their illness a secret might feel shame, isolation and fear. The opportunities of staying overnight with friends, going to parties and school trips can be denied because of fear of disclosure.
- Other children are curious and notice differences in their classmates. Lack of an explanation is more likely to lead to bullying and teasing.
- Other children may spread rumours about why medication is being taken. These might be much more upsetting than the truth.
- Even if a child is healthy so that secrecy can be maintained, the need for clinic visits and unpredictable acute medical complications usually makes secrecy impractical in the long term (Fowler, Johnson & Atkinson 1985).

When starting a new school or changing teachers, it is important for the child and the parents to discuss exactly what they want the other pupils to know. This is particularly important for secondary school pupils. CF now appears in parts of the National Curriculum and there have been instances of teachers asking CF pupils to explain about their condition to their class, without prior consultation.

Evolving independence

School can provide the child with their first opportunity to take responsibility for their treatment. Remembering to take enzymes correctly at lunchtime and before snacks can demonstrate growing independence (Angst 1993). Indirect supervision can confirm this and allay parent's fears. Most schools will not take legal responsibility for supervising children taking medication. Parents must discuss this with staff. The CF Team can provide additional advice.

Children should be encouraged to participate in all aspects of school life. They should take part in physical education. If they have limitations this should be discussed.

Outings and overnight trips

Children might be denied such opportunities for fear of jeopardising treatment. Outings and overnight trips should be encouraged. Benefits usually outweigh any temporary lapse in optimal treatment. The CF Team might usefully advise about short-term modifications to routine treatment regimes. Schools may be concerned about:

- Physiotherapy – if independent treatment is not appropriate it is usually possible to train a helper to assist the child.
- Medication – the school will probably be familiar with enzyme administration. Other medication might be unfamiliar and explanations about how and when it is taken, as well as any storage requirements, should be given. Staff should be given a list of medication and contact details.
- Equipment – compressors and feeding pumps can usually be provided in a portable form.

Treatment during the school day

Some aspects of treatment cannot be avoided during the school day but it is preferable to keep as much of the daily treatment regime out of school as possible. Treatment other than enzymes will result in the child being excluded from other aspects of the normal school day and might single them out as being 'different'. This is generally disliked and can result in compliance problems. In general, treatment undertaken by specific staff only occurs when these staff members are available and will not occur during weekends and holidays.

If a treatment is needed during the school day but only for a short time, schools can usually accommodate this within their special needs facilities. Special funding will be needed for long-term treatments to ensure their continued provision. Obtaining the necessary support can be a lengthy process.

Children may wish to attend school whilst receiving intravenous antibiotics. Head teachers have the right to refuse to take a child back whilst receiving intravenous treatment. Open discussion, prior to the event, should prevent problems and ensure appropriate arrangements are made to cover all aspects of the school day.

While most schools try to be supportive, parents must realise there are legal restrictions about how much physical care staff can undertake. Requests need to be realistic and supported by written and verbal information.

Absence from school

Time off school, if only to attend clinics, is inevitable (Ellerton 1996). If the amount of time starts to create educational difficulties, the followings options can be explored:

- Work can be transferred to the home setting.
- Work planned for the time of clinic appointments can be rescheduled.
- In-patients should receive educational provision from the hospital school service. This is most successful when linked to their school. If the admission is pre-planned an appropriate work programme should be arranged.
- Examinations can be arranged within the hospital setting or rearranged for when the child is well. Extra time for exams can be granted, but this needs close liaison between school and examination board and must be arranged in advance.

- A formal statement of special educational needs (Department for Education and Employment) might clarify a child's specific medical or educational requirements and thus their access to resources.
- Whilst the National Curriculum contains specific subjects that must be included, it is possible to obtain permission to drop a subject. This can allow catch-up time in the school day and time for treatment or rest.

> **Note**
>
> Information for staff is available from the CF Trust.

GAP YEARS

CF should not prevent the opportunity of a gap year but it is vital that health needs are taken into account. Individuals need to be realistic about the challenges their illness might cause. They should not rely on travelling companions as their only form of help and support.

Obtaining a regular supply of medication

Once a person has been out of the UK for more than three months they are no longer eligible to receive medication on prescription via the NHS (National Health Service Regulations 1992). GPs are obliged to remove patients from their register if absent from the UK for more than three months. One solution is to use private prescriptions, but this is at the GP's discretion. On returning to the UK, individuals are automatically re-entitled to prescriptions via the NHS but have to re-register.

Transporting medication

Carrying several months' supply of medication may not be physically possible because of the volume and storage needs of individual items. Whilst some products can be purchased in some countries this might not always be possible and can be very expensive. Arrangements to receive regular supplies from home are often the best solution but need careful planning and negotiation with the GP. Storage of medication in transit needs consideration, especially if it needs refrigeration.

Sending medication abroad

Whilst making arrangements to send parcels might seem the best solution, some countries require drug import licences to permit this. Students should contact the appropriate embassies to check the documentation required. Some countries might not permit the importing of medication if it is similar to one produced in their own country – even if only for personal use.

Medical cover when away

Consideration must be given about how medical help will be obtained and what medical facilities are available. Comprehensive travel insurance is vital but a realistic look at what the countries offer when planning a route can prevent problems. Students likely to require intravenous antibiotics are probably best discouraged from spending months in an area where there are no CF centres. Shorter visits, using bases in areas where such treatments are available, are a better option.

FURTHER EDUCATION

CF should not be an obstacle to academic success (Adult CF Association 1995). Many students leave home to pursue further education. This is a major change in lifestyle and whilst moves to independence should be encouraged, support is often needed (McLaughlin 2001).

Where are they going to live?

It is often possible to stay in university or college accommodation for the entire duration of the course on medical grounds. Many institutions of higher education have special provision for people with health needs and these should be looked into when making a choice.

Is there a local adult CF centre?

Most students return home between terms and CF centres in university cities will usually operate a shared care system to maintain links with the local referring unit.

What provisions are there to assist with treatment?

Most students need additional help with their care at some time. Strategies to achieve this should be discussed when considering a university or college – support should not rely entirely on other students. Most universities have medical centres that are able to offer support and this should be discussed during informal open day visits.

What are the physical demands of the course?

It might not be obvious how physically demanding a particular course is going to be. Careful consideration should be given to courses involving foreign travel or multiple field trips. Being realistic at the start is more likely to result in successful completion.

> **Note**
>
> There are special allowances, such as the Disabled Students Allowance, that can assist with the costs of higher education. Individuals should speak with the CF team social worker to find out more about specific allowances.

DRINKING, DRUGS, AND SEX

CF patients should not be denied the rich varieties of life. There are some considerations:

- Those with liver disease should be advised about safe drinking levels.
- Solvents and other volatile inhaled substances might have a more profound effect than on someone without lung problems. Their use should be discouraged.
- Females need to know they can get pregnant. Males are generally infertile (see Chapter 16) (Gilljam, Antoniou & Shin 2000).
- Both sexes should be advised about using condoms to protect against sexually transmitted diseases.

EMPLOYMENT

Consider:

- Certain occupations such as the Armed Forces and some Police Forces exclude anyone with a chronic medical condition.
- A heavily polluted environment should be avoided. The smoking policy for the workplace should be considered.
- The physical and time demands of the job must be matched with health and treatment needs.
- Finding a job that can be flexible can be difficult but worthwhile.

Leaflets advising about employment are available from the CF Trust.

Informing a prospective employer

Individuals are often reluctant to disclose their condition to prospective employers. Technically, if they are not specifically asked about health problems, they do not have to disclose them. However, employers are more likely to be sympathetic about health issues if they are aware of the problem from the beginning. If an employee is asked directly about their health status they must declare any medical problems. Failure to do so could result in dismissal if a problem is later revealed (Walters, Britton & Hodson 1993). Written information, enclosed with an application form, will ensure that an employer is able to make a judgement based on up-to-date knowledge. Whilst leaflets for employers are available from the CF Trust, applicants may find it useful to enclose their own information explaining exactly how the disease affects them.

Ensuring health needs

- If physical adaptations to the work environment are needed it may be possible for local councils to provide an employer with financial assistance.
- If treatment needs are discussed with an employer it may be possible to negotiate flexible working hours and time off. The CF Team can assist with negotiations by talking to an employer if requested.

> **Remember**
>
> In the UK, the Disability Discrimination Act ensures that people with health needs should not be discriminated against.

FINANCE AND INSURANCE

This information applies to individuals in the UK only. Those living outside of the UK might find it applies to them but they are advised to contact their local CF Association for further details.

People with CF commonly experience difficulties securing reasonable terms for personal insurance (Baker 1997). They should be advised about the following:

- The CF Trust and The Diabetic Association have lists of companies willing to provide policies to cover people with medical needs.
- Premiums are generally higher but can vary considerably from company to company. Shop around.

- Full disclosure of medical information, including associated problems such as diabetes and liver disease, is necessary. Failure to disclose information might result in the policy being null and void.
- Immediately inform your company about any changes to health status.

Mortgages (Input 1996)

- Endowment mortgages are often difficult to obtain and have higher premiums. Many financial institutions are no longer offering this type of mortgage and so costs to 'higher risk clients' have increased.
- Mortgage protection policies are recommended if a repayment mortgage is being considered as well as the necessary life insurance.

Buildings and contents insurance

- Premiums should not be affected by the policy holder's health.
- Extra individual cover might be needed if expensive medical equipment is used, even if it is on loan.
- The insurance company must be notified if oxygen is installed and there might be an increase in the premium.

Motor insurance and driving licence (DVLA website 2003)

- Those in receipt of high rate motability are eligible to apply for a provisional car driving licence a year earlier, at the age of 16 years. Insurance can be difficult to obtain and is extremely expensive, unless the person is using a motability vehicle.
- There are no driving test concessions for disabled drivers other than allowing them to take their test in a specially adapted vehicle.
- Drivers who take and pass their test in specially adapted vehicles will only be eligible to drive specially adapted vehicles and no other vehicle.
- CF is not a listed disorder requiring compulsory notification to the DVLA but individuals should be encouraged to disclose their medical condition when applying for a licence.
- There are several restrictions to licences for vehicles other than cars or motorcycles and individuals applying for these types of licences should be encouraged to discuss their health with the DVLA.
- There should be no additional loading for vehicle insurance policies unless the driver has a restricted licence.
- A medical is not usually necessary for vehicle insurance but notification of medical conditions is required. Any restrictions must be declared.
- Patients with diabetes must notify the Drivers Medical Branch of the DVLA upon diagnosis. They will be issued with a restricted licence and this will affect their insurance premiums. Better rates can be obtained by using specialist companies (contact The British Diabetic Association).
- Patients receiving continuous oxygen might still be able to drive but should contact the DVLA first. They must also notify their insurance company who may increase the policy premium. Similar recommendations apply to parents transporting children requiring oxygen.
- If oxygen is being carried in a vehicle a 'compressed gas' label must be clearly displayed on the back of the vehicle.

- Seat belt exemption certificates can be obtained from the General Practitioner. These certificates are only issued under exceptional circumstances and those holding such certificates must disclose this when taking out life and motor insurance or notify the company holding existing policies.

FINANCIAL SUPPORT AND ENTITLEMENTS (CF Trust 2000)

There are several benefits a person with CF, or their carer, may be entitled to claim. The two main ones are the Disability Living Allowance and the Invalid Care Allowance.

The disability living allowance (CF news 1996)

This is designed for all those under 65 years of age who need help looking after themselves and/or have difficulty getting around. It is not means tested and can be paid on top of other benefits.

Key features include:

- Payable in two parts – personal care and mobility
- Claimants can receive one or both parts
- Each part is divided into different levels of payment according to need
- The care component has three rates of payment. Recipients of the middle or high rates are eligible to claim for the invalid care allowance.

The application form for this allowance is lengthy and CF does not fit easily into many of the categories. Families usually need help to complete the form. The CF Trust can provide additional help via the benefits helpline. The application form should reflect how severely the individual can be affected, as well as how they are on a daily basis. Families should be reminded that it is an offence to make false representations on the application form and that if this is discovered they risk a criminal prosecution resulting in a large fine or even a prison sentence.

Whilst there is an official scoring system used to assess applications, there is often a wide variation in the level of allowance awarded. Those turned down completely or who receive an award at a lower rate than considered appropriate, should be encouraged to appeal. They can receive help with this via the CF Trust or local Citizens Advice Bureau.

Invalid care allowance

This is payable to anyone spending at least 35 hours a week caring for someone with special needs. The carer does not have to be a relative or live with the person who has the disability.

- The allowance is not means tested.
- The claimant must not be in full time education, working full time or have part time earnings over £50 per week.

Families can be eligible for a variety of other benefits or awards depending on social circumstances and income. Further information can be obtained from:

- Social Service Departments
- Citizens Advice Bureaux
- CF Trust booklet 'A Guide to Government Help'
- CF Trust Helplines.

Motability

Those receiving the top rate mobility component of the DLA can use it to lease a car using the Motability scheme. This allowance is available to the individual, if old enough and able to drive, or to their carer. Parents of children aged under 3 years are not eligible to receive motability.

Blue badge schemes (Hickey 1997)

These badges have replaced the 'orange badges' enabling the badges to be used in some parts of Europe as well as the UK. They permit car-parking concessions to disabled drivers or passengers. To qualify the person must be aged over 3 years and fulfil one of the following:

- Receive high rate mobility component of DLA
- Use a car supplied on the motability scheme
- Have a permanent and substantial disability.

Badges are available through local council offices, post offices or social services offices. Drivers planning to use them abroad should contact the relevant embassy to check the validity and permitted concessions.

Prescription charges

- Children under the age of 16 or those in full time education are exempt.
- Adults in the UK do not qualify for exemption on the basis of CF but do if they develop diabetes. Receipt of certain allowances or low income can mean that adults are entitled to exemption.
- Adults should check the prescription exemption criteria very carefully because there are some that can legitimately 'fit' certain aspects of CF. Those with ports or gastrostomies are exempt under the 'permanent fistula' exemption criteria.
- Exemption forms (FP92A) can be obtained from most adult CF centres, GPs or the Post Office. They have to be endorsed by a consultant or GP.
- Pre-paid certificates can be purchased (known as 'season tickets') either four monthly or annually. Application forms are available from Post Offices.
- Individuals with difficulties affording certificates can apply for a loan from the CF Trust.

TRAVELLING ABROAD

More individuals are travelling overseas. They need to consider how their care might best be provided away from home.

Before travelling

Discuss travel plans with the CF Team before booking, especially if recently unwell or health status has changed since last travelling. When considering possible destinations, remember that standards of health care vary throughout Europe and the rest of the world. It is possible to find out about specific CF centres and their services via the internet (see Chapter 25) or the CF Trust.

Considerations

- Medical cover for Europeans travelling within Europe is available using an E111 form obtained from Post Offices or Government Offices.

This will entitle the traveller to care at the same level available to the countries' own nationals. Individuals should not travel with this as their only form of medical cover.

- Medical Certificates – most airlines require a letter stating the person's 'fitness to fly'. Some airlines have their own medical assessments that have to be authorised before they will confirm the booking. Bookings made without this authorisation are unlikely to be refunded in the event of rejection on medical grounds.
- Fitness to fly can be assessed by spirometry or simulating the effects of altitude. See section below on air travel for full flying considerations.
- Immunisation – patients should receive all recommended vaccinations. Anti-malarial medication is normally well absorbed.
- A letter from the CF Centre giving information about medical needs and suggested treatment regimes in the event of illness should be carried. The letter should also list any allergies and previous drug reactions. It is possible to get this letter translated into another language – the CF Trust can assist with this.
- Some might find high altitude makes them breathless and physically limited. The same might occur in extreme temperatures. Many find it harder to breathe in high humidity.

Holiday insurance
- Check that the level of medical cover offered is appropriate for all eventualities.
- Always use policies that cover medical repatriation as well as expenses occurred whilst away.
- Ensure that cover includes accommodation and travel expenses for a parent to stay with children.
- Personal property cover should include compressors and other equipment.
- Some insurance companies will require letters from medical staff stating fitness to travel.

Medication
- There are some restrictions regarding medication imported into some countries. Check with the appropriate embassy and obtain necessary documentation.
- It is often difficult and costly to obtain medication in another country. Ensure sufficient supplies to last throughout the holiday, taking into account the risk of loss and changes in diet.
- Consider the need for a standby course of antibiotics and discuss with CF Team.

Equipment
- Those using needles and syringes for any aspect of their treatment must ensure they can be disposed of in 'sharps bins'. It might be possible to dispose of the bins at the resort. Discuss with the tour operator.
- If using compressors, remember plug adaptors. Portable equipment can run off its own batteries but will need re-charging. Nebulisers should be washed in bottled or sterilised water.

Air travel

Considerations

Flying might be inadvisable after pneumothorax. Discuss with the CF doctor.

The need for supplemental oxygen must be discussed prior to any booking and well in advance of travel. An FEV1 of less than 50% is predictive of the need for oxygen during flight. Fitness to fly can also be assessed by simulating the effects of altitude. Reduced oxygen saturations whilst breathing an FiO_2 of 15% indicates the likely need for oxygen. Hypoxia tests can be carried out in a body box titrating the oxygen requirement using nasal cannula (Air travel working party 2002).

The cost of supplemental oxygen varies considerably between airlines with some making no charges. It is vital to check with the airline before booking as the additional cost can be more than the flight.

Some airlines will not take passengers who require oxygen and if the information is given after the booking they might not refund the ticket price. Whilst all airlines carry some oxygen for emergency use, never rely on this supply if likely to require it.

Smaller aircraft are not pressurised to the same level as larger craft. This might increase the need for oxygen.

Individuals might still require oxygen during flight even if they have passed a 'fitness to fly' test. Symptoms indicating this include:

- Breathlessness
- Tightening of the chest
- Loss of colour
- Feeling generally unwell
- Feeling dizzy or confused.

When packing, medication should be divided between hand and hold luggage, to allow for delays or loss of luggage.

Some medication (e.g. insulin) is affected by extreme cold and should not be transported in the hold. Check packaging for information about individual medication. Some airlines will provide refrigeration facilities.

Compressors must be carried as hand luggage because they can be damaged by heavy handling. They often weigh more than the hand luggage allowance. Discuss with the airline on booking.

Seats offering more leg room can be requested especially if treatment is needed during the flight. These should be booked as soon as possible.

Airports usually involve walking long distances. Wheelchairs or buggies can be arranged to meet passengers at the entrance to the terminals and throughout the journey. Special arrangements can be made for boarding and leaving the aircraft if adequate notice is given.

Aircraft can get cold during a flight. Take extra clothing. Consider temperature changes on arrival.

Remember

Whilst most flights are on time, there is always a risk of delay. Take snacks, drinks and some medication in hand luggage.

If individuals become unwell during a flight the aircraft will, if necessary, land at the nearest available airport. Unscheduled landings cost airlines considerable amounts of money. If the airline has reason to believe the medical problem could have been foreseen they might claim this expense against the person(s) involved.

Patients with diabetes should discuss the timing of insulin injections with the Diabetic or CF Teams when crossing multiple time zones. They should carry a supply of snacks as well as glucose tablets or Hypostop.

Care whilst abroad

Eating and drinking

- Dehydration can precipitate distal intestinal obstruction syndrome. Drink bottled or boiled water. Check the seal is intact before purchasing.
- Oral rehydration fluids such as Dioralyte are recommended for gastroenteritis.
- Be generous with enzyme dosing. It is sometimes hard to tell exactly how food has been prepared and malabsorption from under dosing might be difficult to distinguish from other stomach complaints.
- Extra salt will be needed in hot climates. Salt supplements are recommended.

Medication

- Book a refrigerator for the room to store medication. Medication requiring low temperatures should be transported in cool bags.
- Do not leave medication to overheat in a vehicle.
- Ciprofloxacin and tetracyclines cause photosensitivity. Total sun block might be necessary.

Becoming unwell whilst abroad

- Ring the CF centre in the UK – this can be difficult if there are time differences.
- Contact the travel company's representative at the resort. Ask for advice about obtaining medical assistance. They will usually be able to provide help with translators.
- Ask to see a hotel doctor.
- Contact the nearest CF centre. If this is close to the resort, visiting the centre might be possible but avoid arriving without making contact first as staff might not be available.
- Contact a local hospital or medical centre.

When seeing a doctor, have all documentation from the local CF centre available as well as medication. Take passport, E111 and travel insurance documentation. Obtain receipts for all payments and ask for letters detailing treatment received.

Those with ports should not allow them to be accessed unless certain that staff are properly trained and using the correct equipment. Those who can access ports may feel happier taking and using their own equipment. Contact the CF centre as soon as possible on return. This is important if symptoms persist.

CF HOLIDAYS

There are several specialist organisations providing charitable holidays for families. They offer different types of holidays and can cater for most circumstances. The expenditure covered depends on the charity concerned and individual circumstances. Whilst some offer foreign holidays, most will be in the UK.

Although the charities try to help all those who apply, resources are limited, and they will prioritise families who have not had a holiday before or who have been through a difficult time. Referrals should be clear about the family's status.

Risks of cross infection prohibit group holidays.

FURTHER INFORMATION

The following are available from the CF Trust unless otherwise indicated (see Chapter 25).

For schools
CF Teachers and School – information sheets.
CF and School – A Guide for Teachers and Parents – booklet
Starting School with CF – audio cassette
Secondary School Pack – information pack.

Adolescents to Adulthood
Getting on with CF – the Move to Adulthood – booklet
Insurance/Assurance Policies – information sheets
An Employers Guide to CF – information sheet
Finding Employment 1 & 2 – information sheet
Growing up with CF – A Guide for Young People – booklet.

Travel
Holidays and Travel Abroad – information sheet
Planning a Holiday – Directions Education Programme, Forest Laboratories
A–Z of Travel – Available from Chiron as part of the TOBI drug information package.

Allowances
CF – A Guide to Financial Help – information pack.

References

Air travel working party 2002 Managing passengers with respiratory disease planning air travel: British Thoracic Society recommendations. Thorax 57:1–15

Angst D B 1993 The school-aged child with CF. Pediatric Pulmonology 9:104–105

Baker T 1997 How assured is insurance. CF News Summer Edition

Department for Education and Employment Special Educational Needs 2002 a guide for parents. The Publications Centre, London

DLA – are you getting it? CF News Winter 1996

DVLA Website. www.dvla.gov.uk.

Ellerton M L, Steward M J, Ritchie J A et al 1996 Social support in children with a chronic condition. Canadian Journal of Nursing Research 28:15–36

Fowler M G, Johnson M P, Atkinson S S 1985 School achievement and absence in children with chronic health conditions. Journal of Pediatrics 106:683–687

Gilljam M, Antoniou M, Shin J 2000 Pregnancy in CF – fetal and maternal outcome. Chest 118:85–91

Hickey L 1997 Have badge will travel. Input – Adult CF Association 13:51

McLaughlin R 2001 Off to Iowa. In: Bluebond-Langner M, Lask B, Angst D B (eds) Psychosocial aspects of CF. Arnold, London, p 59–60

Moving out – Part 1. Input – Adult CF Association 1996 7:47.

Nicholson K G, Hammersley V, Kent J 1996 Effects of upper respiratory tract infections in patients with CF. Thorax 51:1115–1123

Regulation 19 part iv of the national Health service (General Medical Services) Regulations 1992.

Simmons R J, Goldberg S 2001 ….. In: Bluebond-Langner M, Lask B, Angst D B (eds) Psychosocial Aspects of CF. Arnold, London

Special Educational Needs and Disability Act – 2001

The benefits of education – part 1&2. Input – Adult CF Association. 1995 Issue 7. No 45.

Walters S, Britton J, Hodson M E 1993 Demographic and social characteristics of adults with CF in the UK. British Medical Journal 306:549–552

Chapter **22**

Transition to adult services

Mary Carroll, Gary Connett

INTRODUCTION

The majority of CF individuals maintain good health throughout child-hood and will be referred to an adult specialist centre. This is best achieved through transition in an adolescent clinic.

Successful transfer depends upon:

- Good relationships between adult and paediatric CF Teams
- A seamless approach to treatment. Ideally, demonstrated in a joint clinic
- An expectation of adult care from shortly after diagnosis
- Allowing the individual concerned to dictate the pace.

Generally individuals should not move across at times of acute illness or social upheavals such as starting a new school, leaving home or parental break-up. Once the teenagers are nearing the end of secondary school (but not during exams) arrangements should be made to visit the adult ward and outpatient department. They should have the opportunity to discuss all aspects of their care with the adult team in a suitable setting – usually not a formal clinical environment. They should be encouraged to express their expectations and concerns about moving services. Parents some-times have different agendas to those of their child and it can be useful to provide an opportunity to speak to them alone to explore these issues.

Joint adolescent transfer clinics for teenage patients offer many advantages:

- Time for the teenager to consider transfer without pressure and to get to know the adult team.

- The adult team gain insights about family dynamics and how the individual and their family relate to the paediatric team.
- The adult team has several opportunities to assimilate complex information relating to medical care without direct responsibility for its delivery.
- The adult team begins to contribute ideas about management.
- Paediatricians gain insight into the differing needs of CF adults and can work towards preparing their patients for these changes.
- Both teams clarify that specific issues such as suitability for lung transplantation, smoking, contraception, the need for PERT with alcohol etc. have been addressed.
- The adolescent feels in control of the process and can make an informed choice about when they want to transfer after their 16th birthday.

Paediatricians need to:

- Remember to make eye contact with the teenager and address questions to them directly.
- When parents answer for them, acknowledge the parent but check the response with the teenager.
- If the teenager gives a response and parents start pulling faces, acknowledge their disagreement but continue to direct the consultation to the teenager.
- Involve the teenager in making decisions, be prepared to compromise and give options when appropriate.
- Whenever possible, give the teenager ways to back down without loss of face.
- Ensure that transfer is perceived as a positive event.

Adult physicians need to:

- Appreciate the strong bond between patients, families and the paediatric team.
- Introduce changes gradually.

ADULT CARE ISSUES

Practical considerations include:

- The transfer of responsibilities for adherence from the parent to the young adult.
- Increased psychology input.
- The CF social worker's role to facilitate the take up of educational, housing and financial entitlements.
- Eligibility for mobility benefit which, if individuals pass their driving test, might include help with the purchase of a car.

It is important that the adult team acknowledges the care previously given by the paediatric service. Treatment changes should be gradual and clearly explained. The adult service will communicate directly with the individual. Parents often take longer to feel comfortable with the new team, especially as they might feel that they have lost part of their role.

Paediatric teams are used to dealing with families as whole units. Most consultations will have several people present and the needs of the family are balanced with the needs of the child. In adult medicine most clinicians are used to addressing just the patient during a consultation and other family members' needs are not usually of concern. In CF, adult physicians have had to adapt their approach. Whilst remaining focused on the individual, they need to acknowledge the role of other family members and the impact they have on overall care. Young adults might still be very dependant upon parents for much of their treatment and parents may need considerable persuasion before finally letting go. Very ill individuals, who had previously left home, might have to return home and their parents once again become their main carers. Parents' roles vary with time but very few have no continuing involvement in their child's care.

Chapter **23**

Terminal care

Claire Forsyth, Judi Maddison

INTRODUCTION

Even with optimal medical care, CF remains a life limiting condition. The terminal phase can occur at any time. It is usually heralded by increased frequency and severity of respiratory exacerbations, oxygen dependence and declining function although sudden deterioration and unexpected deaths can also occur.

> **Remember**
>
> There is no right or wrong way to cope with death. Every family will handle it in their own unique way.

CHANGING THE EMPHASIS OF CARE

Acknowledging that an individual is moving into a terminal phase can be difficult for team members. Ensuring there is a unified team view is important before discussions with the family. When discussing the change in treatment with families it is important to avoid euphemisms. Conveying the news that death is expected is difficult and many parents may consciously or subconsciously block out what is being said. Use clear, concise language including the words 'death' and 'dying' to avoid misunderstandings.

Involving the expertise of a palliative care team to work 'hand in hand' with the CF Team has many benefits but families should not be given the impression that familiar professionals are withdrawing.

The teams should agree clear plans of management using appropriate treatment options for individual needs.

The patient on a transplant programme

Changing the emphasis of care can be difficult in this situation. Acceptance on an active waiting list acknowledges that without transplant life expectancy is severely limited. The transplant centre and the local CF Team should communicate to ensure appropriate care without jeopardising the chances of a late transplant.

Failure to acknowledge impending death in the hope of rescue by transplantation can leave families bewildered and doubly bereft if no donor becomes available. It can deny individuals the opportunity to say their farewells, and exacerbate feelings of alienation and loneliness.

SUPPORT AND COMMUNICATION

Whilst drugs and technology can ease the physical pain of dying, emotional support for the individual and their family is vital. Common questions such as 'How long do I have to live?' and 'How will I die?' should be anticipated. It is usually impossible to predict the timing of death. The terminal phase can be prolonged. Guessing about how long individuals will survive should be avoided. Explanations about the mode of death in simple terms about 'drifting off and stopping breathing through the retention of waste gases' can help overcome fears and provide reassurance.

CF Team members and ward staff will all need increased support and time should be put aside at regular meetings to address people's needs.

The dying child

Parents should be seen together (if appropriate) and away from their child to discuss what is going to be said to them and by whom. Regular meetings enable opportunities for subjects to be revisited, questions asked and views expressed by all those involved. Children often have more insight than their carers realise. Parents sometimes wish to protect children from the reality of their situation. This can deny children the opportunity to express their fears and might exacerbate them. Advice about openness and honesty should be given, but ultimately the family's decisions should be respected whenever possible. Parents need to know they can always change their minds and re-explore issues that they have previously settled.

A move to palliative treatment can sometimes enable families to regain control of their child's care. CF Teams must be aware of the pressure this can put on the family and intervene if signs of stress are evident. Some parents wish to be less active in administering treatments and emphasize their 'Mum' or 'Dad' role.

Children sometimes have clear ideas about things they would like to achieve and friends they would like to see before they die. Some even like to give their toys and possessions to siblings and friends. Older children may have already thought about their own funeral arrangements and it is important that they are given an opportunity to discuss this.

It is usually possible to reassure with confidence that death will occur with minimal pain or distress. Discussions need to be carefully timed and appropriate to the child's understanding. Few children below the age of 6 years understand fully the irreversibility of death. Between the ages of 6 and 10 years they begin to understand the permanence of death but often see it as having a reason, for example, a punishment for some misdemeanor. This may cause siblings of this age to think that they 'caused' the death through personal actions. Above the age of 10, most understand that death is a permanent, natural event. The use of games, books or videos or the help of a trained play therapist can be useful.

The dying young adult

This can be hard to accept. Those with dependent partners or children might be burdened by practical worries. Some have a mature and realistic attitude to dying, after years of anticipation through declining health. Others remain fearful and angry, particularly when treatments such as transplant have not transpired. Some have difficulty handling their relatives and caregivers. Staff of a similar age may find this situation particularly emotionally charged and identify with the patient.

Maintaining an honest, open dialogue and respecting individual wishes are crucial. Many will want to write a will and have firm ideas about funeral arrangements. Sometimes families find these subjects difficult to discuss and caregivers can help.

PRACTICAL CONSIDERATIONS
Symptom control

Open discussion about the limits to invasive treatment and what is achievable are vital. In general, palliative care should occur on a familiar hospital ward.

Breathlessness

This is often the most distressing symptom. Individuals often feel as if they are breathing through a straw. It is important to discuss individual worries about breathlessness.

Treatment options include:

- Humidified oxygen. This should be given according to symptomatic relief rather than to achieve specified oxygen saturations.
- An electric fan blown across the face often provides some relief.
- BIPAP ventilation. Nasal and or facemask set ups can be used with low pressures initially adjusted according to patient comfort for up to 24 hours a day as desired.
- Anxiolytics. Levomepromazine titrated according to symptoms can be highly effective. This can be given by continuous infusion plus oral or IV boluses. Infusions of 12–24 mg/24 hours can be used. Both drugs can be mixed in an infusion pump. Doses of oral or IV midazolam and sublingual lorazepam can also be used.
- A diamorphine infusion, 10–20 mg plus cyclizine 50–100 mg over 24 hours can be of benefit as a second line option. Up to 15 mg/ml of either drug is compatible with sterile water. Additional doses of Oramorph can be given. Enquire about the need for laxatives.
- Correct electrolyte imbalances and trace element deficiencies that might be exacerbating respiratory muscle weakness.
- Continue IV antibiotics to ease symptoms.
- Give diuretics to try and improve secondary heart failure.
- Cognitive behavioral therapy might be appropriate for older children and adults.

- Consider non-pharmacological measures such as music, relaxation techniques, aromatherapy, acupuncture, reflexology and optimal positioning.
- Remove intrusive monitoring equipment.

Nausea
- Slow infusions might be preferable to bolus feeds in those with gastrostomies. If there are swallowing difficulties, Pancrex powders can be given in 10–20 ml of water via the tube although these might be less effective than microspheres.
- IV feeding is a consideration for severe nausea but the aim should be to prevent dehydration and metabolic disturbance rather than weight gain.
- Artificial salivas such as Glandosane can help keep the mouth moist and aid swallowing.
- Effervescent vitamin C tablets can 'de-fur' a coated tongue.

Pain

Severe pain is not usually a major issue if distress related to breathlessness can be adequately addressed. Back pain can be a problem. Consider:

- Sheep skins.
- Heat pads.
- Regular massage.
- Transcutaneous Electrical Nerve and Muscle Stimulators (TENS machines).
- Non steroidal anti-inflammatory drugs.
- Opiates for more severe symptoms.

Acetazolamide might be of benefit for headache caused by hypercarbia.

Religious beliefs

Whatever the religious or moral views it is important to discuss beliefs and wishes before death. Families need to be aware of legal issues and procedures that might have to take place. Discussion and planning can help ensure that appropriate people are summoned at the right time, thus avoiding mistakes that can cause offence.

Place of death

The wishes of the individual and their family should determine this. In practice most patients die in hospital in a familiar CF unit where their needs can best be met. Twenty-four hour in-patient cover by experienced and familiar staff ensures the adequate use of treatment for symptom control and rapid appropriate responses to changes in clinical status. Individuals can be particularly fearful at night. The management plan for symptom control and resuscitation status must be clearly documented in the case notes. Dying at home is often not practical and is physically and emotionally exhausting for the family. Hospice involvement is rare and probably not appropriate given the lack of involvement from such services prior to the terminal phase.

The moment of death

- This should not be rushed.
- The needs of the family should come before ward routines.

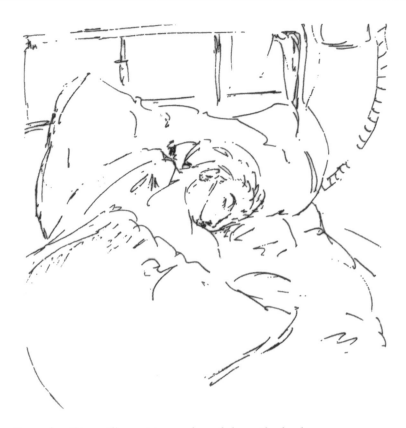

Figure 23.1 'We held her in silence and were deeply moved. It seemed to us a beautiful going ... We had no desire to part with that moment so peaceful and now with the machinery and pumps all stilled'.

OTHER CONSIDERATIONS

- Some families will want to wash and dress the body.
- The needs of other CF ward patients must be considered. It might be appropriate to move these individuals, ensuring that this does not make the affected family feel ostracized.
- Post mortem examination may be required and families can find the report findings helpful.
- Practices will differ between cultures but advice on registering the death, employing an undertaker and options for disposal of the body might be required.
- Heart, corneas, kidney, skin and bone donations are a possibility.

Funeral arrangements

- Families need to choose a funeral director.
- It is generally preferable for families to receive practical information in advance.
- Funerals currently cost from around £3000. The CF Trust and social services can provide some financial assistance to meet these costs.
- CF teams should decide which team members will attend the funeral and have insight into reasons for these decisions.
- The CF Team and ward staff should be debriefed.

Aftercare

The death of a CF individual can result in loss of:

- The support network of professional carers and other CF families.
- The parents' role as carers.

- Financial support. Allowances including a motability vehicle will be withdrawn shortly after death. This could deny a family their only means of transport.

Maintaining contact to provide support leading up to and after the funeral, through home visits and regular phone calls, can cushion some of these losses. The CF Team should maintain contact with the family according to their perceived needs. Some CF centres run bereavement support groups although families might seek help from other groups (see Useful Organisations, Chapter 25).

Other family members with CF

A death in a family where others have CF needs special attention. Usually this is a sibling but it can be a cousin, niece or nephew. The affected individual has to deal not only with grieving but with fears about their own premature death. Staff should be particularly sensitive and the surviving individual should be offered counselling. If the death was in hospital the same bed space must be avoided and the option of alternative ward accommodation considered. The first anniversary of the death should be acknowledged and admission or outpatient visits avoided on this date. The age at which the relative died may assume particular significance and explain changes in attitude or compliance.

The effect on the rest of the clinic

Deaths during childhood are increasingly rare. A death reminds everyone about the seriousness of the disease and might reawaken individual fears. CF Teams should acknowledge the effect a death has on other individuals and families and help address their fears.

USEFUL RESOURCES

Books and videos for children

Badger's Parting Gifts by Susan Varley. Published by Collins. Age 3–7. A warm forward-looking story, good to help young children.

Water Bugs and Dragonflies by Doris Stickney. Published by Mowbray. Age 3–7. Deals gently with the permanence of death.

Someone Special Has Died by St Christopher's Hospice. Age under 12. Explains emotions of bereavement.

Books for teachers

Death and Loss – Compassionate Approaches in the Classroom by Oliver Leaman. Published by Cassell.

The Forgotten Mourners by Sister Margaret Pennells and Susan C Smith. Published by Jessica Kingsley.

Good Grief 1 (for under 11s) and *Good Grief 2* (for over 11s), by Barbara Ward and Associates. Published by Jessica Kingsley.

Books for professionals

Care of the dying child, edited by Ann Goldman.

Living in the Shadow of Illness, by Myra Bluebond Langner. Published by Priceton Publications.

Chapter 24

Pharmacopoeia

Amanda Bevan

CHAPTER CONTENTS

INTRODUCTION

> **Note**
>
> Drug doses are given as mg/kg/dose followed by the number of times the dose should be given each day and the route of delivery.
>
> od   once a day
> bd   twice a day
> tds   three times a day
> qds   four times a day
> PO   orally
> IV   intravenous

ANTIBACTERIAL DRUGS

Continuous anti-staphylococcal prophylaxis

Flucloxacillin

Child:	25–50 mg/kg bd PO
Adult:	500 mg–1 g bd PO
Available preparations:	125 mg/5 ml and 250 mg/5 ml suspensions
	250 mg and 500 mg capsules
Administration:	Give on an empty stomach

| | Side effects: | Gastrointestinal upset and rarely sensitivity reactions, hepatitis and cholestatic jaundice have been reported and may occur up to 2 months after stopping treatment |
| | Note: | Low doses can be given initially, for example 250 mg/day, and adjusted upwards if positive isolates occur despite these measures having ensured good compliance. |

Treatment of asymptomatic staphylococcus isolates or minor exacerbations

Flucloxacillin	Child:	25–50 mg/kg bd PO (max dose 2 g bd)
	Adult:	1–2 g bd PO
	(See above for properties.)	
Sodium Fusidate	Child:	16 mg (fusidic acid)/kg tds PO
	Adult:	750 mg tds PO
	Available preparations:	250 mg/5 ml fusidic acid suspension, 250 mg sodium fusidate tablets (equivalent to 240 mg fusidic acid)
	Administration:	Use in combination with another antibiotic, e.g. flucloxacillin, to prevent resistance
	Side effects:	Gastrointestinal disturbances, skin rashes, jaundice. Avoid in liver disease.
Azithromycin	Child:	10 mg/kg od for 3 days PO
	Adult:	500 mg od for 3 days PO
	Available preparations:	200 mg/5 ml suspension, 250 mg capsules
	Administration:	Give on an empty stomach
	Side effects:	Gastrointestinal disturbances, allergic reactions
	Note:	Repeat course 1 week later and again if necessary. Check the sensitivity of isolates. Resistance can occur after repeat dosing.
Clindamycin	Child:	5–7 mg/kg qds PO
	Adult:	300 mg qds PO (can be doubled if severe infection)
	Available preparations:	75 mg/5 ml suspension, 75 mg and 150 mg capsules
	Administration:	Absorption is not affected by food
	Side effects:	Nausea and vomiting, diarrhoea and pseudo-membranous colitis (advise to discontinue and contact doctor if diarrhoea occurs), blood dyscrasias, dermatitis and hypersensitivity

reactions. Monitor liver and renal function if treatment is prolonged.

Rifampicin	Child:	10–20 mg/kg od PO
	Adult:	300–600 mg bd PO
	Available preparations:	Syrup 100 mg/5 ml, 150 mg and 300 mg capsules
	Administration:	Use in combination with another antibiotic to prevent resistance. Give on an empty stomach
	Side effects:	Flushing and itching, gastrointestinal reactions, hepatitis, thrombocytopenia, reddish discolouration of urine, sputum and tears (soft contact lens may be permanently stained). Use with caution in liver impairment, monitor liver function if treatment is prolonged. Liver enzymes are induced and the elimination of other drugs can be increased, e.g. oral contraceptives.

Treatment of more severe staphylococcal exacerbations

Flucloxacillin	Child:	25 mg/kg qds IV
	Adult:	1–2 g qds (max 8 g daily) IV
	Available preparations:	250 mg, 500 mg and 1 g vials
	Administration:	By slow intravenous injection over 3–4 minutes
	Side effects:	See above. Reduce dose in renal impairment.

Cefuroxime	Child:	50 mg/kg tds-qds IV
	Adult:	750 mg–1.5 g tds-qds IV
	Available preparations:	250 mg, 750 mg and 1.5 g vials
	Administration:	Slow IV injection
	Side effects:	See above. Reduce dose in renal impairment.

| *Aminoglycosides* | | See treatment of *Ps. aeruginosa* below. |

Teicoplanin	Child:	10 mg/kg bd for 3 doses, then od IV
	Adult:	400 mg bd for 3 doses, then od IV
	Available preparations:	200 mg and 400 mg injection
	Administration:	Inject over 2–5 minutes or infuse over 30 minutes
	Side effects:	Gastro-intestinal disturbances, rash, Stevens-Johnson syndrome, blood disorders, hearing loss, tinnitus
	Note:	Monitor renal and liver function if prolonged treatment.

Vancomycin	Child: Adult:	10 mg/kg qds or 20 mg/kg bd IV 1 g bd IV. These are starting doses, amend according to levels
	Available preparations: Administration:	250 mg, 500 mg and 1 g vials IV infusion over at least one hour. Must be given slowly (10 mg/min)
	Side effects:	Infusion related events: 'red man' syndrome if infusion given too quickly, nephrotoxicity, ototoxicity, reversible neutropenia and thrombocytopenia
	Note:	Reduce dosage or avoid in renal impairment. Monitor level prior to 3rd dose, trough level 5–10 mg/l.
Linezolid	Child: Adult: Available preparations:	<5 y 10 mg/kg tds PO/IV >5 y 10 mg/kg bd PO/IV 600 mg bd PO/IV 600 mg tablets, 100 mg/5 ml suspension, 600 mg infusion
	Administration: Side-effects:	IV infusion over 30–120 minutes Gastro-intestinal effects, headaches, dry mouth, fatigue, blood dyscrasias, pruritis
	Note:	Monitor full blood counts weekly. Linezolid is a reversible mono-amine oxidase inhibitor, give appropriate dietary advice.

Treatment of asymptomatic H. influenzae isolates or mild exacerbation

Amoxycillin	Child: Adult: Available preparations:	16–32 mg/kg tds PO 500–1000 mg tds PO 25 mg/1.25 ml, 125 mg/5 ml, 250/5 ml syrup or suspension, 250 mg and 500 mg capsules
	Administration: Side effects: Note:	Absorption not affected by food Nausea, diarrhoea and rashes Check isolates for sensitivity.
Cefaclor	Child: Adult: Available preparations:	1 month–1 year 125 mg tds PO 1–7 years 250 mg tds PO >7 years 500 mg tds PO 500 mg tds PO or 750 mg SR bd PO 125 mg/5 ml, 250 mg/5 ml suspension, 250 mg and 500 mg capsules, 375 mg CR tablets
	Administration: Side effects:	Absorption is not affected by food Diarrhoea, nausea and vomiting, headache, allergic reactions and blood dyscrasias.

Cefixime	Child:	6 months–1 year 75 mg od PO
		1–4 years 100 mg od PO
		5–12 years 200 mg od PO
		>12 years 400 mg od PO
	Adult:	400 mg od PO
	Available preparations:	100 mg/5 ml suspension, 200 mg tablets
	Administration:	Absorption not affected by food
	Side effects:	Similar to those of cefaclor
	Note:	Reserve for resistant cases.

Treatment of severe exacerbation of H. influenzae infection

| *Cefuroxime* | | See treatment of *S. aureus* above |

Cefotaxime	Child:	50 mg/kg tds-qds IV
	Adult:	2 g tds IV
	Available preparations:	500 mg, 1 g, 2 g vials
	Administration:	Slow IV injection
	Side effects:	See cefaclor
	Note:	Less active against *S. aureus* than cefuroxime.

Treatment of atypical infections, e.g. Mycoplasma

| *Azithromycin* | | See treatment of *S. aureus* above |

Clarithromycin	Child:	7.5 mg/kg bd PO
	Adult:	500 mg bd PO
	Available preparations:	125 mg/5 ml and 250 mg/5 ml suspension, 250 mg and 500 mg tablets
	Administration:	Not affected by food
	Side-effects:	See under azithromycin.

Treatment of Ps. aeruginosa infection: treatment of asymptomatic isolates or mild exacerbation

Ciprofloxacin	Child:	15–20 mg/kg bd PO
	Adult:	750–1000 mg bd PO
	Available preparations:	100 mg, 250 mg, 500 mg, 750 mg tablets
	Administration:	Avoid alcohol
	Side effects:	Side effects include nausea, vomiting, joint pain, abdominal pain, headache, rash, dizziness,

	pruritus, photosensitivity (use high factor sun screen), hepatitis and jaundice. Nausea commonly resolves after continuation with lower doses.
Note:	Use with caution in epileptic individuals. Reduce dose in severe renal impairment. Arthropathy has developed in weight bearing joints after use in young animals but used widely to treat children with good effect.
Antimicrobial sensitivity:	Activity against gram positive infections, but a high incidence of *S. aureus* resistance after repeat dosing.

Treatment of moderate or severe exacerbations of Ps. aeruginosa infection or those resistant to ciprofloxacin

Antibiotic choice will be guided by:

- Antibiotic sensitivity of infecting organisms
- Ease of administration of drug, particularly for home therapy
- Risk of side effects or known hypersensitivity
- Cost.

First line treatment

An anti-pseudomonal penicillin or third generation cephalosporin in combination with an aminoglycoside is recommended. Combination therapy might reduce the emergence of resistant organisms and produce useful synergistic effects.

Third generation cephalosporins

These have short-term efficacy as monotherapy but administration in combination with an aminoglycoside reduces the emergence of resistant organisms and improves efficacy. They are not active against *S. aureus*.

Ceftazidime

Child:	50 mg/kg tds IV (max 6 g/day)
Adult:	2–3 g tds IV (max 9 g/day)
Available preparations:	250 mg, 500 mg, 1 g, 2 g and 3 g vials
Administration:	Slow IV injection
Side effects:	Rash, hypersensitivity reactions, diarrhoea, nausea and vomiting, headache and bad taste
Note:	Reduce dose in renal impairment.

Anti–pseudomonal penicillins

Anti-pseudomonal penicillins have activity against *H. influenzae* but not *S. aureus*. The addition of a beta lactamase inhibitor (tazobactam) to piperacillin (Tazocin) and clavulanic acid to ticarcillin (Timentin) confer activity against *S. aureus*.

Piperacillin + Tazobactam

Child:	90 mg/kg tds IV (Tazocin)
Adult:	4.5 g tds IV
Available preparations:	2.25 g (piperacillin 2 g and tazobactam 250 mg) 4.5 g (piperacillin 4 g and tazobactam 500 mg) vials

	Administration:	Slow IV injection
	Side effects:	Gastrointestinal upset, rash, hepatitis and chloestatic jaundice
	Note:	Can be given qds if necessary.

Ticarcillin + clavulanic acid

Child:	82.5–100 mg/kg (max 6 g) qds IV (Timentin)
Adult:	3.2 g qds IV
Available preparations:	1.6 g (ticarcillin 1.5 g and clavulanic acid 100 mg) 3.2 g (ticarcillin 3 g and clavulanic acid 200 mg) vials
Administration:	IV infusion over 30–40 minutes
Side effects:	See Tazocin
Note:	Reduce dosage in renal impairment.

Second line treatments

Other beta lactam antibiotics can be considered if hypersensitivity reactions have occurred following anti-pseudomonal penicillins and cephalosporins, provided organisms are sensitive.

Meropenem

Child:	20–40 mg/kg tds IV (max 2 g tds)
Adult:	1–2 g tds IV
Available preparations:	250 mg, 500 mg and 1 g vials
Administration:	Slow IV injection
Side effects:	Skin reactions, gastrointestinal reactions, blood dyscrasias and headache
Antimicrobial sensitivity:	Also active against *S. aureus* and *H. influenzae*.

Aztreonam

Child:	50 mg/kg qds IV (max 8 g in 24 hours)
Adult:	2 g qds IV
Available preparations:	500 mg, 1 g and 2 g vials
Administration:	Slow IV injection
Side effects:	Rash, blood dyscrasias diarrhoea, nausea, vomiting, jaundice and hepatitis
Note:	Reduce dose in moderate to severe renal impairment
Antimicrobial sensitivity:	A narrow spectrum of activity against gram negative pathogens including *H. influenzae*. No gram positive activity therefore usually used in combination with an aminoglycoside.

Imipenem and cilastin

Child:	15 mg/kg qds (max 2 g/day)
Adult:	0.5–1 g qds (max 4 g/day)
Available preparations:	250 mg imipenem with 250 mg cilastin, 500 mg imipenem with 500 mg cilastin
Administration:	500 mg or less infuse over 30 minutes >500 mg infuse over 60 minutes

Side effects:	Rash, nausea, and vomiting (can be helped by reducing infusion rate), blood dyscrasias, confusion, dizziness
Note:	Use with caution in those with CNS disorders and reduce dosage or avoid in renal impairment. Bacterial resistance commonly induced when used as monotherapy
Antimicrobial sensitivity:	See meropenem.

Polymyxins

Useful for multiresistant organisms. Only active against gram negative organisms.

Colistin

Child up to 60 kg:	16,667 units/kg tds IV
Adult:	2,000,000 units (2 megaunits) tds IV
Available preparations:	0.5 megaunit, 1 megaunit, and 2 megaunit vials
Administration:	By slow injection into a TIVAD or slow IV infusion over 30 minutes if given peripherally
Side effects:	Sensory disturbances, vasomotor instability, visual disturbance, confusion and neurotoxiticy
Note:	Reduce dosage in renal impairment and when used in combination with nephrotoxic drugs. Monitor renal function
Antimicrobial sensitivity:	No activity against *S. aureus*.

Aminoglycosides

These are used in combination with other antibiotics (see above) and can have synergistic effects. Higher doses are required than in non cystic fibrosis individuals due to poorly defined mechanisms of increased plasma clearance. Consider hearing tests for those receiving repeated courses.

Tobramycin/gentamicin

Child:	3–4 mg/kg tds IV
Adult:	3–4 mg/kg tds IV
All:	10 mg/kg od IV
Available preparations:	Tobramycin 20, 40, 80 and 240 mg vials. Gentamicin 20 and 80 mg ampoules
Administration:	IV injection for three times a day but infuse over 30 mins for once daily. Do not mix with other antibiotics in the same syringe
Side effects:	Nephrotoxicity and ototoxicity
Note:	Monitor blood levels after the third dose. Recheck levels during the second week. Aim for: trough <1 mg/l and peak 8–12 mg/l (at 60 minutes) for three times a day dosing. Aim for a trough of <1 mg/l for once daily dosing. Reduce dose in renal impairment and if

		individuals have had high trough levels during a previous course.
	Antimicrobial sensitivity:	Also active against *S. aureus* and *H. influenzae*. There are differences between individual aminoglycosides in activity against *Ps. aeruginosa*. Tobramycin has superior activity and sputum penetration and does not easily induce bacterial resistance. Tobramycin might cause less renal toxicity.

Amikacin	Child:	10 mg/kg tds IV
	Adult:	350–450 mg bd IV
	Available preparations:	100 mg and 500 mg vials
	Administration:	As above
	Side effects:	As above
	Note:	Aim for trough <10 mg/l. Peak levels should not exceed 30 mg/l at 60 minutes.

Long-term oral therapy

Azithromycin		<40 kg: 250 mg three times per week PO
		>40 kg: 500 mg three times per week PO
	Available preparations:	See above
	Administration:	See above
	Side effects:	See above.

Nebulised anti-pseudomonal antibiotics

The polymyxin colistin either as monotherapy or in combination with tobramycin or gentamicin can be used to treat individuals chronically infected with *Ps. aeruginosa*. These drugs have also been used in combination with oral ciprofloxacin to eradicate early infection.

Colistin	Child:	<1 year: 0.5 megaunits bd nebulised
		>1 yrs: 1–2 megaunits bd nebulised
	Adult:	2 megaunits bd nebulised
	Available preparations:	0.5, 1 and 2 megunit vials
	Administration:	Dissolve in 2–4 ml water or 0.9% sodium chloride and give via a suitable nebuliser
	Side effects:	Bronchospasm can be relieved by mixing with a B-2 agonist nebuliser solution as the diluent or, in less severely affected individuals, by pre-dosing with a B-2 agonist via an MDI and spacer. In some cases bronchospasm can be minimised by using a more hypotonic solution. Transient sensory disturbances can occur.
	Note:	Give first dose in hospital and measure lung function pre and post dose. There are 2 branded

products of colistin available; Colomycin and Promixin.

Gentamicin	Child:	<5 yrs: 40 mg bd nebulised
		5–10 yrs: 80 mg bd nebulised
		>10 yrs: 160 mg bd nebulised
	Adult:	160 mg bd nebulised
	Available preparations:	As above. Use preservative free formulations
	Administration:	Can be mixed with colistin but must be used within 24 hours. As monotherapy, dilute to 4 ml with 0.9% sodium chloride if needed
	Side effects:	Local effects.

Tobramycin	Child >6 y/adult:	300 mg bd nebulised alternating 28 days on and 28 days off
	Available preparations:	300 mg nebuliser solution (TOBI®)
	Administration:	Give using a Pari LC nebuliser
	Side effects:	Local effects.

Options for oral treatment of B. cepacia

Co-trimoxazole	Child:	6 wks–6 months 120 mg bd PO
		6 months–5 yrs 240 mg bd PO
		6 yrs–12 yrs 480 mg bd PO
	Adult:	960 mg bd PO
	Available preparations:	240 and 480 mg/5 ml syrup and suspension 480 mg, 960 mg tablets and 480 mg dispersible tablets
	Administration:	Absorption not affected by food
	Side effects:	Gastrointestinal disorders, rash (discontinue immediately) blood disorders (discontinue immediately), jaundice
	Antimicrobial spectrum:	Also active against *S. aureus* and *H. influenzae*
	Note:	Can be given in higher doses as used to treat pneumocystis to eradicate early *B. cepacia* infection.

Doxycycline	Child:	<12 years contraindicated
		>12 years 100–200 mg od PO
	Adult:	200 mg od PO
	Available preparations:	50 and 100 mg capsules, 100 mg dispersible tablets
	Administration:	Swallow whole with plenty of water while sitting or standing
	Side effects:	Gastrointestinal disorders, erythema (discontinue treatment), headache and visual disturbances, hepatotoxicity
	Antimicrobial spectrum:	Also active against *H. influenzae*.

Chloramphenicol	Child:	25 mg/kg qds PO
	Adult:	25 mg/kg qds PO
	Available preparations:	250 mg capsules
	Administration:	Absorption not affected by food
	Side effects:	Blood disorders including aplastic anaemia. Monitor blood counts before and during treatment. Also gastrointestinal disturbances, peripheral and optic neuritis.
	Note:	Monitor levels in children under 4 years and in liver impairment, trough <15 mg/l, and peak 1 hour after IV 15–25 mg/l.
	Antimicrobial spectrum:	Also active against *H. influenzae*.

IV treatment of B. cepacia infection

Ceftazidime		See treatment of *Ps. aeruginosa*
Carbapenems		See treatment of *Ps. aeruginosa* (Imipenem/Meropenem)

Nebulised antimicrobials for B. cepacia infection

Ceftazidime	Child:	1 g bd nebulised
	Adult:	1 g bd nebulised
	Available preparations:	250 mg, 500 mg, 1 g, 2 g and 3 g vials.
	Administration:	Dissolve in 3 ml water for injection.
	Side effects:	Sensitivity reactions. Local effects.

OTHER COMMONLY USED DRUGS

Treatment of allergic bronchopulmonary aspergillosis

Prednisolone	Child:	1–2 mg/kg od PO
	Adult:	40–60 mg od PO
	Available preparations:	5 mg and 25 mg tablets, 5 mg soluble tablets
	Administration:	Give with or after food
	Side effects:	Moon face, weight gain, glucose intolerance, growth retardation, osteoporosis
	Note:	Reduce dose gradually (see Chapter 3).
Itraconazole	Child:	100–200 mg bd PO
	Adult:	200 mg bd PO
	Available preparations:	100 mg capsules, 10 mg/ml sugar-free liquid

	Administration:	Give an hour before food or on an empty stomach
	Side effects:	Nausea, headache, dizziness, allergic reactions, peripheral neuropathy (stop treatment), liver dysfunction, monitor liver function tests if on prolonged therapy (>1 month)
	Note:	Monitor itraconazole levels with prolonged treatment. Avoid in liver impairment. Interacts with many other drugs, check current SPC for details. Absorption might be more consistent with the liquid preparation.
Amphotericin	Child:	5–10 mg bd nebulised
	Adult:	5–10 mg bd nebulised
	Available preparations:	50 mg vial, reconstitute with 10 ml water for injection to give 5 mg/ml
	Administration:	Dilute up to 5 ml with normal saline
	Side effects:	Sensitivity reactions, cough, unpleasant taste.

Mucolytics

Hypertonic saline	Child:	4.5% bd nebulised
	Adult:	4.5% bd nebulised
	Available preparations:	Hospital special
	Administration:	As 5 ml through standard nebuliser system
	Side effects:	Can cause bronchospasm. Administering a beta agonist prior to dose can prevent this.
rhDNase (dornase alpha)	Child:	2.5 mg od nebulised
	Adult:	2.5 mg od nebulised
	Available preparations:	1 mg/ml, 2.5 ml vials.
	Administration:	Give undiluted via a jet nebuliser at least 2 hours prior to physiotherapy.
	Side effects:	Pharyngitis, voice changes, laryngitis, rashes, urticaria.
	Note:	Not licensed in children <5 years.

Vitamin supplements

The following are UK recommendations correct at the time of writing. This is an area of active research and recommendations might change. All doses are once daily PO.

Vitamin A	Child:	<6 wks 600 μg (2,000 IU) 6 wks–6 mths 1,200 μg (4,000 IU) >6 mths 2,400 μg (8,000 IU)

	Adults:	2,400 µg (8,000 IU)
	Available formulations:	Vitamin A + D BPC: 1 capsule = 4,000 IU
		Halibut Cold Liver Oil (LAB – UK)
		1 capsule = 4,000 IU
		Dalivit 1.2 ml = 10,000 IU

Vitamin D   Child: <6 weeks 200 IU (5 µg)
                            6 weeks to 6 months   400 IU (10 µg)
                            >6 months 800 IU (20 µg)
              Adult: 800 IU (20 µg)
              Available formulations: Vitamin A + D BPC 1 capsule = 400 IU
                            Halibut Cold Liver Oil 1 capsule = 400 IU
                            Dalivit 1.2 ml = 800 IU

Vitamin E   Child: <12 months 50 mg
                            1–10 years 100 mg
                            >10 years 200 mg
              Available formulations: Alpha-tocopherol acetate chewable tablets
                            100 mg tablets, capsules various strengths,
                            suspension 100 mg/ml.

Liver disease

Ursodeoxycholic acid Child: 7.5–12.5 mg/kg bd PO
                        Adult: 7.5–12.5 mg/kg bd PO
                        Available preparations: 150 mg tablets, 250 mg capsules, 250 mg/5 ml
                                    suspension
                        Administration: Give with or after food
                        Side-effects: Gastro-intestinal disturbances, pruritis
                        Note: Adjust doses to normalise liver function tests.

Vitamin K   Child and adult: 10 mg od PO
              Available preparations: Menadiol phosphate 10 mg, phytomenadione
                            10 mg

Pancreatic enzyme supplements   See Table 24.1
The current Committee on Safety of Medicines recommendations (UK) are that:

- Pancrease HL, Nutrizym 22 and Panzytrat 25,000 are contraindicated for children with cystic fibrosis aged 15 years or below although Creon 25000 is considered safe.
- An intake in excess of 10,000 units of lipase/kg/day should be avoided where possible.

Proton–pump inhibitors

Lansoprazole   Child: 15 mg od
                 Adult: 15–30 mg od-bd

Table 24.1 Types of enzymes available.

Product (Manufacturer)	Composition (per granule or per capsule/tablet/sachet) BP units		
	Lipase	Protease	Amylase
Enteric Coated Microspheres			
Creon Micro (Solvay) (Per 100 mg)	5000	200	3600
Pancrease (Cilag)	5000	350	3000
Nutrizym GR (Merck)	10000	650	10000
Creon 10000 (Solvay)*	10000	600	8000
Higher strength enteric coated minitablets			
Pancrease HL (Cilag)	25000	1250	22500
Nutrizym 10 (Merck)*	10000	500	9000
Nutrizym 22 (Merck)	25000	1100	19800
Higher strength enteric coated microspheres			
Creon 25000	25000	1000	18000
Creon 40000	40000	1600	25000

*Smaller capsule size

	Available preparations:	15 and 30 mg capsules and fastabs, 30 mg sachets
	Administration:	Fast-tabs melt in the mouth, capsules should be swallowed whole, suspension should not be used down an NG tube
	Side effects:	Gastro-intestinal disturbances, headache, hypersensitivity reactions, dizziness, Stevens-Johnson syndrome, alopecia, blood dyscrasias
	Note:	Not licensed for use in children.
Omeprazole	Child:	0.7–1.4 mg/kg od PO
	Adult:	10–20 mg od PO
	Available preparations:	10 mg, 20 mg and 40 mg capsules or MUPS® tablets
	Administration:	Swallow whole or disperse tablets in water, capsule contents may be mixed with yoghurt
	Side effects:	See above.

Distal intestinal obstruction syndrome

Acetylcysteine	Orally:	1–2, 200 mg sachets, or up to 30 ml of 20% solution administered with a flavoured cordial 4–8 hourly.
	Enema:	50 ml of 20% solution in 50 ml of water.
Gastrografin	Orally:	Children <8 years: 50 ml in 200 ml of water (preferably flavoured).

	Adults and children >8 years: 100 ml in 400 ml of water
Enema:	100 ml bd
Note:	Gastrografin is powerfully osmotic and administration should always be supported with oral or intravenous fluids.

Balanced intestinal lavage solutions, for example GoLytely

This must be taken at high volumes up to 750–1000 ml/hour to a total of 4–6 litres. Few patients can tolerate this orally and most require a nasogastric tube.

Oral contraceptives

It is recommended that individuals are started on a tablet containing 30 microgram of oestrogen. If they have breakthrough bleeding, they can be converted to a higher strength (50 microgram) product.

Standard strength (30 microgram)

e.g. Microgynon 30, Ovranette, Eugynon 30, Loestrin 30, Marvelon, Femodene, Minulet.

Medium strength (35 microgram)

e.g. Cilest, Ovysmen, Norimin, Brevinor

High strength (50 microgram)

e.g. Norinyl 1

Side-effects:	Gastro-intestinal disturbances, headache, changes in body-weight, breast tenderness, fluid retention, thrombosis, changes in libido, depression, skin reactions.
Note:	Contra-indicated in individuals with a history of thromboembolism, pulmonary hypertension and liver disease.

Chapter 25

Useful organisations for families and professionals

Judi Maddison

INTRODUCTION

There are many charities, societies, support groups and Government Departments accessible to health care professionals and the general public. This list is not comprehensive but includes some of the agencies used by the authors in writing this book and in their daily work.

There are now thousands of websites about CF and a few of these have been included. Beware – not all web-based information comes from reputable sources. Individuals should always discuss with their CF Team before following any advice from a website.

USEFUL ORGANISATIONS

Action for Sick Children
Argyle House
29–31 Euston Road
London
NW1 2SD
Tel: 020 7833 2041

A charity dedicated to improving standards and quality of childhood services at home, in hospital and in the community. Also lists local support groups. Professionals or parents can apply for grants.

ACT – Association for Children with Life Threatening Conditions and their Families
65 St Michaels Hill
Bristol
BS2 8DZ
Tel: 0117 922 1556

A national information resource for parents and key workers. They campaign to highlight the care needs of these children, attempting to increase service provision and support for terminally ill children. Also produce 'Guide to Children's Palliative Care Services'.

Arthritic Association
First Floor Suite
2 Hyde Gardens
Eastbourne
East Sussex
BN21 4PN
Tel: 01323 416550
(Mon–Fri 10–13:00 & 14–16:00)
Fax: 01323 639793
www.arthriticassociation.org.uk

A charitable organisation aiming to relieve the pain of arthritis by natural methods. They promote natural drug-free treatment based on dietary guidance, homoeopathic and herbal preparations – suitable for individuals of all ages.

Diabetes UK (formerly the British Diabetic Association)
10 Parkway
London
NW1 7AA
Tel: 020 7424 1000
Fax: 020 7424 1001
www.diabetes.org.uk

A charity helping people with diabetes and supporting diabetes research. Provides practical help and information. Organises educational and activity holidays for young people.

Insulin Dependent Diabetes Trust
PO Box 294
Northampton
Northamptonshire
NN1 4XS
Tel: 01604 622837 (10 am–10 pm)
Fax: 01604 622838
www.iddtinternational.org

Supports diabetics and their families – especially those who experience adverse effects from 'human insulins'.

CF Holiday Fund for Children
Woodrow High House
Cherry Lane
Woodrow
Amersham

Bucks
HP7 QG
Tel: 01494 725433
Fax: 01494 7222280

Provides holidays for affected children in the UK and abroad. The child has to be aged between 7–18 and must be nominated by a hospital or social services. Strict precautions against cross infection are in place.

Children's Chronic Arthritis Association
47 Battenhall Avenue
Worcester
WR5 2HN
Tel: 01905 763556

Provides a support network for children with arthritis and their families. Practical help and support providing various educational and recreational opportunities.

Children's Liver Disease Foundation
36 Great Charles Street
Birmingham
West Midlands
B3 3JY
Tel: 0121 212 3839
Fax: 0121 212 4300
www.childliverdisease.org

Specialises in providing emotional support to children who suffer from liver disease and their families. It provides literature, as well as a helpline and locally based volunteer support workers. Contactable directly by the family.

British Liver Trust
Ransomes Europark
Ipswich
Suffolk
IP3 9QG
Tel: 01473 276 326
Fax: 01473 276 327
www.britishlivertrust.org.uk

This is a national charity assisting adults with liver disease. They endeavour to inform, support and advice people who are concerned about or living with liver disease, to enable them to make informed decisions about their lives.

In Contact
United House
North Road
London

N7 9DP
Tel: 0870 770 3246
Fax: 0870 770 3249
www.incontact.org

For information and advice about coping with incontinence.

CF Trust
11 London Road
Bromley
Kent
BR1 1BY
Tel: 020 8464 7211
Fax: 020 8313 0472
CF helpline: 0845 859 1000
Benefits advice: 0845 859 1010
Welfare grants: 0845 859 1020
www.cftrust.org.uk

The only national charity funding research into a cure for CF. It also provides advice and support for families, friends, etc. They provide literature on all aspects of CF, both for individuals and health care professionals. They have an excellent website containing comprehensive and accurate information.

DLA Helpline: 0800 882200

ICA Helpline: 0800 000100

Disabled Person's Tax Credit: 0800 597 5976

Working Families Tax Credit: 0800 597 5976
Freephone helpline for advice about the disability living and invalid care allowances.

Motability
Goodman House
Station Approach
Harlow
Essex
CM20 1HR
Tel: 01279 635 999
Admin: 0845 456 4566
Helpline: 01279 632 000
www.motability.co.uk

Blue Badge Scheme
RADAR 12 City Forum
250 City Road
London

EC1V 8AF
Tel: 020 7890 6800

For information about the disabled parking badge scheme. Badges are issued via local authorities.

Dream Flight
3 Saxeway
Chartridge
Bucks
HP5 2SH
Tel: 01494 792991
Fax: 01494 775211
www.dreamflight.org

A national charity that takes seriously ill children on a trip of a lifetime to Disneyland in Florida. All children are accompanied by a team of health care professionals.

Make a Wish Foundation
329–331 London Road
Camberley
Surrey
GU15 3HQ
Tel: 01276 24127
Fax: 01276 683727
www.make-a-wish.org.uk

A national charity to help grant special wishes for children with life threatening illnesses. The wish can be as big or as small as the child wants – but they won't provide animals.

Eating Disorders Association
First Floor
Wensum House
103 Prince of Wales Road
Norwich
Norfolk
NR1 1DW
Tel: 01603 664915
Adults: 0845 6341414
(Mon–Fri 8:30–20:30)
Youthline: 0845 6347650 (Mon–Fri 4–6 pm)
www.edauk.com

Provides help and support for individuals with an eating disorder and their families. Includes advice about anorexia nervosa, bulimia nervosa, binge eating and other eating related disorders.

ERIC (Enuresis, Resources & Info Centre)
34 Old School House
Britannia Road

Kingswood
Bristol
BS15 8DB
Helpline (Mon–Fri 9.30–5.30): 0117 960 3060
www.enuresis.org.uk

A national organisation that provides specific information for children, teenagers, parents and health care professionals about all aspects of continence. They also provide practical advice about products that are available in this field.

Family Welfare Association
501–505 Kingsland Road
London
E8 4AU
Tel: 020 7254 6251
Fax: 020 7249 5443
www.fwa.org.uk

Aims to create a caring and secure society. They provide numerous services for children and their families, including financial support for essential needs. Also advice on educational grants.

Family Fund
PO Box 50
York
YO1 2ZX
Tel: 0845 130 4542
www.familyfundtrust.org.uk

A charity that provides financial assistance for a variety of reasons for example, washing machines, driving lessons. Families can apply direct, but will need some medical backing to support their request.

Family Holiday Association
16 Mortimer Street
London
W1N 7RD
Tel: 020 7436 3304
Fax: 020 7323 7299

A charity providing family holidays for socially deprived families. Referrals must come from a welfare/health agency and the family should not have had a holiday for at least four years.

British Homoeopathic Association
27A Devonshire Street
London
W1N 1RJ
Tel: 020 7935 2163

Provides lists of practitioners, including postgraduate doctors. Also provides further information about homoeopathy.

Enteral Feeding Companies
Nutricia Clinical Care Homeward
Tel: 01225 711531 – Information Hotline

Fresenius Home Care
Tel: 01928 579333 – Patient Services

Abbott Nutrition Hospital to Home
Tel: 0800 0183799 – Patient Services

Heart Transplant Families Together
c/o Cardiomyopathy Association
40 The Metro Centre
Talpits Lane
Watford
WD1 8SB
Tel: 01923 249977
Tel: 0800 018 1024
Fax: 01923 249987
www.htft.org.uk

A voluntary self-help group made up of parents and carers whose children have had, or are awaiting, heart or heart–lung transplants.

The Patient Association
PO Box 935
Harrow
Middlesex
HA1 3YJ
Tel: 020 8423 9111
Fax: 020 8423 9119
www.patients_association.com

Campaigns for patients' rights in the NHS. Also provides educational material on illnesses and treatments.

National Portage Association
127 Monks Dale
Yeovil
BA21 3JE
Tel: 01935 471641
www.portage.org.uk

For advice about the provision of home learning schemes for pre-school children.

Rainbow Trust Children's Charity
Claire House
Bridge Street

Leatherhead
Surrey
KT23 3PU
Tel: 01372 363438
Fax: 01372 363101
www.rainbowtrust.org.uk

Specialises in helping families with a terminally ill child throughout the UK. Experienced carers offer extensive support to families in their own home. The Trust also offers short breaks for the whole family in two respite centres. Contact should be made by professionals initially.

React
St Lukes House
270 Sandycombe Road
Kew
Richmond
Surrey
TW9 3NP
Tel: 020 8940 2575
Fax: 020 8940 2050
www.reactcharity.org

A charity supporting children with a life-threatening illness and their families. They assist with grants for a wide variety of needs including domestic appliances, bedding and holidays. Contact can be made by professionals, or directly by the family.

SKILLS: National Bureau for Students with Disabilities
336 Briton Road
London
SW9 7AA
Tel: 0171 274 0565

Information on allowances for disabled students.

The Compassionate Friends
53 North Street
Bristol
BS3 1EN
Helpline: 01727 539639 (9.30 am–5 pm Mon–Fri)
Tel: 01272 665202
Fax: 01272 665202

A nationwide (and international) self-help organization of parents whose child of any age, including adult, has died through accident, illness, murder or suicide. The organisation offers friendship and understanding from other bereaved parents through personal or group support. A postal library is also available.

Cruse (Bereavement Care)
Cruse House
126 Sheen Road
Richmond
Surrey
TW9 1UR
Tel: 0181 9404818
Helpline: 0181 332 7227 (9.30 am–5 pm Mon–Fri)
Fax: 0181 940 7638

Cruse offers free help to all bereaved people through 194 local branches, by providing individual and group counselling, opportunities for social contact and practical advice.

Child Death Helpline
Freephone: 0800 282986
Open 7.00–10.00 pm every day and Monday, Wednesday and Friday 10 am–1 pm.

For anyone affected by the death of a child. All calls answered by parents who have themselves lost a child.

Life-time Project
The Lifetime Service
Room 20
Child Health Department
Newbridge Hill
Bath
BA1 3QE
Tel: 01225 420785

WEBSITE ADDRESSES

International CF Association and the International Association of CF Adults: www.cfww.org

Driving licenses: www.dvla.gov.uk

Travel information: www.fitfortravel.nhs.uk

Patient information: www.patient.uk

European CF Society: www.ecfsoc.org

CF Foundation: www.cff.org

International Nurses Group: www.cfnurses.net

British Thoracic Society: www.brit-thoracic.org.uk

Cochrane CF and Genetic Disorders Group: www.liv.ac.uk/cfgd

Index

Page numbers in *italics* refer to figures; note that figures are only indicated when they are separated from their text references.